Care of the Newborn:

A Handbook for Primary Care

Edited by

David E. Hertz, MD

Associate Professor of
Clinical Pediatrics
Indiana University School of Medicine
Indianapolis, Indiana

LIPPINCOTT WILLIAMS & WILKINS
A **Wolters Kluwer** Company

Philadelphia • Baltimore • New York • London
Buenos Aires • Hong Kong • Sydney • Tokyo

Acquisitions Editor: Anne M. Sydor
Developmental Editor: Louise Bierig
Managing Editor: Nicole Dernoski
Project Manager: Nicole Walz
Senior Manufacturing Manager: Ben Rivera
Senior Marketing Manager: Kathy Neely
Design Coordinator: Holly McLaughlin
Cover Designer: Christine Jenny
Production Services: Laserwords Private Limited
Printer: Edwards Brothers

© 2005 by LIPPINCOTT WILLIAMS & WILKINS

530 Walnut Street
Philadelphia, PA 19106
www.lww.com

Printed in the United States

Library of Congress Cataloging-in-Publication Data
Care of the newborn : a handbook for primary care / [edited by] David E. Hertz.
  p. ; cm.
  Includes bibliographical references and index.
  ISBN 0-7817-5585-9 (alk. paper)
  1. Infants (Newborn)--Medical care--Handbooks, manuals, etc. 2. Infants (Newborn)--Diseases--Handbooks, manuals, etc. 3. Primary health care--Handbooks, manuals, etc. I. Hertz, David E. [DNLM: 1. Infant, Newborn--Handbooks. 2. Infant Care--methods--Handbooks. 3. Infant, Newborn, Diseases--Handbooks. 4. Primary Health Care--Handbooks.]
RJ254.C373 2005
618.92'01--dc22

2005003405

Care has been taken to confirm the accuracy of the information presented and to describe generally accepted practices. However, the authors, editors, and publisher are not responsible for errors or omissions or for any consequences from application of the information in this book and make no warranty, expressed or implied, with respect to the currency, completeness, or accuracy of the contents of the publication. Application of this information in a particular situation remains the professional responsibility of the practitioner.

The authors, editors, and publisher have exerted every effort to ensure that drug selection and dosage set forth in this text are in accordance with current recommendations and practice at the time of publication. However, in view of ongoing research, changes in government regulations, and the constant flow of information relating to drug therapy and drug reactions, the reader is urged to check the package insert for each drug for any change in indications and dosage and for added warnings and precautions. This is particularly important when the recommended agent is a new or infrequently employed drug.

Some drugs and medical devices presented in this publication have Food and Drug Administration (FDA) clearance for limited use in restricted research settings. It is the responsibility of health care providers to ascertain the FDA status of each drug or device planned for use in their clinical practice.

The publishers have made every effort to trace copyright holders for borrowed material. If they have inadvertently overlooked any, they will be pleased to make the necessary arrangements at the first opportunity.

The websites that appear throughout this text were accessible at the time of publication. The authors and the publisher cannot accept responsibility for the content or functionality of the websites.

To purchase additional copies of this book, call our customer service department at (800) 638-3030 or fax orders to (301) 824-7390. Lippincott Williams & Wilkins customer service representatives are available from 8:30 am to 6:30 pm, EST, Monday through Friday, for telephone access. Visit Lippincott Williams & Wilkins on the Internet: http://www.lww.com.

10 9 8 7 6 5 4 3 2 1

Dedication

To my wife, Leesa, and my children, Grace and Grant.

Contents

Contributing Authors

Matthew E. Abrams, MD, FAAP

Neonatologist, Phoenix Children's Hospital, Phoenix Perinatal Associates, Pediatrix Medical Group, Phoenix, Arizona

Kimberly E. Applegate, MD, MS

Associate Professor, Department of Radiology, Indiana University School of Medicine; Radiologist, James Whitcomb Riley Hospital for Children, Indianapolis, Indiana

David W. Boyle, MD, FAAP

Associate Professor, Department of Pediatrics, Indiana University School of Medicine; Staff Neonatologist, Department of Pediatrics, James Whitcomb Riley Hospital for Children, Indianapolis, Indiana

William F. Buss, BS, PharmD

Affiliate Professor, Department of Pharmacy Practice, Purdue University College of Pharmacy, School of Pharmacy, West Lafayette, Indiana; Clinical Pharmacist, Neonatal Intensive Care, Department of Pharmacy, James Whitcomb Riley Hospital for Children, Clarian Health Partners, Indianapolis, Indiana

Randall L. Caldwell, MD

Director, Pediatric Cardiology, Department of Pediatrics, Indiana University School of Medicine; Director, Pediatric Cardiology, Department of Pediatrics, Riley's Children's Hospital, Clarian Healthcare, Indianapolis, Indiana

Mary R. Ciccarelli, MD

Associate Professor of Clinical Medicine and Pediatrics, Department of Pediatrics, Indiana University School of Medicine; James Whitcomb Riley Hospital for Children, Indianapolis, Indiana

Scott C. Denne, MD

Professor, Department of Pediatrics, Indiana University School of Medicine; Department of Pediatrics, James Whitcomb Riley Hospital for Children, Indianapolis, Indiana

Mark Lawrence Edwards, PhD, MD

Fellow, Neonatal/Perinatal Medicine, Department of Pediatrics, Indiana University School of Medicine, Indianapolis, Indiana

William A. Engle, MD

Eric T. Ragan Professor of Pediatrics, Department of Pediatrics, Indiana University School of Medicine, Indianapolis, Indiana

Scott A. Engum, MD

Associate Professor, Department of Surgery, Indiana University School of Medicine; Associate Professor, Department of Pediatric Surgery, James Whitcomb Riley Hospital for Children, Indianapolis, Indiana

Anne G. Farrell, MD

Assistant Professor of Clinical Pediatrics, Department of Pediatrics, Indiana University School of Medicine; Pediatric Cardiologist, Department of Pediatric Cardiology, James Whitcomb Riley Hospital for Children, Indianapolis, Indiana

Julia Foster, MD

Assistant Professor of Clinical Pediatrics, Department of Pediatrics, Indiana University School of Medicine; Department of Pediatrics, James Whitcomb Riley Hospital for Children, Indianapolis, Indiana

Jay L. Grosfeld, MD

Lafayette Page Professor of Pediatric Surgery, Department of Surgery, Indiana University School of Medicine; Surgeon-in-Chief, James Whitcomb Riley Hospital for Children, Indianapolis, Indiana

Mitchell A. Harris. MD

Associate Professor of Clinical Pediatrics, Department of Pediatrics, Indiana University School of Medicine, Indianapolis, Indiana

David E. Hertz, MD

Associate Professor of Clinical Pediatrics, Department of Pediatrics, Indiana University School of Medicine; Medical Director of Nurseries, Community Hospitals of Indianapolis, Indianapolis, Indiana

Alan P. Ladd, MD

Assistant Professor, Department of Surgery, Indiana University School of Medicine; Faculty, Department of Surgery, James Whitcomb Riley Hospital for Children, Indianapolis, Indiana

James A. Lemons, MD

Hugh McK. Landon Professor, Department of Pediatrics, Indiana University School of Medicine; Director, Section of Neonatal-Perinatal Medicine, Department of Pediatrics, James Whitcomb Riley Hospital for Children, Indianapolis, Indiana

Diane Estella Lorant, MD

Associate Professor of Pediatrics, Department of Pediatrics, Indiana University School of Medicine; Attending Neonatologist, James Whitcomb Riley Hospital for Children, Indianapolis, Indiana

Jo Ann E. Matory, MD

Associate Professor of Clinical Pediatrics, Department of Pediatrics, Indiana University School of Medicine; Attending Neonatologist, Department of Pediatrics, James Whitcomb Riley Hospital for Children, Indianapolis, Indiana

Caroline Rose Paul, MD

Assistant Professor of Clinical Pediatrics, Department of Pediatrics, Indiana University School of Medicine, Indianapolis, Indiana

Brenda B. Poindexter, MD

Assistant Professor of Clinical Pediatrics, Department of Pediatrics, Indiana University School of Medicine; Attending Neonatologist, James Whitcomb Riley Hospital for Children, Indianapolis, Indiana

Maureen Shea, MSW

Pediatric Social Worker, Department of Pediatrics, James Whitcomb Riley Hospital for Children, Indianapolis, Indiana

Neal Simon, MD

Associate Professor of Clinical Pediatrics, Department of Pediatrics, Indiana University School of Medicine, Indianapolis, Indiana

Deborah K. Sokol, PhD, MD

Associate Professor of Clinical Neurology, Section of Neurology–Pediatrics, Indiana University School of Medicine; Pediatric Neurologist, Section of Neurology–Pediatrics, James Whitcomb Riley Hospital for Children, Indianapolis, Indiana

Gregory M. Sokol, MD

Associate Professor of Clinical Pediatrics, Department of Pediatrics, Indiana University School of Medicine, Indianapolis, Indiana; Attending Neonatologist, James Whitcomb Riley Hospital for Children, Indianapolis, Indiana

Vicki Powell-Tippit, RNC, NNP

Neonatal Nurse Practitioner, Neonatal Intensive Care, Community Health Network, Indianapolis, Indiana

Michael Stone Trautman, MD

Associate Professor of Clinical Pediatrics, Department of Pediatrics, Indiana University School of Medicine; Attending Neonatologist, James Whitcomb Riley Hospital for Children, Indianapolis, Indiana

Mervin C. Yoder, MD

Richard and Pauline Klingler Professor of Pediatrics, Professor of Biochemistry and Molecular Biology, Departments of Pediatrics, Biochemistry, and Molecular Biology, Indiana University School of Medicine; Attending Neonatologist, Department of Neonatal-Perinatal Medicine, James Whitcomb Riley Hospital for Children, Indianapolis, Indiana

Foreword

When we started working on the first edition of *Care of the Newborn* 25 years ago, our vision was to offer a book for professionals that presented the essentials of neonatal care in a relatively simple text. There are excellent comprehensive neonatology texts that serve as reference books, but our goal was to provide basic, essential information, focusing on the most common clinical problems of the newborn. Shorter "manuals" of newborn medicine attempt to abbreviate all of neonatology into a few pages, frequently in outline form, a format that is difficult to read and retain. The premise of *Care of the Newborn* has always been to be comprehensive, yet straightforward and easy to read. The contents in this current text can easily be read in a one-month neonatal rotation by a resident, nurse, or medical student. Practicing general pediatricians and family physicians can update their knowledge in neonatology by reading *Care of the Newborn: A Handbook for Primary Care*.

After more than 30 years of working in neonatology and academic medicine, I am convinced that if every family physician, pediatrician, and neonatal nurse practitioner mastered the information in *Care of the Newborn: A Handbook for Primary Care*, excellent care would be provided to all neonates, both healthy and ill. This book will be of particular interest to general pediatricians, family practitioners, and obstetricians; family practice, pediatric, and obstetric residents; neonatal nurse practitioners; neonatal nurses and neonatal respiratory therapists; and medical students who are on a neonatology rotation. Dr. David Hertz and his fellow clinicians and authors are to be congratulated on a masterful job with this current edition.

Richard L. Schreiner, MD
Edwin L. Gresham Professor and Chairman
Department of Pediatrics, Indiana University School of Medicine
Physician-in-Chief, James Whitcomb Riley Hospital for Children

Preface

Care of the Newborn: A Handbook for Primary Care was written at the request of Dr. Richard Schreiner, Physician-in-Chief of James Whitcomb Riley Hospital for Children in Indianapolis, Indiana. Dr. Schreiner was the editor of a text that was written several years ago with the goal of providing a simple, practical approach to common clinical problems faced by any practitioner caring for newborn infants. He saw the need for a similar, current text and this book is the result. We would like to acknowledge and thank the authors of the prior text for their timeless contributions that serve as a foundation for the current publication.

In this text, the reader will find a comprehensive guide to caring for newborn infants, both healthy and ill. Normal newborn care, neonatal disease processes, and neonatal procedures are discussed and illustrated in a straightforward, concise manner that will provide the pediatrician, family practitioner, resident, neonatal nurse practitioner, and medical student with the core of knowledge required to provide comprehensive neonatal care. We hope that the final chapter will provide guidance in one of the most difficult aspects of newborn care, caring for the family with a neonatal loss.

David E. Hertz, MD

Acknowledgments

We would like to thank Deb Parsons and Louise Bierig whose tireless efforts saw this project to completion.

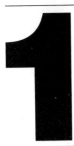

Care of the Normal Newborn and Family

Mitchell A. Harris and
Mary R. Ciccarelli

I. **Description of the issue.** Ideally, the care of the newborn infant begins during the prenatal period. The prenatal visit, which optimally includes both parents, offers an opportunity to establish a relationship between the family and physician. At this time the physician can collect important information about the pregnancy, as well as discern the needs and concerns of the parents. Advice and anticipatory guidance, particularly about breastfeeding, may be discussed. A full prenatal visit may not be necessary for each pregnancy. Certainly, the multiparous woman who is familiar with her children's physician and is experiencing an uncomplicated pregnancy may not benefit as much as the primiparous woman or the woman who will be taking her infant to a new physician. The prenatal visit should be scheduled approximately 4 to 6 weeks before the expected date of confinement. If the mother is at risk for delivering prematurely (e.g., a multiple gestation), the visit may be scheduled earlier.

When the prenatal visit does not occur, the aforementioned topics may be discussed during the hospitalization after delivery. When a mother is hospitalized antenatally because of medical complications, a visit by the infant's physician will promote a good family–physician relationship and can also serve as the prenatal visit.

II. **Medical history.** At the prenatal visit, the medical history of the mother (Table 1-1) should be reviewed. In addition, it is important to address the parents' relationship, their concerns, and their parenting experience. The family's feelings and expectations concerning this pregnancy should be explored, and the parents should be provided the opportunity to express any anxiety and fears that they might have. Posing the question "Was this a planned pregnancy?" may reveal that an abortion had been considered, that this child is seen as a solution to marital turmoil, or that the pregnancy precipitated the marriage. Identifying and providing any further resources that the family may need can help decrease stress and provide encouragement to the family.

III. **Parental topics.** A general discussion of the routine hospital care of the mother and infant makes the parents more at ease during the hospital stay (Table 1-2). Included in this discussion should be topics such as the policies of the hospital, rooming-in options, sibling visitation, and discharge plans.

   A. **Feeding.** The prenatal visit is the ideal time to discuss infant feeding and the advantages of breastfeeding (see Chapter 6). The mother has often thought about this prior to the visit. If the mother has made the decision to breastfeed, then suggestions can be given regarding reading material and preparation for breastfeeding. Questions may arise about nursing and returning to work, supplementation with formula, the use of vitamins, and support services for breastfeeding mothers. It has been shown that supportive and knowledgeable hospital personnel influence the lactating mother positively. If the mother is still undecided about whether to nurse or formula feed her infant, then it is important to explore all reasons for doing either. If she is asking permission not to breastfeed her infant, then her decision should be supported. Questions may then arise about formula types, bottle types, and methods of preparation. Mothers often ask about frequency of feeding. Most infants will do well with a demand-feeding schedule, although there may be some advantage to adjusting the schedule by feeding an infant before bedtime or by awakening a twin for a feeding simultaneously with the other infant.

   B. **Skin care.** Parents should be instructed to postpone tub bathing until after separation of the umbilical cord. A mild soap or clear water should be used. Skin creams, lotions, harsh soaps, and detergents should be avoided. Reviewing this information with parents prior to the birth can help them avoid making unnecessary purchases.

   C. **Bowel habits.** The variability in number and consistency of stools in the normal newborn should be explained to the parents. The breastfed infant may have one to six yellow, seedy stools per day or, once breastfeeding is established, may not stool for a few days at a time. The stools of the formula-fed infant are slightly firmer, more rancid in

1

Table 1-1. Information to be obtained from parents and/or obstetrical records

Maternal history
General health
  Age
  Presence of chronic disease
  Medications
  Alcohol, smoking, substance abuse
  Genetically transmitted diseases
Present pregnancy
  Estimated date of confinement
  Exposures to communicable diseases
  Maternal illnesses during pregnancy (e.g., gonorrhea, syphilis, herpes)
  Complications of this pregnancy (e.g., pre-eclampsia, bleeding, multiple gestation)
  Outcome of previous pregnancies (e.g., type of delivery, gestational age and weight of infants, postnatal complications)

Paternal history
General health
Genetically transmitted diseases

Social history
Support systems
Problems with past children (e.g., failure to thrive, neglect, abuse, removal of other children)
Parental expectations

> odor, pale yellow to light brown, and occur with an average frequency of one or two per day; however, this number may be quite variable, and a frequency of one to seven per day may be normal.
>
> **D. Umbilical care.** The umbilical stump can be expected to detach by 7 to 10 days of age. Alcohol applied to the cord two or three times a day facilitates the detachment by drying and will decrease bacterial colonization. Parents can be reassured that the

Table 1-2. Topics of discussion with parents-to-be

Routine hospital care
Labor and delivery including presence of father and/or siblings
Routine visitation including siblings
Rooming-in options
Discharge plans

Routine baby care
Feeding: breastfeeding versus formula
Skin care
Bowel habits
Umbilical care
Circumcision
Sleeping
Home safety
Vitamins and fluoride

Family life
Parental expectations
Parental plans for returning to work
Child-care arrangements
Support systems

Physician–family relationships
Routine well-child care and immunizations
Emergencies
Phone calls

small amount of bleeding that may occur when the cord does separate may be stopped with gentle pressure and should not be of great concern. Purulent drainage and erythema require the attention of the physician.

E. Circumcision. In 1999, the American Academy of Pediatrics Task Force on Circumcision stated that current evidence demonstrates potential medical benefits of circumcision, but that these potential benefits are not sufficient to recommend routine neonatal circumcision. The incidence of complications has been low—reported to be between 0.2% and 0.6%—with the most frequent being bleeding. Circumcision on religious grounds is still performed. Decisions regarding circumcision ideally should be made prenatally. Circumcision is always an elective procedure and, when desired, should be performed only on term, healthy infants. Parents should be made aware that there may be contraindications to circumcision. Parents who elect not to have their infant circumcised should be taught that nonretractability is the normal condition of an infant's foreskin. Forcible retraction should be avoided, and the glans may not be completely exposed until adolescence. This is not an indication for therapeutic circumcision. Newborn infants who are circumcised demonstrate a physiologic response to circumcision pain. If circumcision is performed, a procedural anesthesia should be provided. Options for anesthesia include EMLA cream, dorsal penile nerve block (DPNB), and subcutaneous ring block. After circumcision, a small amount of petroleum jelly or antibiotic ointment (and gauze) should be placed around the end of the penis to prevent the skin edges from sticking to the diaper. Alcohol should not be applied to the circumcision.

F. Sleeping. Infants should be placed to sleep on their backs to reduce the risk of sudden infant death syndrome. For the same reason, soft sleep surfaces, pillows, and loose bedding should be avoided, as should bed sharing or co-sleeping on sofas. Positional skull deformities (flattening of the occiput) that may result from supine sleeping may be prevented by a certain amount of prone positioning while awake, or by alternating the supine head position between the right and left occiputs nightly.

G. Safety. Safety is an important issue often overlooked by new parents. Because car accidents are the number-one killer of children, the importance of the appropriate use of child-restraint devices should be discussed. Many hospitals, public health departments, and service organizations will rent car seats to families. Correct use and positioning of the restraint system should be demonstrated to the parents. Many municipalities have car seat checkpoints set up to assist families with proper installation. Infants from birth to one year of age should be placed in an infant-only or rear-facing convertible safety seat that is placed in the back seat, with the seat in the rear-facing position only.

Before the birth, parents should begin "childproofing" the home. If there are older siblings, there may be inappropriate toys with small pieces that will be choking hazards. The use of a pacifier on a string around the infant's neck should be discouraged. If there are pets in the home, parents should be reminded that animals will also notice the addition of a new family member, and the infant should be kept safe from a pet that may be curious or aggressive.

H. Vitamins and fluoride. Vitamin supplementation is provided in commercial formulas. Formula with iron is recommended during the first year of life. In the breastfed baby, a supplemental product containing vitamins A, C, and D is recommended to provide vitamin D to prevent rickets (there is currently no product containing only vitamin D). If a baby is receiving supplemental formula in excess of one pint (500 mL) per day, then additional vitamin D is not necessary. Fluoride supplementation (0.25 mg per day) is indicated for the exclusively breastfed infant or the infant receiving no fluoridated water.

I. Family life. At some point, the needs of the parents should be discussed. If this is the first baby, the changes in the family routine that may result should be noted. The plans of the parents to return to work, as well as the planned child-care arrangements, should be discussed. These future plans are very important to discuss with single and adolescent mothers. Parents may not be prepared for the overwhelming demands a newborn can make on their time, and they may also not be prepared for the change this creates in their relationship with each other. Support systems for the family should be identified. The family with no identifiable support systems may need closer attention from the physician.

J. Physician–family relationships. The prenatal visit is a good time to inform the parents of the routine the physician follows regarding well-child care and immunizations. How to contact the physician for an emergency and some of the indications for seeking medical attention should be discussed. Often physicians will have a time set aside every day to handle phone inquiries regarding routine questions or concerns. Use of this time should be discussed with the parents.

IV. **Hospital routine.** The immediate newborn period, during which time the baby recovers from the stress of labor and delivery, is a time for close observation. The use of selected screening procedures permits the early recognition or avoidance of serious disorders.

   A. **Initial assessment and stabilization.** Thermal stability is essential for neonatal stabilization. The infant is dried and placed under a radiant warmer to maintain a skin temperature of 36°C to 36.5°C (97°F to 97.7°F). Once thermal stability is established, the infant is transferred to an open crib. In addition to temperature, heart rate and respiratory rate need to be monitored. Vitamin K (0.5 to 1 mg) is given intramuscularly as prophylaxis for hemorrhagic disease. Erythromycin ophthalmic ointment is instilled into the conjunctival sac to prevent gonococcal ophthalmia neonatorum. Hepatitis B vaccination is generally given to all newborn infants. It is given within the first 12 hours of birth along with hepatitis B immune globulin for an infant whose mother is infected with hepatitis B virus or to an infant weighing less than two kilograms whose mother's hepatitis status is unknown.

   B. **Glucose and hematocrit screening.** A screening test for glucose may be obtained during the first hours of life. Any infant at risk for hypoglycemia may need further screening tests (see Chapter 7). A hematocrit performed on a small sample of blood may provide useful information to the physician. A capillary hematocrit greater than 70% suggests polycythemia, which may require a partial plasma exchange transfusion. The capillary or "peripheral" hematocrit is usually higher than the "central" hematocrit, and therefore a venipuncture may be indicated to obtain a "central" hematocrit to verify an abnormal peripheral value.

   C. **Initiation of feeding.** Feedings are initiated shortly after birth in a healthy newborn infant. The infant is either breastfed or offered formula by bottle. Most infants have relatively little interest in feeding during the first 24 hours of life. Breastfed infants may begin nursing immediately after birth and *ad libitum*. Neonates commonly lose 5% to 7% of their body weight during the first days of life; however, after the first week, weight gain of approximately 250 g (8 oz) per week may be anticipated.

   D. **Physical examination and assessment.** The physician performs a detailed physical examination of the infant and completely reviews the perinatal history and the infant's chart prior to 24 hours of age. The growth parameters of weight, length, and head circumference are plotted on standard curves. The time of the first void and stool should be noted, and if more than 24 hours has elapsed without passage of stool or urine, the physician is notified.

   E. **Metabolic screening.** Prior to discharge or some time soon after discharge, most states require that infants have blood tests performed to screen for certain inherited diseases, such as phenylketonuria (PKU), hypothyroidism, galactosemia, homocystinuria, hemoglobinopathies, and maple syrup urine disease. Each state has different laws requiring which screening tests are to be performed, but it is the responsibility of the physician and the hospital to see that the tests are performed. The American Academy of Pediatrics has endorsed universal newborn hearing screening, and Early Hearing Detection and Intervention (EHDI) programs exist in many states.

   F. **Early discharge.** More patients are requesting discharge from the hospital within the first day of life. Families to be considered for early discharge (hospital stay <48 hours) should meet a predetermined set of criteria placing them in a low-risk situation. The American Academy of Pediatrics established recommendations for considering early discharge in a policy statement in 2004 on Hospital Stay for Healthy Newborns (Table 1-3). Parents should understand when to contact a physician and should have easy access to medical care. An office or home visit and/or telephone call the next day and again at 3 to 7 days of age are recommended to evaluate the progress of the mother and the baby. All breastfed infants should be evaluated by a health care professional 48 hours following discharge. Close attention should be paid to the development of jaundice and the fluid status of the infant. Metabolic screening tests may need to be repeated on infants discharged soon after delivery.

V. **Clinical pearls.** Prenatal visits provide the opportunity to do the following:

   A. **Establish relationships.**
   1. The family learns what the doctor is like. They can observe the doctor's style of communication, explore how the patient–doctor relationship works, and test the "fit" between the office and the family.
   2. The family learns the "rules" of the practice, such as for sick calls, referrals, and hospital(s) used by the practice.

Table 1-3. Criteria to consider for early discharge

A. **Uncomplicated antepartum, intrapartum, and postpartum course for baby and mother**
1. Vaginal delivery
2. Single birth
3. Term
4. Appropriate weight-for-gestational-age and normal physical examination
5. Normal, stable vital signs
6. Maintains thermal regulation for 12 h in an open crib
7. Baby has voided and had a bowel movement
8. If circumcised, no excessive bleeding
9. Has fed normally, at least twice
10. Newborn screen sample follow-up arranged and hearing screen protocol completed
11. Hepatitis B vaccine given or scheduled indicated

B. **No risk factors**
1. If jaundice is present prior to discharge, appropriate evaluation, management, and follow-up plans are made
2. Family, environmental, and social risk factors assessed
   a. Includes substance abuse, history of neglect or child abuse, domestic violence, mental illness, teen mother, lack of social support, inadequate housing arrangements
3. Laboratory data normal
   a. Includes maternal infectious screens, infant blood type, and a direct Coombs test if indicated

C. **Adequate support**
1. Mother has adequate knowledge to care for the baby
   a. Includes knowledge and training in breastfeeding or bottle feeding
   b. Knowledge of normal urine and stool frequency
   c. Knowledge of care of cord, skin, genitals
   d. Recognition of common signs of illness, especially jaundice
   e. Knowledge of infant safety issues (car seat, sleep position)
2. Family members and health care providers available to the mother and familiar with newborn care including lactation and are able to identify dehydration, jaundice, and signs suggesting sepsis
3. Physician continuing care identified
   a. If discharged at <48 h, definite appointment within the next 48 h
   b. Barriers to follow-up (e.g. transportation, language, telephone access) are addressed

From American Academy of Pediatrics, Committee on Fetus and Newborn. Policy Statement: Hospital Stay for Healthy Term Newborns. *Pediatrics* 2004;113:1434–1436, with permission.

    3. The physician learns what the parents' experiences are as a family.
  B. Address the decisions and preparations that should be made prebirth. This includes topics such as circumcision, breastfeeding, and purchasing equipment for the home.

BIBLIOGRAPHY

Texts

Green M, ed. *Bright futures: guidelines for health supervision of infants, children, and adolescents.* Arlington, VA: National Center for Education in Maternal and Child Health, 1994.
Shelov S, Hannemann R, eds. *Caring for your baby and young child: birth to age 5*, 4th ed. New York: Bantam, American Academy of Pediatrics, 1998.

WEBSITE

http://brightfutures.aap.org

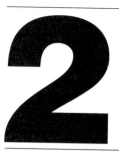

Resuscitation

David W. Boyle and
William A. Engle

I. **Description of the issue.** Perhaps no other group benefits more from the rapid initiation of a skilled resuscitation than newly born infants in the delivery room. The ability to perform such resuscitation requires an understanding of the unique and dramatic physiologic events that occur during the transition from fetal to postnatal life. Major physiologic changes occur in cardiopulmonary dynamics, which, if interrupted because of maternal disease, perinatal complications, neonatal illness, or congenital anomaly, may result in delayed transition, hypoxemic or ischemic injury, or death. Both hypoxemia and delayed transition to postnatal life may require immediate life-support interventions. Unlike the adult or even older child, successful resuscitation of the newly born infant is almost entirely dependent on *establishment of adequate ventilation.*

The purpose of this chapter is to review the physiologic transitions and resuscitation/stabilization measures that are most frequently encountered during the immediate postpartum period of life. Although the principles of neonatal resuscitation and the individual techniques used in the resuscitation of the newly born infant will be discussed in this chapter, the skills required for successful implementation of neonatal resuscitation can only be gained through completion of a course designed specifically for this purpose, such as the American Heart Association/American Academy of Pediatrics Neonatal Resuscitation Program.

The guidelines from which the Neonatal Resuscitation Program is developed present the consensus on science of the International Liaison Committee on Resuscitation (ILCOR). Thus, whenever possible, evidence-based recommendations are made following a comprehensive review of the scientific literature. However, many aspects of neonatal resuscitation continue to be controversial, and many have not been studied sufficiently to formulate an evidence-based recommendation.

A. **Epidemiology.** Approximately 5% to 10% of newborn infants require active resuscitation after birth and, depending on the hospital delivery population, 1% to 10% of newborns will require some period of assisted ventilation. It is estimated that the outcome of more than 1 million newborns throughout the world can be improved with implementation of the relatively simple resuscitative measures outlined in the Neonatal Resuscitation Program developed collaboratively by the American Academy of Pediatrics and American Heart Association (Fig. 2-1).

B. **Purpose of resuscitation.** The purpose of neonatal resuscitation is straightforward:
- Reduce the risk of central nervous system damage.
- Reduce the difficulty of resuscitation through early and skillful intervention.

C. **Consequences of ineffective resuscitation.** The consequences of a delayed or ineffective resuscitation are equally simple:
- Increased likelihood of central nervous system damage.
- Resuscitation becomes more difficult.

D. **Performance of effective resuscitation.** Effective resuscitation requires that delivery room personnel not only have the knowledge and skills necessary to carry out a complete resuscitation, but also that they be capable of working as a team. Competency to perform neonatal resuscitation should be developed through simulation as well as under direct supervision in the delivery room. Maintenance of resuscitation skills requires that they be practiced frequently. Although the need for neonatal resuscitation may be anticipated in most cases, there are always some infants who unexpectedly require resuscitation at birth. Therefore, at least one person capable of initiating neonatal resuscitation should be present at every delivery. An additional skilled person capable of carrying out a complete resuscitation should be immediately available for low-risk deliveries and in attendance for any delivery considered to be high risk.

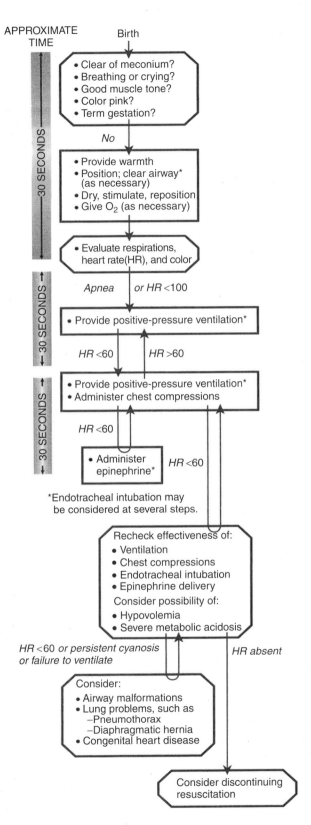

Figure 2-1. Flow diagram of neonatal resuscitation. (From The American Academy of Pediatrics and American Heart Association, *Textbook of Neonatal Resuscitation*, 4th edition. Elk Grove Village, IL: American Academy of Pediatrics, 2000:6–14, with permission.)

II.   **Physiologic transitions at birth.**
  A.   **Normal transition.** Physiologic transition for the neonate following birth is highly de-
       pendent upon a series of complex events. Prior to birth, the fetus is dependent on the
       maternal–placental circulation for oxygen, nutrients, and waste removal. Prenatally,
       the fetal lungs are fluid filled and low amplitude "breathing" movements occur. The
       fetal cardiopulmonary circulation is characterized by blood flow through a series of
       vascular shunts and cardiac structures (Fig. 2-2). Beginning at the level of the pla-
       centa, nutrient- and oxygen-rich fetal blood flows through the umbilical vein and
       ductus venosus into the right atrium. Most of this blood is diverted through the fora-
       men ovale and passes from the left atrium, left ventricle, and aorta to supply the
       heart, brain, and right upper extremity with the most well-oxygenated and nutrient-
       dense blood from the placenta. Blood that has traveled through the brain and other
       body organs returns to the right atrium by way of the superior and inferior vena
       cava. This carbon dioxide/waste-rich and oxygen/nutrient-depleted blood in the right
       atrium is directed into the right ventricle/pulmonary artery to be diverted across the
       ductus arteriosus into the descending aorta. The diversion of blood flow from the
       right ventricle through the ductus arteriosus occurs because of high pulmonary vas-
       cular resistance generated in the fetus by active pulmonary vasoconstriction. In the
       aorta distal to the ductus arteriosus, blood supplying the rest of the body is a mix-
       ture of oxygen/nutrient-rich and depleted blood, most of which flows through the um-
       bilical arteries back to the placenta.
            After birth, the *series* circulatory pattern of the fetus must transition to the *par-
       allel* circulatory pattern that characterizes the normal neonate, child, and adult
       (Fig. 2-3). This transition rapidly progresses with the onset of breathing. *Normal
       cardiopulmonary transition after birth requires clearance of fetal lung fluid from
       alveoli and an increase in pulmonary blood flow.* With the first breaths, fluid within
       the airways and alveoli is forced into the lung tissue where it is absorbed and car-
       ried away from the lungs by the lymphatics and pulmonary veins. Fluid within the
       alveoli is replaced with air. Oxygen diffuses into the blood raising arterial PO_2 and
       leading to relaxation of the pulmonary arterioles. Separation of the placenta results
       in loss of the low-resistance placental circulation and is accompanied by an increase
       in systemic vascular resistance. A fall in pulmonary vascular resistance following the
       onset of ventilation results in increased pulmonary blood flow, improved oxygena-
       tion, and increased blood pressure in the left atrium. Right atrial pressure falls with

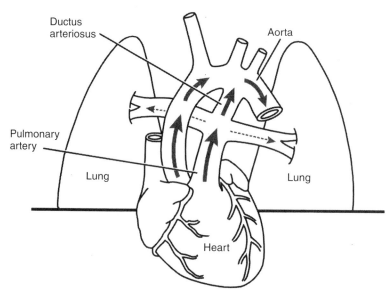

Figure 2-2. Fetal circulation. (From The American Academy of Pediatrics and American Heart Association, *Textbook of Neonatal Resuscitation*, 4th edition. Elk Grove Village, IL: American Academy
of Pediatrics, 2000:1–4, with permission.)

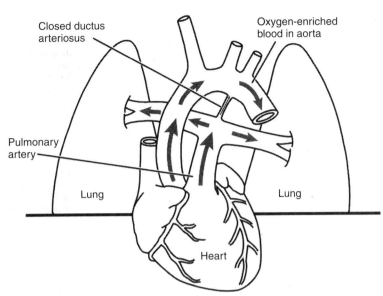

Figure 2-3. Adult circulation. (From The American Academy of Pediatrics and American Heart Association, *Textbook of Neonatal Resuscitation*, 4th edition. Elk Grove Village, IL: American Academy of Pediatrics, 2000:1–5, with permission.)

loss of blood flow from the umbilical vein/ductus venosus associated with placental separation and ductus venosus closure. With increased left atrial pressure and lower right atrial pressure, the foramen ovale functionally closes. An increase in oxygen tension in blood flowing through the ductus arteriosus from approximately 30 mm Hg in the fetus to 80 mm Hg in the newly born infant triggers functional closure of the ductus arteriosus. Therefore, the fall in pulmonary vascular resistance sets in motion a number of rapidly evolving physiologic changes that close the ductus venosus, foramen ovale, and ductus arteriosus, effecting separation of the pulmonary and systemic circuits into parallel circulations. These transitions predominantly occur during the first minutes to hours of life with completion by 2 to 4 weeks of age.

Clearance of fluid from the lungs at the time of birth is enhanced by labor prior to delivery and is facilitated with effective initial breaths. Infants who are apneic at birth or those with shallow, ineffective respirations have impaired clearance of fluid. Apnea and ineffective respiration are common clinical findings in preterm infants and infants who have experienced a peripartum hypoxic insult (see below). Failure to clear fluid from the lungs delays normal cardiopulmonary transition and may result in transient tachypnea of the newborn (TTN). Many pathophysiologic events will delay the normal fall in pulmonary vascular resistance, impairing the increase in pulmonary blood flow and resulting in failure of closure of the foramen ovale and ductus arteriosus. Continued admixture of pulmonary and systemic circulations through these open channels maintains fetal hypoxemic levels. This inability to effect a fall in pulmonary vascular resistance is termed persistent pulmonary hypertension of the newborn (PPHN), a common pathophysiologic pathway in many diseases that compromise the pulmonary and cardiac systems of newly born infants. These entities are described in detail in Chapter 9.

Metabolic and endocrine changes precipitated at birth include a surge in cortisol, catecholamine, and thyroid hormone levels; nonshivering thermogenesis; and loss of nutrient supply from the placenta, especially glucose. Cold stress and its associated increase in metabolic activity can be minimized by preventing heat loss; this is accomplished by drying the newly born infant immediately after birth, removing wet linen, placing the infant in warmed blankets, or placing the infant skin-to-skin on the mother's chest or abdomen. A wet newborn will lose as much as two degrees Farenheit in core temperature in 20 minutes if left wet and exposed to air temperature. For newborns requiring resuscitation, placement under a preheated radiant warmer maintains thermoregulatory balance.

Loss of nutrient supply, especially when stores are deficient (e.g., prematurity, intrauterine growth restriction), may result in hypoglycemia and symptoms of jitteriness, lethargy, hypotonia, and/or seizures. This is more problematic in the cold, stressed newly born infant. For healthy newborns, early feeding helps mitigate the risk for hypoglycemia. For sick newly born infants who cannot enterally feed, intravenous glucose may be needed within the first minutes to hours following birth. Prevention requires knowledge of the clinical findings associated with hypoglycemia and glucose monitoring of newborns at high risk for glucose instability (asphyxia, infant of diabetic mother, small-for-gestational-age, infection, prematurity, respiratory distress).

B. **Pathophysiology of asphyxia.** Asphyxia occurs when there is impairment of function within the organ of gas exchange. In the fetus, asphyxia results from decreased placental blood flow or maternal hypoxia. In the newly born infant, asphyxia occurs either when there is alveolar hypoventilation or impaired pulmonary blood flow. During the process of asphyxia, oxygen concentration falls and carbon dioxide increases in the bloodstream. The pH falls as a result of the increase in PCO_2 (respiratory acidosis) as well as the accumulation of organic acids (metabolic acidosis).

When infants become asphyxiated, they undergo a well-defined series of physiologic adaptive responses including redistribution of cardiac output to the brain, heart, and adrenal glands. Blood flow to other body systems is limited by intense vasoconstriction, which if severe and long-standing, will lead to organ injury and dysfunction. The initial fetal response to hypoxemia includes a vigorous effort to breathe with preservation of heart rate and blood pressure (Fig 2-4). If hypoxemia continues, *primary apnea* with bradycardia but preservation of blood pressure follows. If delivery occurs at this stage, the newly born infant often responds quickly to tactile stimulation. However, if the hypoxemic exposure continues, the fetus will begin gasping followed by *secondary apnea*, bradycardia, hypotension, and early evidence of end organ injury. If the infant is delivered during this stage of secondary apnea, vigorous resuscitative efforts will likely be required. If uninterrupted, secondary apnea will proceed to significant central nervous system damage or death. To avoid this progression, specific fetal complications associated with asphyxia and other perinatal problems (premature labor, maternal illness, maternal medications, and congenital anomalies) must be anticipated, identified, and treated.

It is important to recognize that the sequence of events described above may begin *in utero* and continue after delivery. An infant that presents with apnea may be in primary or secondary apnea and the two cannot be distinguished clinically. The infant must be rapidly evaluated and, if he/she fails to respond promptly to tactile stimulation, assisted ventilation should be initiated to reverse the effects of the asphyxial insult.

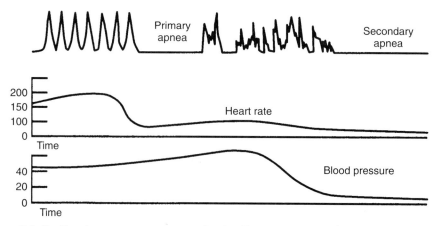

Figure 2-4. Cardiopulmonary response to asphyxia. (From The American Academy of Pediatrics and American Heart Association, *Textbook of Neonatal Resuscitation*, 4th edition. Elk Grove Village, IL: American Academy of Pediatrics, 2000:1–7, with permission.)

III. **Effective resuscitation.** Approximately 60% of necessary resuscitations in newly born infants can be predicted, while 40% of necessary resuscitations are generally unanticipated. This uncertainty requires that the knowledge and skills necessary to perform neonatal resuscitation be learned by all providers responsible for newborns in the delivery room. In the anticipated high-risk delivery, there must be a team of caregivers capable of providing extensive resuscitation. All hospitals that deliver babies should assure the presence of at least one person capable of initiating neonatal resuscitation during all deliveries, with a second person capable of performing all aspects of the resuscitation immediately available.

The primary purpose of neonatal resuscitation is to assist the transition from fetal to postnatal life, thereby preventing asphyxia and its related neurologic and multisystem organ injury. Because delay in cardiopulmonary transition is the most life-threatening obstacle to neonatal survival and well-being during the first minutes following birth, it is essential for all providers to master the steps necessary to assess and support cardiopulmonary transition in the healthy and sick newborn. Anticipation (Table 2-1), preparation for delivery (Table 2-2), accurate evaluation, and prompt resuscitative interventions are the keys to success.

Principles of a successful resuscitation include:
- Personnel adequately trained in neonatal resuscitation are present at every delivery.
- Personnel in the delivery room must not only know what they have to do, but they must be able to do it efficiently and effectively.
- Personnel involved in resuscitating a newly born infant must work together as a coordinated team.

A. **Anticipation and preparation for neonatal resuscitation.** Anticipation of the need for resuscitation requires meaningful communication among the delivering physician, obstetric and nursery staff, and physician(s) responsible for care of the newborn. A high-risk mother or fetus is best managed by delivery at a high-risk obstetric and neonatology center; this may require interhospital transfer of the mother, or, when delivery of a high-risk newborn occurs in a nonspecialty hospital, transfer of the neonate after resuscitation and stabilization. Verbal communication and chart review by the staff and physician(s) responsible for care of the newly born infant should include a determination of gestational age, significant maternal illness, maternal medications and drugs, peripartum complications, maternal screening results, and predelivery fetal evaluations. Parental knowledge, psychosocial issues, and content of counseling by the delivering physician and subspecialists should also be shared and documented.

Anticipation of high-risk deliveries often allows time for prenatal counseling and preparation by the pediatric provider or neonatology staff. If the newly born infant is unexpectedly ill, time for prenatal counseling and preparation often does not exist before the initiation of therapy or a decision for transfer.

Table 2-1. Anticipation of high risk for neonatal resuscitation in newly born infants

Antepartum factors	Intrapartum factors
Chronic maternal illness	Emergency cesarean, forceps, or vacuum-assisted delivery
Pregnancy-induced hypertension	
Isoimmunization	Abnormal presentation
Bleeding or anemia	Abnormal labor: premature, prolonged, or precipitous
Prior fetal or neonatal death	
Preterm or postterm gestation	Chorioamnionitis
Premature rupture of membranes	Prolonged rupture of membranes
Maternal infection	Fetal heart rate abnormalities
Multiple gestation	General anesthesia
Intrauterine growth restriction	Uterine tetany
Fetal macrosomia	Maternal narcotics <4h before delivery
Fetal malformation	Meconium-stained amniotic fluid
Diminished fetal activity	Umbilical cord prolapse
Polyhydramnios or oligohydramnios	
Abruptio placenta or placenta previa	

From The American Academy of Pediatrics and American Heart Association, *Textbook of Neonatal Resuscitation*, 4th edition. Elk Grove Village, IL: American Academy of Pediatrics, 2000:1–12, with permission.

Table 2-2. Preparations for delivery

Communication and consultation

Discussion with obstetric provider

Consultation with physicians and staff responsible for care of the newly born infant

Maternal chart review

Prepartum counseling

Equipment and supplies for neonatal resuscitation

Suction equipment: bulb syringe, mechanical suction and tubing, suction catheters (5 F, 6 F, 8 F, 10 F, 12 F), feeding tube (8 F), 20 mL syringe, meconium aspiration device

Manual resuscitator (bag) and mask equipment: neonatal bag (<750 mL) with pressure-release valve or pressure manometer (must be able to deliver FIO_2 0.9–1.0), newborn and preterm face masks, oxygen with flowmeter

Intubation equipment: laryngoscope with #0 and #1 straight blades, spare batteries and bulbs, endotracheal tubes (2.5–4.0 mm internal diameter), stylet, scissors, tape, alcohol sponges, CO_2 detector, laryngeal mask airway (optional)

Medications:

Antibiotics, surfactant, prostaglandin, emergency red blood cells if indicated

Epinephrine (1:10,000 or 0.1 mg/mL)

Normal saline, Ringer's lactate

Naloxone hydrochloride (0.4 mg/mL or 1.0 mg/mL, use single concentration within an institution to avoid dosing error)

Dextrose (10%, 5%)

Sodium bicarbonate 4.2% (0.5 meq/mL)

Vascular access supplies: umbilical vessel catheterization trays with 3.5 and 5.0 F catheters (2.5 single and 4.0 F double lumen catheters are optional), syringes (1, 3, 5, 10, 20, and 50 mL), intravenous catheters (22, 24, 26, 27 gauge), and tubing connectors

Miscellaneous supplies: 23 and 25 gauge butterfly needles for thoracentesis, 18 and 20 gauge 1.5, 2.0, and 3.0 in. angiocatheters for thoracentesis, paracentesis, or pericardiocentesis, chest tube suction devices, radiant warmer, personal protective equipment and gowns, firm resuscitation surface, warmed linens, stethoscope, cardiac and oxygen saturation monitors, oropharyngeal airways, continuous positive airway pressure device (optional), mechanical ventilator (optional), sterile bowel bags

From Osborn L, Dewitt T, et al eds. *Pediatrics Philadelphia*, PA: Elsevier Moseby, 2005:1253, with permission.

Preparation for resuscitation includes ensuring that all equipment is immediately available and in good working order. In addition, all team members must be competent in providing a complete resuscitation and must work well together in the event of a complicated resuscitation.

B. **Initial evaluation.** Evaluation of the newly born infant begins immediately after birth with visual inspection of several important signs that signal if the transition to the extrauterine environment is proceeding normally (Fig. 2-1). These signs, on which further resuscitative decisions are based, include:

- Meconium in the amniotic fluid or on the skin
- Respiratory effort
- Muscle tone
- Persistent cyanosis
- Preterm birth

In the absence of meconium staining and in the presence of strong respiratory efforts and cry, appropriate muscle tone, pink color, and term gestation, routine care with wiping the mouth and nares to clear the airway, drying, warmth, and reunion with mother and family is generally advocated. Early breastfeeding and skin contact with mother may reduce the risk of temperature and glucose instability and enhance family cohesiveness.

C. **Indications for continuing evaluation and resuscitation.** Signs that indicate the need for further evaluation and the potential need for intervention include the following: presence of meconium staining, weak respiratory efforts, low neuromuscular tone, persistent cyanosis, and prematurity (Fig. 2-1). In the presence of these findings, the infant should immediately be transferred to a radiant warmer with the rapid and simultaneous evaluation of respiration, heart rate, and color. Evaluation of these "vital signs" of neonatal resuscitation occurs concurrently with providing warmth (radiant warmer, drying, removal of wet linen, prewarmed blankets) and establishing the airway (positioning supine or side with the head in a neutral or slightly extended position and clearing the airway). In the absence of meconium staining, gentle suctioning of mouth and then the nasopharynx with either a bulb syringe or suction catheter (8 to 10 F with <100 mm Hg negative pressure) may be indicated. When copious, secretions should be removed with the head positioned to the side. Gentle tactile stimulation is provided simultaneously with drying and removal of wet linen. Initial resuscitation procedures should be initiated promptly, and each further step must be selected on the basis of specific patient response. All of these initial steps in resuscitation should be completed within 30 seconds after birth.

1. **Meconium staining and indications for tracheal suctioning.** In the presence of meconium staining of amniotic fluid or skin, the caregiver(s) must decide whether tracheal suctioning is indicated to prevent postnatal meconium aspiration syndrome. This decision is frequently required because 12% of deliveries are complicated by meconium staining. Intrapartum suctioning of the mouth, nose, and pharynx after delivery of the infant's head by the delivering physician has been used to reduce the risk of postnatal meconium aspiration syndrome. Despite suctioning the upper airway at the perineum, approximately 25% of newly born infants who are meconium stained and depressed [absent or depressed respiratory efforts, hypotonia, and/or bradycardia (heart rate <100 beats per minute)] will have meconium within the trachea. In this situation, intubation of the trachea and use of a "meconium aspiration" device until the trachea is clear is indicated. Tracheal suctioning may need to be repeated to completely clear the airway. If the infant's heart rate and oxygen saturation fall significantly, tracheal suctioning may need to be aborted and bag-mask ventilation initiated despite the persistent presence of some airway meconium. If meconium staining is present and the infant is not depressed, tracheal suctioning is not recommended because of risk for inducing bradycardia, apnea, vomiting and aspiration, and upper airway trauma. Thick or particulate meconium in the presence of a vigorous, active infant is no longer an indication for tracheal suctioning. The exception to this recommendation is the initially vigorous, meconium-stained infant who becomes apneic or develops respiratory distress soon after birth; in this circumstance, intubation and suctioning the trachea for meconium before positive-pressure ventilation is recommended. Gastric suctioning should be delayed until tracheal suctioning has been completed and respiration has been stabilized in order to prevent aspiration of swallowed meconium.

2. **Indications for oxygen and positive-pressure ventilation.** Once the airway is clear, regular and unlabored respiratory efforts that support a heart rate >100 beats per minute and pink color of oral mucus membranes is expected. If respiratory distress (retractions, tachypnea, grunting, increased work of breathing) or apnea are present, repositioning the infant's head and placement of a towel under the shoulders may help open and clear the airway. Drying the infant is usually sufficient to stimulate the onset of spontaneous ventilation in infants experiencing primary apnea or poor respiratory drive. Further tactile stimulation may be provided by gently rubbing the feet or back. Blow-by oxygen (5 to 10 L per minute) may help the transition once respiratory efforts are established in infants with cyanosis of the oral mucous membranes. Irregular gasping may be present in a newly born infant who has experienced an asphyxial insult. This pattern of respiration is ineffective in establishing spontaneous ventilation. Newly born infants with gasping respirations should be managed as those who remain apneic following tactile stimulation. Ventilation is the key to successful resuscitation in newly born infants.

    Positive-pressure ventilation may be provided with either a bag and mask or with a mask connected to a t-piece device capable of delivering positive-pressure ventilation. The two basic types of resuscitation bags used are the self-inflating bag and the flow-inflating, or anesthesia, bag. Commercially available t-piece devices that attach to a mask and to a flow-controlled pressure limited delivery system are also available for use in neonatal resuscitation. Regardless of which device is used, it should be equipped with a pressure-release valve or manometer to avoid delivery of excessive pressure. Each of these pieces of equipment has advantages and disadvantages. The self-inflating bag is easy to use and will always refill after being squeezed even if there is no compressed gas source. The disadvantages are that it will inflate even if there is not a seal between the mask and the patient's face and it requires a reservoir attachment to deliver close to 100% oxygen. The flow-inflating bag requires a compressed gas source to inflate and a tight seal between the mask and the patient's face to remain inflated. The advantages of the flow-inflating bag are the ability to deliver continuous positive airway pressure and the ability to provide any concentration of oxygen desired when connected to an oxygen blender. T-piece devices have the ability to control the peak inflation pressure and end expiratory pressure as well as the inspiratory time and concentration of oxygen delivered. Similar to the flow-inflating bag, the t-piece devices require a compressed gas source. Using mechanical models, these devices have been shown to be easy to use and to deliver more consistent pressures from one breath to the next. There is insufficient evidence at this time to recommend one piece of equipment over another.

Indications for positive-pressure ventilation:
- Apnea or gasping respirations unresponsive to gentle tactile stimulation
- Bradycardia (heart rate <100 beats per minute) even when breathing
- Persistent central cyanosis despite 100% free-flow oxygen

Positive-pressure ventilation using a bag and mask (40 to 60 breaths per minute, FIO_2 1.0 for 30 seconds) is indicated in the following circumstances: when tactile stimulation is unsuccessful in establishing ventilation; bradycardia (heart rate <100 beats per minute) is present; or, central cyanosis (blue oral mucus membranes) persists despite blow-by oxygen administration. The decision to provide bag and mask ventilation is generally made within 30 seconds of birth. If positive-pressure ventilation using a bag and mask is required, the goal is to correct ineffective respiration, bradycardia, and/or cyanosis. *An increase in the heart rate to >100 beats per minute is the best indicator of effective positive-pressure ventilation.* Secondary confirmation is made by listening for breath sounds and observing chest wall movement. Overventilation, as evidenced by large chest wall excursion with positive-pressure ventilation, increases the risk for pneumothorax, other air leaks, and barotrauma that may lead to chronic lung disease, particularly in the premature infant. It can also result in compromise of venous return and cardiac output. If bag-mask ventilation is ineffective, care should be taken to check for an adequate seal, to reposition the head, and to suction the oropharynx. If still ineffective, opening the mouth may be beneficial. The use of higher ventilatory pressures may ultimately be necessary. Most often, bradycardia and cyanosis respond to establishment of ventilation. If respiratory efforts significantly improve, then bag and mask ventilation can be withdrawn as tolerated.

It is recommended that positive-pressure ventilation should be provided using 100% oxygen. The goal of supplemental oxygen use should be to achieve normoxia. This can be assessed with the use of pulse oximetry or by observation of the color of the mucous membranes. Recent studies have suggested that providing <100% oxygen is equally as effective and may be more beneficial than the use of 100% oxygen in neonatal resuscitation. However, until further evidence is reported, 100% oxygen should be used when given by positive-pressure ventilation with a bag and mask. In circumstances where supplemental oxygen is not available, positive-pressure ventilation can be initiated using room air. *Establishment of ventilation remains the most important and effective step in neonatal resuscitation.*

Most infants can be ventilated and oxygenated adequately with a bag and mask. However, if bag and mask ventilation is ineffective, intubation and bag and endotracheal tube ventilation or mechanical ventilation is indicated. Endotracheal intubation may be considered at several points during neonatal resuscitation (Fig. 2-1, Table 2-3). The primary reasons for placement of an endotracheal tube are for tracheal suctioning of meconium, ineffective or prolonged bag-mask ventilation, airway stabilization for chest compressions, or for specific clinical problems that will require prolonged mechanical ventilation (congenital diaphragmatic hernia, extreme prematurity, severe hydrops, hyaline membrane disease, surfactant administration, apnea, pulmonary hypoplasia, etc.). Unsuccessful or prolonged attempts at intubation that result in cyanosis and bradycardia should be avoided.

Laryngeal mask airways can be effective in ventilating newly born term infants in whom bag-mask ventilation is ineffective or if endotracheal intubation is not successful. In infants with respiratory distress in whom high peak inspiratory

Table 2-3. Indications for endotracheal intubation and use of laryngeal mask airways

1. Endotracheal intubation
   a. Suctioning meconium from trachea if meconium-stained skin or amniotic fluid and absent/depressed respiratory efforts, hypotonia, or heart rate <100 beats/min
   b. Ineffective or prolonged bag-mask ventilation
   c. Improved coordination of positive pressure ventilation and chest compressions
   d. Epinephrine administration
   e. Special situations: extreme prematurity, surfactant administration, congenital diaphragmatic hernia, apnea unresponsive to bag-mask ventilation
2. Laryngeal mask airway (optional due to limited information about use during neonatal resuscitation)
   a. Ineffective bag-mask ventilation
   b. Failed endotracheal intubation

From Osborn L, Dewitt T, et al eds. *Pediatrics Philadelphia*, PA: Elsevier Moseby, 2005:1254, with permission.

pressures may be necessary for adequate ventilation and in preterm infants (especially those weighing <2000 g), laryngeal mask airways may not be effective. Laryngeal mask airways are not intended to replace tracheal suctioning in the meconium-stained and depressed neonate. Additional evidence is needed before recommending routine use of these devices in the delivery room.

Placement of an orogastric tube is recommended if positive-pressure ventilation using a bag and mask is required for more than 2 minutes or if marked gastric distension occurs. Gastric distension can significantly compromise ventilation, especially in newly born infants with significant lung disease in whom gastric ventilation occurs because of lower resistance to gas flow. In preterm infants, gastric decompression with an orogastric tube may be beneficial before 2 minutes of bag-mask ventilation have occurred.

   3. **Indications for chest compressions.** If effective positive-pressure ventilation is established and bradycardia (heart rate <60 beats per minute as determined by palpation of the base of the umbilical cord and/or auscultation) persists during resuscitation of the neonate, chest compressions are usually indicated. Rarely, a newborn may have congenital heart block that will not respond to positive-pressure ventilation and most of these infants will have adequate cardiac output, perfusion, and oxygen saturation without chest compressions. Unless prenatal testing indicates congenital heart block, bradycardia should generally be attributed to continued hypoxemia and chest compressions should be initiated while positive-pressure ventilation is continued. Chest compressions are indicated if the heart rate is <60 beats per minute despite 30 seconds of effective positive-pressure ventilation. The goal is to establish perfusion, especially to the brain, and reverse myocardial insufficiency, acidemia, peripheral vasoconstriction, and tissue hypoxia.

   To establish adequate perfusion, chest compression to a depth of one-third the anterior–posterior diameter of the chest is required. The force should be of sufficient magnitude to generate a palpable pulse. The magnitude of this force may be underestimated because of concern for rib and sternum injury. Of the two techniques for chest compressions, the two-thumb-encircling-hands technique is recommended, although the two-finger technique is acceptable. Coordination of ventilation and chest compressions is recommended with a 3:1 ratio of chest compressions to ventilations, so that 90 compressions and 30 ventilations are performed each minute. This half second per event is a more rapid pace than that used in older children and adults. When the heart rate responds and exceeds 60 beats per minute, chest compressions should be discontinued; positive-pressure ventilation is continued until the heart rate is >100 beats per minute and spontaneous respirations are reestablished.

   4. **Indications for medications during neonatal resuscitation.** If the heart rate remains <60 beats per minute despite a further 30 seconds of combined positive-pressure ventilation with 100% oxygen and chest compressions, medications should be given (Table 2-4). The primary drug used during neonatal resuscitation is epinephrine given as a 1:10,000 solution (versus 1:1,000 solution utilized for adults). Epinephrine is particularly beneficial in elevating peripheral vascular

Table 2-4. Medications for neonatal resuscitation and stabilization

A. Acute phase of resuscitation

Medication	Concentration	Dose/Route	Rate/Precautions/Caveats
a. Epinephrine	1:10,000	0.1–0.3 mL/kg ET or IV	Rapid injection Flush ET tube with 0.5–1.0 mL saline
b. Volume expansion Normal saline Ringer's lactate O-negative RBCs		10 mL/kg IV	Infuse over 5–10 min

B. Postresuscitation phase and stabilization

Medication	Concentration	Dose/Route	Rate/Precautions/Caveats
a. Sodium bicarbonate	0.5 meq/mL	2 meq/kg IV	Slow infusion (1 meq/kg/min) Give only after effective ventilation has been established
b. Naloxone	0.4 or 1.0 mg/dL	0.1 mg/kg IV, IM, SQ	Maternal narcotics within 4 h of delivery **Do not give if maternal narcotic abuse is suspected**
c. Glucose	D10W (10% glucose)	2 mL/kg IV	Follow with continuous IV glucose infusion
d. Phenobarbital		20 mg/kg IV	Slow infusion (1 mg/kg/min) Watch for respiratory depression
e. Dopamine		2–15 μg/ kg/min IV	For hypotension unresponsive to volume expansion
f. Surfactant		Dose according to manufacturer's directions	For surfactant deficiency with hyaline membrane disease; perhaps meconium aspiration, persistent pulmonary hypertension, and congenital diaphragmatic hernia
g. Prostaglandin E1	500 μg in 100mL D5W, D10W, or saline solution	0.03–0.1 μg/ kg/min	Risks: apnea, hypertonia, seizures, hyperthermia

From Osborn L, Dewitt T, et al eds. *Pediatrics Philadelphia*, PA: Elsevier Moseby, 2005:1255, with permission.

resistance, cardiac contractility, and heart rate, all of which improve perfusion pressure to the brain and heart. The drug is administered by intravenous (peripheral or low umbilical venous line) or intratracheal routes at a dose of 0.1 to 0.3 mL/kg (0.01 to 0.03 mg/kg) every 3 to 5 minutes. When given through an endotracheal tube, distribution may be improved by following with 0.5 to 1.0 mL normal saline or diluting the dose to a total 1.0 mL prior to placement into the endotracheal tube. Epinephrine should not be given by intramuscular route and not more frequently than every 3 to 5 minutes to avoid postresuscitation hypertension. High-dose (>0.03 mg/kg) epinephrine is not recommended in the neonate.

Hypovolemia may result in the need for or complicate resuscitation efforts in the delivery room. Clinical findings of hypovolemia include pallor, diminished peripheral and central pulses, tachycardia, and slow capillary refill. Perinatal risk factors include placenta previa, abruptio placenta, hydrops fetalis, vasa previa, twin–twin transfusion syndrome, and neonatal bleeding following a traumatic delivery. Volume expansion with normal saline, Ringer's lactate, or O-negative uncrossmatched red blood cells (if blood loss suspected) is recommended. Although not generally preferred, albumin-containing solutions may be acceptable alternatives during the acute phase of resuscitation. The umbilical vein is the easiest and most accessible vascular access during a resuscitation. Peripheral veins and umbilical artery and intraosseous sites may also be considered. The initial dose of a volume expander is 10 mL/kg given intravenously over 5 to 10 minutes. This dose may be repeated as needed; however, caution is warranted when volumes >30 mL/kg are needed, because this may predispose to volume overload, pulmonary edema, heart failure and, perhaps, intracranial hemorrhage in preterm neonates.

Naloxone is recommended for newly born infants with respiratory depression whose mothers received narcotics within 4 hours of delivery. Naloxone may be given by three routes: intravenous, intramuscular, or subcutaneous each at a dose of 0.1 mg per kg. It is important to note that naloxone solution is supplied in two concentrations, 0.4 mg/mL and 1.0 mg/mL; therefore, the dose administered may be 0.25 mL per kg or 0.1 mL per kg, respectively. *For infants whose mothers have used narcotics chronically, naloxone may be contraindicated because of the potential risk for acute withdrawal symptoms in the infant.* Additionally, newly born infants who receive naloxone should be monitored for recurrent respiratory depression because the duration of naloxone action may be shorter than the duration of the narcotic effect. Cardiorespiratory monitoring in the transitional or special care nursery for a minimum of 4 hours is advisable in these infants.

Sodium bicarbonate is not generally recommended during the acute phase of resuscitation. Paradoxical intracellular acidosis may further depress cardiac and neuronal activity and in the absence of controlled ventilation may worsen carbon dioxide retention and further depress the pH. Once ventilation is established, sodium bicarbonate may be given judiciously by intravenous route (1 to 2 meq/kg over at least 2 minutes) during a prolonged resuscitation unresponsive to other therapy. The efficacy of epinephrine is not enhanced with alkalinization.

IV. **Special circumstances in the delivery room.** Greater than 95% of newly born infants who require resuscitation in the delivery room will respond to appropriate airway management and the initiation of effective positive-pressure ventilation. A small number of babies, however, will remain apneic, bradycardic, and cyanotic even after receiving chest compressions and epinephrine. For these infants, further resuscitative efforts will depend on their clinical presentation (Fig. 2-1). The process of evaluation, decision, and action must be repeated frequently throughout resuscitation. If there is inadequate response to resuscitation, it is necessary to recheck the effectiveness of ventilation, chest compressions, and epinephrine administration. If not already done, endotracheal intubation should be considered. If epinephrine has been administered via the endotracheal route, placement of an umbilical venous catheter for intravenous administration should be considered.

A. **Central apnea.** In the delivery room, the newborn may suffer from central apnea due to asphyxia, prematurity, respiratory exhaustion, intracranial anomalies or bleeding, metabolic imbalances, hypothermia, or hyperthermia. Central apnea may also be associated with maternal narcotics, hypermagnesemia, or general anesthesia. The most important interventions for central apnea are gentle tactile stimulation and positive-pressure ventilation. Other interventions may include naloxone, correction of temperature and metabolic disturbances, continuous positive airway pressure, and mechanical ventilation.

B. **Prolonged bradycardia.** Conditions to consider when there is prolonged bradycardia unresponsive to resuscitation are outlined in Table 2-5. Prolonged bradycardia associated with inadequate ventilation may result from mechanical obstruction of the airways or impaired lung function. Obstructive apnea will present with cyanosis with or without bradycardia associated with increased work of breathing, poor air movement, or absent breath sounds. Absence of air movement through the nares by auscultation, inability to pass a catheter through the nares, or cyanosis and respiratory distress during initial oral feedings or when the mouth is closed suggest choanal atresia. If the newborn cannot compensate for the choanal obstruction by mouth breathing, an oral airway or endotracheal intubation may be lifesaving. Stridor or increased work of breathing with inadequate or absent breath sounds may indicate vocal cord paralysis (may follow difficult vaginal delivery and brachial plexus injury or may be the result of injury during intubation), vocal cord edema (may follow endotracheal intubation for meconium), laryngotracheal anomaly/malacia, or significant micrognathia with pharyngeal obstruction by the tongue. If respirations are labored and accompanied by cyanosis or bradycardia, endotracheal intubation is indicated.

Table 2-5. Special circumstances in resuscitation of the newly born infant

Condition	History/Clinical signs	Actions
Mechanical blockage of the airway		
Meconium or mucus blockage	Meconium-stained amniotic fluid	Intubation for suctioning/ventilation
	Poor chest wall movement	
Choanal atresia	Pink when crying, cyanotic when quiet	Oral airway
		Endotracheal intubation
Pharyngeal airway malformation	Persistent retractions, poor air entry	Prone positioning, posterior nasopharyngeal tube
Impaired lung function		
Pneumothorax	Asymmetrical breath sounds	Needle thoracentesis
	Persistent cyanosis/bradycardia	
Pleural effusions/ascites	Diminished air movement	Immediate intubation
	Persistent cyanosis/bradycardia	Needle thoracentesis, paracentesis
		Possible volume expansion
Congenital diaphragmatic hernia	Asymmetrical breath sounds	Endotracheal intubation
	Persistent cyanosis/bradycardia	Placement of orogastric catheter
	Scaphoid abdomen	
Pneumonia/sepsis	Diminished air movement	Endotracheal intubation
	Persistent cyanosis/bradycardia	Possible volume expansion
Impaired cardiac function		
Congenital heart disease	Persistent cyanosis/bradycardia	Diagnostic evaluation
Fetal/maternal hemorrhage	Pallor; poor response to resuscitation	Volume expansion, possibly including red blood cells

From *Pediatrics* 2000;106(3). URL: http:www.pediatrics.org/cgi/contents/full/106/3/e29.

C. **Pneumothorax.** Spontaneous or acquired pneumothorax may present with respiratory distress, overexpansion of one lung, absent/diminished breath sounds (often unilateral in location), and shift of the heart sounds to the contralateral chest cavity. The likelihood of a pneumothorax is increased if positive-pressure ventilation has been required, especially if there has been aspiration of meconium or in the presence of a lung malformation, for example, congenital diaphragmatic hernia or pulmonary hypoplasia. Transillumination using a fiberoptic light and/or chest radiograph may be helpful diagnostic studies. Transillumination allows immediate bedside assessment, eliminating the time inherent in obtaining a portable chest radiograph. Once diagnosed, thoracentesis and/or chest tube placement may be required. If not associated with severe respiratory distress or bradycardia, treatment with nitrogen washout by placing the infant in an oxyhood with FIO_2 1.0 for up to 24 hours may facilitate spontaneous resolution. Pneumothoraces are discussed in detail in Chapter 10.

D. **Congenital diaphragmatic hernia.** Congenital diaphragmatic hernia commonly presents with severe respiratory distress, unilateral absence of breath sounds, shift of heart sounds to the contralateral chest cavity (usually to the right because 80% of diaphragmatic hernias are left-sided) or the presence of bowel sounds in the chest. Clinical clues to this diagnosis include scaphoid abdomen and absent transillumination on the ipsilateral side of the hernia; chest radiographs are often diagnostic. If diaphragmatic hernia is suspected in the delivery room, immediate intubation and placement of an orogastric tube is recommended. Congenital diaphragmatic hernias are discussed in detail in Chapter 10.

E. **Pulmonary hypoplasia.** Pulmonary hypoplasia, like diaphragmatic hernia, also presents immediately in the delivery room. The infant will exhibit severe respiratory distress with symmetric but diminished breath sounds. High positive pressures to attain adequate oxygenation and ventilation are required in the most severe cases. Transillumination is negative unless pneumothorax complicates the resuscitation.

Pulmonary hypoplasia should be anticipated when oligohydramnios, renal anomalies, abdominal mass, congenital diaphragmatic hernia, ascites, hydrops, pleural effusions, or lung mass are recognized prenatally.

F. Hyaline membrane disease, transient tachypnea, meconium aspiration, and pneumonia. These entities may present with varying degrees of respiratory distress in the delivery room and are discussed in detail in Chapter 9. Supportive care and specific treatments such as oxygen, intravenous fluids, and antibiotics may be indicated. Consultation should be obtained to determine whether continuous positive airway pressure, mechanical ventilation, and surfactant are indicated.

G. Shock. Impaired cardiac function should be considered in those infants who remain bradycardic or cyanotic despite good ventilation. Pulses that are difficult to palpate, pallor, delayed capillary refill, and bradycardia are often indicative of shock in the delivery room. Hypovolemic shock associated with acute blood loss during delivery, asphyxia, or overwhelming sepsis will require volume expansion with normal saline, Ringer's lactate, and/or red blood cell transfusion. The volume of fluid administered to expand intravascular volume and the time frame to add dopamine must be based on clinical response and physician judgment.

Pneumothorax, congenital diaphragmatic hernia, excessive mean airway pressure with positive-pressure ventilation, pneumopericardium, and other respiratory disorders may lead to compromise of cardiac output and venous return and diminished pulses with acidemia. Cardiogenic shock associated with asphyxia, septic cardiomyopathy, and congenital heart disease may require volume expansion and dopamine infusion. When central cyanosis persists following initial resuscitation with 100% oxygen and effective ventilation, cyanotic congenital heart disease should be considered and may require the initiation of prostaglandin infusion (see Chapter 14). Subsequent therapies will be determined on the basis of the underlying etiology for shock.

H. Bowel obstruction. Bilious or copious gastric secretions and/or abdominal distension should prompt concern about bowel obstruction. When suspected, orogastric tube placement to low intermittent (feeding tube) or continuous (Replogle tube) suction is warranted until a diagnosis is established.

If oral secretions are copious, swallowing dysfunction or esophageal atresia should be considered. Esophageal atresia can be confirmed by an inability to pass a catheter into the stomach and chest radiograph that includes the neck; the catheter is often curled in the proximal esophageal pouch. Because the most common type of esophageal atresia includes a fistula from the trachea to the distal esophagus, gastric distension may occur, especially in neonates who require positive-pressure ventilation; prompt referral for gastric decompression with a gastrostomy tube is recommended.

I. Abdominal wall defects. Gastroschisis and omphalocele are obvious anomalies in the delivery room and require immediate intervention with orogastric tube placement, fluid resuscitation (150 to 200 mL/kg/day), heat maintenance, antibiotics, and placement of the lower body into a sterile "bowel bag" at the time of delivery. Because omphalocele is associated with other anomalies in about 50% of cases, a complete physical examination, careful evaluation of midline structures, and monitoring of blood glucose (Beckwith-Wiedemann Syndrome) are warranted. When gastroschisis exists, careful positioning of the infant to maximize bowel perfusion is especially important because the bowel is unsupported and has a tendency to twist and kink the vascular supply. Latex precautions and immediate referral for surgical intervention are indicated. These entities are discussed in greater detail in Chapter 18.

J. Meningmyeolocele. If a meningomyelocele is open, prone positioning, temperature maintenance, and placement of the lower body and meningomyelocele into a sterile "bowel bag" to minimize infection and fluid loss is recommended. An alternative is to place a protective sterile dressing moistened with normal saline over the meningomyelocele. Evidence for hydrocephalus and other anomalies should be sought. Latex precautions and referral are particularly important in these infants.

K. Dysmorphic features. Neonates with multiple dysmorphic features or ambiguous genitalia require referral to a tertiary center for extensive subspecialty evaluation and consultation. At this time, sensitive, honest parental counsel is often helpful for families in crisis. In the delivery room, resuscitation should be provided unless a lethal diagnosis has been established prenatally and a plan of comfort care established by parents and caregivers. Following stabilization, a complete physical examination, radiographic studies, and parental counseling regarding suspected diagnoses and potential outcomes should be provided. Often a specific diagnosis and outcomes prediction must await further investigation and consultation. If a newborn has ambiguous genitalia, it is recommended to defer choosing a first name or consider names that are gender neutral. Bladder and cloacal extrophy are rare disorders but require a "bowel bag," and latex precautions in the delivery room.

    L. **Prematurity.** Premature infants are at an increased risk for perinatal asphyxia both as a consequence of complications arising from premature labor as well as from physiologic immaturity. Premature and immature development of the lungs leads to a significant increase in the need for positive-pressure ventilation. The appropriate use of surfactant and continuous positive airway pressure (CPAP) are among the specific interventions that are still debated by experts in the field of neonatology. Special emphasis should be placed on thermal management of preterm infants as they are more likely to suffer from cold stress. In addition, care should be taken when providing volume resuscitation, because these infants are at increased risk for developing intracranial hemorrhage.

V.   **Discontinuation of resuscitation.** For those infants in whom there is no heart rate following 15 minutes of complete and adequate resuscitation (Apgar 0), it is reasonable to discontinue resuscitative efforts due to an extremely high likelihood of mortality or severe disability. In infants who are severely depressed (apnea or respiratory distress, bradycardia, hypotonia) but show signs of initial recovery, continued resuscitative efforts are warranted. Approximately 60% of infants with Apgar scores of 1 at one minute will survive and 60% are reported to be neurodevelopmentally normal.

VI.   **Postresuscitation evaluation and management.** Most newborn infants respond to early and efficient resuscitative measures. Infants who have been delivered through meconium-stained amniotic fluid, have initial respiratory depression and/or cyanosis, and who have required some resuscitation at birth are at risk for developing problems associated with their perinatal compromise. These infants should be evaluated frequently during the immediate neonatal period. Those infants who have required positive-pressure ventilation or more extensive resuscitative efforts are at high risk for developing complications associated with abnormal cardiopulmonary transition. These infants should be managed in an environment where close observation with frequent evaluation and monitoring is available.

    Neonates who require resuscitation are at risk for complications from their underlying illness, or from the hypoxemia that led to their resuscitative need (Table 2-6). Following the initial resuscitative measures, the effectiveness of ventilation should be reevaluated. In some cases, endotracheal intubation may be appropriate. If hypotension is present and does not respond adequately to volume expansion, a dopamine infusion (5 to 10 micrograms/kg/minute) should be initiated. On occasion, hypotension is a complication of a pneumothorax or other intrathoracic air leak; in this situation, thoracentesis may be lifesaving. Seizures may complicate hypoxic-ischemic encephalopathy, central nervous system bleeding, or trauma and may require phenobarbital administration (20 mg/kg intravenously by slow push). Hypoglycemia, hypocalcemia, anemia, polycythemia, disseminated intravascular coagulation, and acidemia should be identified and treated. Hypoglycemia is usually responsive to the initiation of intravenous glucose administration such as a slow bolus of 2mL/kg of D10W followed by a continuous infusion of D10W at 60 to 100 mL/kg/day. Calcium gluconate (1 to 2 mL/kg) or calcium chloride (0.35 to 0.7 mL/kg) will provide 10 to 20 mg/kg/dose of elemental calcium when given by intravenous infusion over 10 to 30 minutes. If total calcium levels are low, ionized calcium levels, if available, should be assessed before calcium supplementation is initiated. The benefits versus risks (bradycardia, subcutaneous infiltrate) of intravenous calcium supplementation should also be weighed before administration, especially if given through a peripheral vein. Calcium is not indicated during the acute phase of neonatal resuscitation.

    Acidosis must be determined to be respiratory, metabolic, or mixed. Mild to moderate respiratory acidosis may improve cerebral blood flow, whereas metabolic acidosis unresponsive to ventilation and volume expansion is likely detrimental. Therefore, blood gas values will help guide adjustments in ventilation and the decision to treat metabolic acidosis with sodium bicarbonate. Ventilation must be acceptable before giving sodium bicarbonate.

    A limited number of studies have investigated the use of hypothermia as a neuroprotective strategy in the management of the severely asphyxiated neonate. Insufficient data exist at this time to make a specific recommendation. The use of hypothermia as a neuroprotective strategy in preterm infants has not been studied. Moreover, hypothermia in preterm babies immediately after birth has been shown to be an independent risk factor for death. Hyperthermia postdelivery should be avoided as it is associated with perinatal respiratory depression, neonatal seizures, increased mortality, and cerebral palsy.

    Vitamin K prophylaxis, eye care, and hepatitis B vaccination should be provided as per hospital protocols.

Table 2-6. Postresuscitation care

Organ system	Potential complication	Postresuscitation action
Brain	Apnea	Monitor for apnea
	Seizures	Support ventilation as needed
		Monitor glucose and electrolytes
		Avoid hyperthermia
		Consider anticonvulsant therapy
Lungs	Pulmonary hypertension	Maintain adequate oxygenation and ventilation
	Pneumonia	Consider antibiotics
	Pneumothorax	Obtain x-ray if respiratory distress
	Transient tachypnea	Consider surfactant therapy
	Meconium aspiration syndrome	Delay feedings if respiratory distress
	Surfactant deficiency	
Cardiovascular	Hypotension	Monitor blood pressure and heart rate
		Consider inotrope (e.g., dopamine) and/or volume replacement
Kidneys	Acute tubular necrosis	Monitor urine output
		Restrict fluids if oliguric volume and vascular volume are adequate
		Monitor serum electrolytes
Gastrointestinal	Ileus	Delay initiation of feedings
	Necrotizing enterocolitis	Give intravenous fluids
		Consider parenteral nutrition
Metabolic/hematologic	Hypoglycemia	Monitor blood sugar
	Hypocalcemia; hyponatremia	Monitor electrolytes
	Anemia	Monitor hematocrit
	Thrombocytopenia	Monitor platelets

From The American Academy of Pediatrics and American Heart Association, *Textbook of Neonatal Resuscitation*, 4th edition. Elk Grove Village, IL: American Academy of Pediatrics, 2000:7–16, with permission.

VII. **Documentation.** It is imperative that the assessments and actions employed in the resuscitation of a newly born infant are documented in the medical record. This is essential not only for good care and communication, but also for medico-legal concerns. The Apgar score was developed to communicate the clinical status of newly born infants during the first minutes of life. The five categories scored include respiratory effort, heart rate, color, reflex irritability, and muscle tone (Table 2-7). Although several of these categories are also used to make decisions about neonatal resuscitation, it should be clear that resuscitation begins at the time of birth, if needed. By 90 to 120 seconds of age in depressed newly born infants, resuscitation should be well into its course. Apgar scores were not designed to guide the need for resuscitation! Apgar scores are assigned at 1 and 5 minutes and for an extended period until the Apgar score is >6. The Apgar score is less valid with premature infants. Apgar scores at 15 and 20 minutes correlate with outcome.

VIII. **Ethical considerations in the delivery room.** The ethical principles that guide decision making in the delivery room are no different than those followed in the older child or adult. If resuscitation is initiated in the delivery room, there is no ethical reason prohibiting withdrawal of medical support if indicated. There are situations where noninitiation or discontinuation of support in the delivery room may be appropriate. Under these circumstances, the infant should be treated with dignity and respect. Delayed or partial resuscitations are to be avoided as the outcome of the infant may be worsened if he or she survives. Whenever possible, discussions regarding the approach to resuscitation should take place with the parents before delivery. Parental choice regarding the management of resuscitation and subsequent care should be respected within the limits of medical feasibility and appropriateness.

Noninitiation of resuscitation in the delivery room may be appropriate in situations where it is very unlikely that the infant will survive or survive without severe disability.

Table 2-7. Apgar scores

Sign	Score		
	0	1	2
Heart rate	Absent	<100	≥100
Respiratory effort	Absent	Slow, irregular	Good, crying
Muscle tone	Limp	Some flexion	Active movement
Reflex irritability (catheter in nares or tactile stimulation)	No response	Grimace	Cough, sneeze, cry
Color	Blue or pale	Pink body and blue extremities (acrocyanosis)	Pink body and extremities

From The American Academy of Pediatrics and American Heart Association, *Textbook of Neonatal Resuscitation*, 4th edition. Elk Grove Village, IL: American Academy of Pediatrics, 2000, with permission.

At present, noninitiation of resuscitation is an acceptable consideration for infants with confirmed gestation of <23 weeks or birth weight <400 g, anencephaly, or confirmed trisomy 13 or 18. Prenatal diagnosis of these conditions allows parents and caregivers to plan for care at delivery. For these infants who have extremely high mortality risks, comfort measures, warmth, and family support are suggested.

Although prenatal diagnosis often forewarns of fetal abnormalities or problems so that transfer to specialty facilities can be prospectively arranged, caregivers must be prepared to stabilize, identify, and treat a number of disorders that only become apparent after delivery and may or may not require cardiopulmonary resuscitation. In situations where no prenatal diagnostic evaluation and counseling are possible, it is generally advisable to intervene, gather more information about the problems that the infant is experiencing, and then decide upon further interventions in consultation with the parents. If uncertainty exists about the outcome and candidacy for resuscitation, for example, uncertain gestational age, it is advisable to stabilize and consult with parents, subspecialty pediatricians, and other parental support persons.

IX. **Clinical pearl.**
- Normal cardiopulmonary transition after birth requires clearance of fetal lung fluid and an increase in pulmonary blood flow.
- The basic steps of neonatal resuscitation include preventing heat loss, establishing a clear airway, and initiating ventilation.
- Establishment of adequate ventilation is the most important and effective step in neonatal resuscitation.
- An increase in heart rate to >100 beats per minute is the best indicator of effective ventilation.
- The knowledge and skills necessary to perform neonatal resuscitation must be learned by all personnel responsible for newly born infants in the delivery room through completion of a course specifically designed for this purpose, such as the American Heart Association/American Academy of Pediatrics Neonatal Resuscitation Program.

BIBLIOGRAPHY

Printed Materials

Evidence Evaluation Worksheets. Neonatal Resuscitation Program, 2004.

Gilstrap LC, Oh W, eds. *Guidelines for perinatal care*, 5th ed. Elk Grove Village, IL: American Academy of Pediatrics, 2002.

International Consensus on Science. International guidelines for neonatal resuscitation: an excerpt from the guidelines 2000 for cardiopulmonary resuscitation and emergency cardiovascular care. *Pediatrics* 2000;106(3):e29.

Kattwinkel J, Short J, Niermeyer S, et al., eds. *Textbook of neonatal resuscitation*, 4th ed. Elk Grove Village, IL: American Academy of Pediatrics, 2000.

Kattwinkel J, Niermeyer S, Nadkarni V, et al. An advisory statement from the Pediatric Working Group of the International Liaison Committee on Resuscitation. *Pediatrics* 1999;103(4):e56.

WEBSITES

http://www.aap.org/profed/nrp/nrpmain.html

Physical Examination of the Newborn

Caroline Rose Paul and
Mitchell A. Harris

I. **Description of the issue.** The clinician must rely on knowledge, intuition, and thoroughness to successfully assess a newborn. A key part of the newborn's examination involves differentiating between findings that are variations of normal from abnormal findings. As with the examination of any age group, a complete history is vital to performing a pertinent examination. The history should contain a maternal history, labor and delivery history, and transition history. The maternal history consists of illnesses, drug use, obstetric record, data of prior pregnancies, and data of the current pregnancy. The labor, delivery, and transition histories should include Apgar scores, delivery room complications, laboratory data, and neonatal signs and symptoms that have been noted by the staff thus far.

The examination should be gentle, unhurried, and minimally stressful to the infant. The best time to examine a newborn is in their sleepy, awake state. One should take advantage of the baby's mainly sleeping or quiet resting state to observe those parameters that require a quiet state for evaluation.

II. **Observation.** The examination is begun by quietly observing the infant. First it should be determined if the newborn is in any immediate distress. Recorded vital signs including temperature, respiratory rate, pulse, and blood pressure should be noted. Observation should be made for any evidence of respiratory distress and/or cyanosis. The resting posture should be noted. A normal full-term infant's resting posture is generally symmetrically flexed. Significant deviation from this may suggest abnormalities including clavicle fractures, brachial plexus injuries, preterm gestation, or hypotonia.

The heart and lungs should be auscultated and the abdomen should be evaluated when the baby is quiet. Warm hands and equipment will avoid startling the newborn. The abdomen is best palpated when the baby is quiet, as relaxed abdominal musculature is a prerequisite for an adequate examination. After the cardiac, respiratory, and abdominal systems have been examined, the remaining portions of the examination can be performed on a more awake infant.

III. **Body measurements.** Certain body measurements (weight, head circumference, and length) are obtained on all newborn babies as baseline criteria for future growth and to identify deviations from normal. These determinations must be performed carefully if they are to be useful.

The head circumference is measured with a flexible tape. The largest measurement with the tape wrapped around the occipital and frontal prominences is the occipital frontal circumference (OFC). In a normal full-term infant this is approximately 34 cm. The infant's length is preferably measured with a measuring board specifically designed for this purpose. The normal length of a full-term baby is approximately 50 cm. Once obtained, these measurements, along with weight, are plotted on a standard growth curve so that deviations from normal can be more readily appreciated and growth followed in a prospective manner. A more detailed discussion of maturity and intrauterine growth is presented in Chapter 4.

IV. **Skin.** The skin of the newborn is generally pink and uniform in color. In order to preserve heat, the newborn responds to cold with peripheral vasoconstriction. Because of the relatively transparent newborn skin, the vascular plexus is easily seen. Consequently, vasoconstriction in response to cold may normally result in a mottled appearance. However, mottling may also reflect shock or sepsis.

A. **Normal skin findings.**
   1. **Acrocyanosis.** Acrocyanosis, or cyanosis of the distal extremities, is often a normal finding and thus is not a good indicator of the baby's oxygen status. In contrast to acrocyanosis, central cyanosis reflects true arterial hypoxemia. Central cyanosis is best seen by observing the lips, perioral region, and tongue. Central cyanosis is always abnormal and requires immediate evaluation.

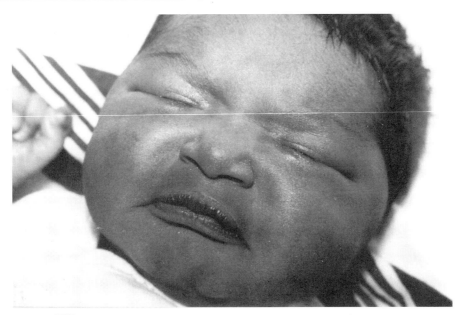

Figure 3-1. Milia.

2. **Milia.** Milia (Fig. 3-1) are small, white, firm papules especially noted on the upper cheeks, nose, and chin. The same type of structure can also appear on the midline of the palate and there they are termed Epstein Pearls. The distribution of milia can be quite extensive. No treatment is necessary as these lesions exfoliate spontaneously in the first weeks of life.
3. **Nevus simplex or "salmon patch."** Nevus simplex (Fig. 3-2), which often involves the eyelids, glabella, and nuchal areas, is a pink/pale-red discoloration of skin. This lesion results from vascular ectasia and can persist for months. The lesion

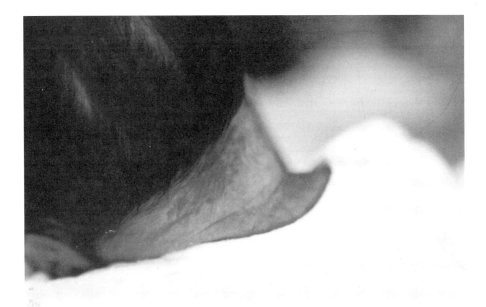

Figure 3-2. Nevus simplex.

tends to get redder with crying. Layperson terminology for nevus simplex includes "storkbite" (occiput) and "angel kiss" (supraorbit). This lesion needs to be distinguished from a port wine stain, which is abnormal and can have systemic implications. Port wine stains tend to be deeper in hue, larger, and unilateral.

4. **Vernix.** Vernix is white, cheese-like material composed of cellular and other debris. It is present on the skin at birth and usually is absent in post-term infants.

5. **Mongolian spot.** A Mongolian spot (Fig. 3-3) is a bluish/green, well-demarcated area of pigmentation that is most commonly noted in black, Native American, and Asian infants. It is a benign lesion that may persist over the first few years. It is often distributed over the buttocks, shoulders, and back. If not familiar with this finding, practitioners may mistake it for a bruise.

6. **Erythema toxicum.** Erythema toxicum (Fig. 3-4), is seen in 30% to 70% of newborns. The rash generally appears after the first 24 hours of life, and usually clears spontaneously within 2 weeks. It begins as an erythematous, macular mark and develops into a small papule on an erythematous base. Sometimes, this lesion may appear simply urticarial in appearance without further progression. The papule can become vesiculopustular and thus may need to be differentiated from serious causes of vesicles in the newborn period, such as herpes simplex and staphylococcal infections. These lesions can occur anywhere on the body but rarely occur on the palms or soles. Wright stains of pustular contents reveal eosinophils.

7. **Transient neonatal pustular melanosis.** This condition (Fig. 3-5A,B) is most common in black infants. The characteristic lesions evolve from small vesiculopustules to collorettes of scaly crust surrounding hyperpigmented macules. The lesions may be present at birth in various stages of evolution and may involve any body surface including palms and soles. The pigmented macules gradually fade over the first few months of life. The condition is benign and requires no intervention.

8. **Lanugo.** Lanugo is fine body hair, which begins to thin after 28 weeks gestation. Between the 32nd and 37th weeks of gestation, it vanishes from the face and between the 38th and 42nd week, it is present only on the shoulders. After the 42nd week, lanugo is absent.

9. **Harlequin color change.** This is a vascular finding and sometimes may be more noticeable when babies are placed on their sides. One side of the body is noted to be pale and the other side a deep red. The line demarcating the two sides can be

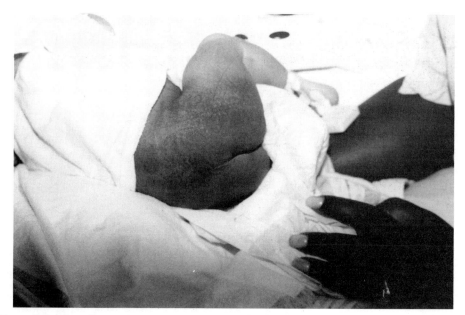

Figure 3-3. Mongolian spot.

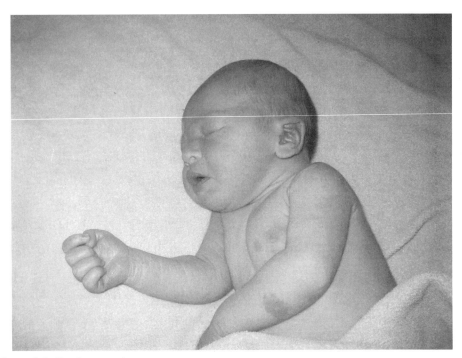

Figure 3-4. Erythema toxicum.

quite distinct and impressive. This color change can last for a few minutes. It is more common in premature infants, but can occur in full-term infants. This is benign and generally does not occur after the third week of life.

B. Abnormal skin findings.

1. **Jaundice.** Jaundice in the term and otherwise healthy newborn is very common (see Chapter 8). However, the presence of jaundice in the first 24 hours of life is considered pathologic and should always be evaluated. Jaundice is more difficult to detect in the neonate than in the older child or adult. The ease of detection of jaundice in the newborn varies, often depending on skin pigmentation and general ruddiness of the infant. Jaundice is best noted in natural light. Applying dermal pressure on the tip of the nose will yield a yellow tinge in the jaundiced newborn. The hard palate is another helpful area to detect jaundice.

   Jaundice usually progresses cephalocaudal in the newborn and serum levels can roughly be estimated depending on the area of the body. Dermal zones of icterus were first described in 1969 and jaundice of the face and neck correlated with bilirubin levels that ranged from 4 to 8 mg/dL. Progression of jaundice to the umbilicus reflected levels between 5 and 12 mg/dL, while further advancement to the groin and upper thighs correlated with bilirubin levels of 8 to 16 mg/dL. Jaundice progressing to the ankles and wrists was consistent with levels of 11 to 18 mg/dL and jaundice of the feet and hands implied levels >15 mg/dL.

2. **Edema.** Edema is seen frequently in premature infants, either as a normal finding or secondary to hypoxia and vascular damage. Edema of the hands and feet may also be seen in Turner syndrome. Diffuse massive edema of the newborn, or hydrops fetalis, is indicative of severe underlying pathology, for example, erythroblastosis fetalis.

3. **Meconium staining.** Meconium can be noted to stain areas of the neonate, especially the nailbeds and umbilical cord. Meconium staining results from the *in utero* passage of stool and may be indicative of fetal distress. Aspiration of meconium can cause a severe aspiration pneumonia (see Chapter 9).

4. **Petechiae.** Petechiae are often noted in areas of pressure in the newborn, such as the face of an infant born in the cephalic presentation or delivered with the umbilical cord wrapped around the neck. Pathologic causes including platelet

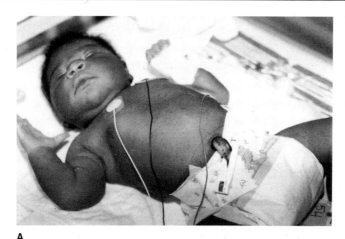

A

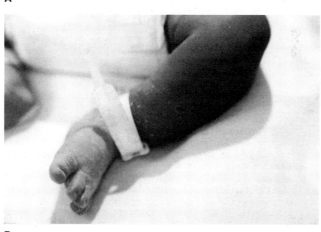

B

Figure 3-5. **(A)** Transient pustular melanosis. **(B)** Transient pustular melanosis.

abnormalities and infection should be considered when petechiae are observed in atypical areas such as the trunk and extremities.

5. **Sacral dimples/dermatologic manifestations of spinal dysraphism.** Dimples (Fig. 3-6) of skin aligned along the spinal processes may indicate spinal dysraphism. It is important to note if a dimple is communicating or superficial. Other findings, which more strongly suggest spinal dysphrasism, include tufts of hair, lipomas, and nevi.

6. **Nevus flammeus or "port wine stain."** Port wine stain (Fig. 16-1) (see Chapter 16), a congenital vascular malformation, tends to be well demarcated, macular, and pink to purple. Mainly unilateral, port wine stains occur most often on the face and neck. This lesion needs to be differentiated from nevus simplex. Unlike the nevus simplex, the port wine stain is a serious finding, which can suggest neurocutaneous disease. When noted in the trigeminal nerve distribution, particularly in the first branch (ophthalmic) distribution, Sturge-Weber disease must be considered. Port wine stain is also associated with syndromes such as Klippel-Trenaunay syndrome.

V.   **Skull.** Measurement and evaluation of the contour of the skull are important parts of the newborn examination. The newborn head is large relative to the body. If the baby is born in a cephalic presentation, considerable molding of the easily malleable skull bones may take place to facilitate passage through the birth canal (Fig. 3-7). Within 2 to 3 days after birth, most of the molding has usually resolved and the head assumes its normal configuration. Molding is not usually present when the infant is born by cesarean section without labor or after breech presentation.

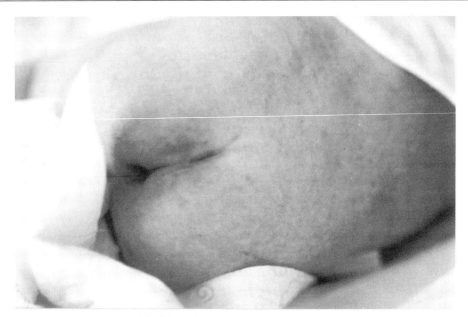

Figure 3-6. Sacral dimple (with skin tag).

The anterior fontanel is diamond-shaped and formed by the convergence of the metopic, coronal, and sagittal sutures (Fig. 3-8). The posterior fontanel, at the convergence of the sagittal and lambdoidal sutures, is fingertip in size in the newborn period. It generally closes by 6 to 8 weeks of age.

The suture lines are often overriding during the immediate newborn period. One can palpate the movable ridges in the benign overriding sutures, unlike the fixed ridges seen in craniosynostosis, a condition resulting from the premature closure of sutures. The most common type of craniosynostosis occurs with the premature closure of the sagittal

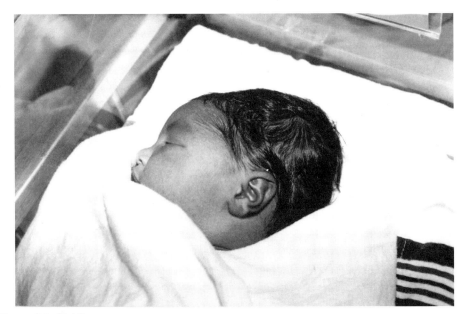

Figure 3-7. Molding.

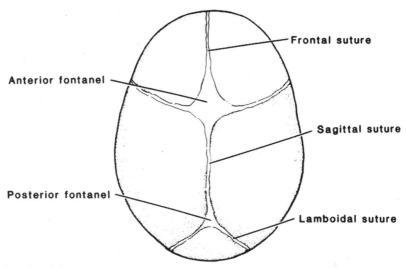

Figure 3-8. Cranial sutures.

suture. Craniosynostosis should be suspected with the presence of a small or closed anterior fontanel, an abnormally shaped skull, and the presence of fixed suture ridges. Craniosynostosis is usually an isolated abnormality but can be associated with syndromes like Aperts and Crouzon.

The anterior fontanel should be examined in both the upright and supine position since the fullness of the fontanel normally varies with position. Also, the anterior fontanel may appear to be relatively full in the normal crying infant. A large, bulging fontanel can suggest hydrocephalus and one needs to investigate for other signs and symptoms of hydrocephalus. The anterior fontanel is usually closed by 2 years of age.

A. Common findings.

    1. Caput succedaneum. Caput succedaneum (Fig. 3-9) is a very common finding in the immediate newborn period. This is a diffuse benign swelling of the soft tissues

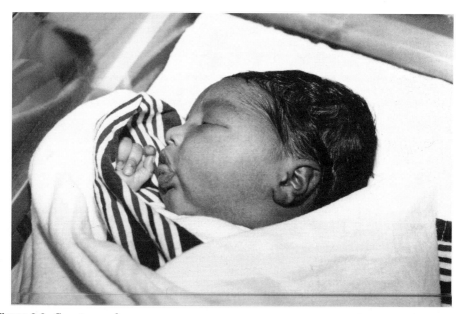

Figure 3-9. Caput succedaneum.

resulting from pressure during delivery. It involves the region of the scalp that is presented during a vertex delivery.

2. **Cephalhematoma.** Cephalhematoma is a subperiosteal hemorrhage. Because it is under the periosteum, it does not cross suture lines and localizes to one cranial bone. A cephalhematoma may not be evident immediately following delivery and may not become evident until several hours or days following delivery. Sequelae of a cephalhematoma include anemia and jaundice.

VI. **Eyes.** Gentle rocking can induce a neonate to open his or her eyes. Also, one can shine a light source directly on the closed eyes and then quickly shut off the light source. Another maneuver that may help induce eye opening is to have the infant suck on a pacifier or gloved finger. The examiner should note the size of the eyes, pupils, and palpebral fissures. Perform a fundoscopic examination, looking for a red reflex and retinal hemorrhages.

It is important to recognize some variances of the newborn's eyes. The eye movements are frequently not coordinated until about 3 to 4 months of age. The sclera of the newborn is thin and bluish in color. The cornea should be clear and any clouding should raise the concern for glaucoma, trauma, or congenital infection. The red reflex should be symmetric and equal. An abnormal red reflex is often seen in retinoblastoma, cataracts, and congenital glaucoma. Early detection is imperative, because early treatment may prevent amblyopia. Also, while often isolated, cataracts can also be associated with intrauterine infections or metabolic disorders. Scleral hemorrhage as a result of the delivery process is not uncommon. These hemorrhages have no significant sequelae and disappear within a few weeks.

While discharge from the eyes may be from a more benign etiology, such as nasolacrimal duct stenosis, any purulent discharge should be investigated for infectious causes. Gonococcal ophthalmia neonatorum tends to manifest itself after the first few days of life; however, it should always be considered in the neonate of any age with significant eye drainage. *Chlamydia trachomatis* is another infectious etiology of eye drainage. It generally presents after the first week of life. Chemical conjunctivitis, especially noted with the use of silver nitrate, presents in the first 2 days.

VII. **Ears.** A considerable amount of information can be obtained from an evaluation of the external ear. Its form and elasticity are helpful guides to the maturity of the newborn as discussed in Chapter 4. Gross anomalies of the exterior aspect of the ear are associated with abnormalities of other body systems, particularly the genitourinary system.

Abnormalities of the external ear include malformation, malposition, preauricular tags, pits, and sinus tracts. Malformations may be familial, isolated findings, or part of a congenital syndrome.

One method to determine if an ear is low-set is to draw an imaginary line between both inner canthi of the eyes and extend that line posteriorly. If the helix of the ear is below this line, the ear is considered low-set. Low-set ears may be associated with other malformations or congenital syndromes.

VIII. **Nose.** An initial examination of the nose for potential obstruction is important since newborns are obligate nose breathers. Inspect externally for nasal septal asymmetry and gross deformities. Nasal septal asymmetry occurs in approximately 1% of newborns. Such asymmetry may be due to compression of the nasal tip. Watchful waiting may be all that is required. In some cases, however, it can be due to nasal dislocation and, in that case, correction may be required in the following few days.

Nasal patency can be assessed by various bedside methods. One can occlude one nostril with a finger and listen for air entry through the other nostril or assess for any respiratory distress. A wisp of cotton can be placed in front of each nostril and checked for movement. One may also pass a 5-French catheter through each nostril. This final maneuver, however, may cause trauma and swelling and should be reserved for cases that are difficult to verify.

IX. **Mouth.** Normal findings of the oral cavity include Epstein pearls and Bohn nodules, which are both the intraoral counterparts of the external milia, and these two terms are now often used interchangeably. Epstein pearls are discrete, round, pearly structures along the midline of the hard palate. Bohn nodules are noted in the gumline distribution.

The oral cavity must be examined for abnormalities such as defects of the palate, masses, micrognathia, natal teeth, a large tongue, and an asymmetric grimace. It is best to perform a clean sweep of the oral cavity with a gloved finger. Palpation of the palate is necessary to detect a submucous cleft.

A. **Abnormal findings.**

1. **Micrognathia.** Micrognathia may be associated with a small, posteriorly positioned tongue that can cause symptomatic airway obstruction and feeding difficulties. This finding is frequently seen in the Pierre Robin sequence.

2. **Natal teeth.** Natal teeth may erupt *in utero* or during the first month of life (neonatal teeth) and have a frequency of about 1 in 2,000 newborns. These teeth may interfere with feeding. Also, there is a risk of detachment and aspiration, especially if the teeth are loose. These teeth should be removed if loose; however, prior to extraction they should be differentiated from normal, prematurely erupted deciduous teeth by x-ray.

3. **Macroglossia or pseudomacroglossia.** Macroglossia or pseudomacroglossia (associated with micrognathia) can interfere with feeding and cause significant airway obstruction. True macroglossia can be associated with congenital hypothyroidism, mucopolysaccharidoses, and Beckwith-Wiedemann syndrome.

4. **Asymmetric grimace.** An asymmetric grimace can be seen with a congenital absence of the orbicularis oris muscle or seventh cranial nerve palsy. With central paralysis, the lower two-thirds of the face is involved and the forehead is intact. With complete peripheral paralysis, the whole side is involved and the mouth is drawn to the nonparalyzed side. Facial nerve palsy may have no readily apparent cause; however, a difficult delivery with or without the use of forceps may result in facial paralysis. Usually no further diagnostic testing is indicated, unless a central nervous system problem is suspected rather than a facial nerve injury. In most cases, observation is the treatment and the paralysis usually resolves in a few weeks to months.

X. **Neck.** While providing nuchal support, examine the neck for webbing, skin folds, torticollis, vertebral anomalies, and neck masses. Fistulas and cysts along the anterior border of the sternocleidomastoid muscle may be manifestations of branchial cleft anomalies. Torticollis noted in the immediate newborn period can result from many disorders, but the most common is fibromatosis coli. Fibromatosis coli refers to a 1 to 2 cm, round, firm, fibrous neck mass within the sternocleidomastoid muscle that may be present at birth but most commonly presents at 2 to 3 weeks of age. It is probably the result of trauma to the muscle during labor and delivery.

XI. **Chest.** The chest wall area should be examined for abnormalities such as wide-spaced nipples, malformation of the rib cage, and supernumerary nipples. Wide-spaced nipples suggest particular syndromes. Malformation of the rib cage may be seen in some of the chondrodystrophies. There may also be failure of fusion of the sternum as well as rib defects. Also, observe carefully any asymmetry during respiration as this may suggest missing ribs or thoracic cage defects. Supernumerary nipples are occasionally observed and usually occur in a line below the existing nipple (they are often small, not well formed, and go unnoticed).

XII. **Cardiorespiratory system.** Evaluation of the cardiorespiratory system is optimal when the newborn is in a quiet resting state. The exam should include observation, palpation, and auscultation. Observe for any chest wall asymmetry. The normal newborn is pink.

While the chest precordium is active because of a relatively anteriorly placed heart and a significant hyperdynamic state, one should still palpate for abnormal heaves and thrills. The femoral pulses should be palpated and compared to the brachial pulses. Weak femoral pulses or decreased blood pressure measured in the lower extremities must be immediately investigated for possible coarctation of the aorta. Very weak peripheral pulses may indicate hypotension or other significant heart disease. Bounding peripheral pulses may indicate hypertension or a patent ductus arteriosus.

The first step in auscultation of the chest is to consciously distinguish between heart and lung sounds, as this can be confusing. For the cardiac portion of the exam, the normal "rapid" rate can be quite distracting to the examiner. One should attempt to note separately the quality of each heart sound and listen for splitting and prominence. Then, attention should be given to the intervals between S1 and S2 and any additional heart sounds. Auscultation should be for at least 30 seconds to obtain a heart rate, due to the heart rate's variability that may be benign or abnormal. The normal heart rate ranges from 120 to 160 beats per minute.

It is common to auscultate early systolic murmurs caused by a persistent patent ductus arteriosus in the first few hours of life. However, any murmur should be carefully evaluated. Given the high pulmonary vascular resistance in the newborn, significant pathologic murmurs may not become evident in the immediate neonatal period. In addition, significant cardiac lesions may not manifest themselves until after the closure of the ductus arteriosus. Thus, it is imperative that careful examinations are performed serially and prior to discharge. Some other signs and symptoms of cardiac pathology are apnea, intermittent or persistent tachypnea, arrhythmias, grunting, cyanosis, abnormal pulses, and poor feeding and activity.

When auscultating the respiratory system, recognize that breath sounds in the newborn are easily referred from the upper airway and from one side to the other. What may sound like significant pathologic rales may only be referred upper airway noise. The normal respiratory rate ranges from 30 to 60 respirations per minute. Observation of the chest wall is the best method to determine a respiratory rate. As with the heart rate, it is important to allow for a longer period than with an adult. Respirations can vary considerably because of periodic breathing when pauses (brief apnea) are followed by a rapid burst of respirations.

XIII. **Abdomen.** Infants' abdomens are best examined when they are quiet. Abdominal palpation of the newborn requires a soft touch so abdominal organs are not pushed out of the way of the examining finger. The newborn liver is normally palpated approximately 1 to 2 cm below the right costal margin. A liver edge more than 3.5 cm below the costal margin is considered abnormal and should be further evaluated. Occasionally, the spleen tip can be palpated, and the kidneys are usually within reach of the examining finger, especially the left kidney. Neonatal abdominal masses may represent a surgical emergency. The most common intraabdominal pathologic mass in the newborn is an enlarged kidney.

Examination of the abdomen includes a close inspection of the umbilical cord. There are normally three vessels present: the two arteries have very small lumens with thick walls, whereas the vein has a large lumen with a very thin wall. If only one artery and one vein are present, there is an associated increased incidence of other congenital malformations.

A. Abnormal findings.

1. **Abdominal distension.** Abdominal distension in the newborn may be secondary to an intestinal obstruction, ruptured viscus, ascites, or a mass. Abdominal distension with or without bilious vomiting requires immediate evaluation. Conversely, when the abdomen is extremely flat, or "scaphoid," and gives the impression of a lack of abdominal contents, diaphragmatic hernia is suspected.

2. **Abdominal masses.** The most common abdominal mass in the newborn is an enlarged kidney caused by hydronephrosis, renal dysplasia, or multiple cysts. Other less common lesions include congenital mesoblastic nephroma, nephroblastoma, renal vein thrombosis, ovarian cyst, hydrocolpos, adrenal hematoma, neuroblastoma, sacrococcygeal teratoma, and gastrointestinal lesions such as a distended loop of bowel.

3. **Prune belly syndrome.** Prune belly syndrome, a condition in which the abdominal muscles are absent, is usually accompanied by genitourinary anomalies such as vesicoureteric reflux. The disorder is most common in males.

4. **Omphalocele.** An omphalocele (Fig. 18-5) (see Chapter 18) is a defect in the umbilicus, with the bowel and possibly other abdominal contents herniated through the umbilical ring. The exposed bowel is covered by peritoneum. There is a high incidence of other congenital malformations in infants with omphalocele.

5. **Gastroschisis.** Gastroschisis (Fig. 18-6) (see Chapter 18) is a defect in the abdominal wall musculature, usually below and to the right of an intact umbilicus. The peritoneal covering is absent and this defect is always associated with peritonitis. There is a low incidence of associated anomalies with gastroschisis.

XIV. **Genitalia.** In the term, female infant, the labia majora are very visible while the labia minora are not prominent (Fig. 4-7) (see Chapter 4). In general, the labia can appear larger than normal in the first day of life because of edema, but this quickly resolves. A whitish vaginal discharge is also common during the first few days of life and is secondary to maternal hormones. Withdrawal vaginal bleeding may also occur during this period. Hymenal tags are common and involute shortly after birth. Clitoromegaly raises the concern of gender identity and metabolic and hormonal derangement.

In the term, male infant, the testes have bilaterally descended into the scrotal sac. However, the testes may "ride high" in the sac. If they can easily be brought down, no intervention is required in the newborn period. The scrotal sac may appear large because of a hydrocele, which is a collection of fluid in the tunica vaginalis. Transillumination of the sac will confirm the presence of a hydrocele and the absence of hernias or testicular abnormalities.

Examine the penis for chordee (ventral penile curvature) and appropriate position of the urethra. When the urethral opening is on the ventral surface, the condition is called hypospadias. Hypospadias is further described on the basis of the position of the meatus (glandular, coronal). In most cases, hypospadias is an isolated finding; however, it can be associated with other genitourinary abnormalities such as undescended testes. It is imperative to diagnose hypospadias in the immediate newborn period, as it is a contraindication for circumcision since the foreskin is often utilized in future surgical repair. Epispadias refers to a urethral meatus that opens on the dorsum of the penis and may be associated with bladder exstrophy.

XV. **Anus.** The anus should be examined for patency and position. An anteriorly placed anus raises suspicion for anorectal anomalies. Failure to pass a meconium stool requires further evaluation.

XVI. **Musculoskeletal system.** Examination of the musculoskeletal system includes observation of the resting posture and observation and palpation of the spine and extremities. The normal resting term infant is usually symmetrically flexed at all extremities. Intrauterine positioning may cause temporary distortion of the extremities, especially the feet. This should not be confused with talipes equinovarus (club foot) or other foot deformities. Mild bowing of the legs is common in the normal newborn, and the newborn's foot is flat.

Examine the extremities for polydactyly and gross deformities. The nailbeds should be examined for hypoplasia as hypoplastic nails can be associated with certain syndromes and maternal drug exposure, for example, diphenylhydantoin.

Positional abnormalities of the feet include metatarsus adductus, calcaneovalgus, and talipes equinovarus. All three may result from *in utero* positioning. Metatarsus adductus and calcaneovalgus usually improve in the first few months of extrauterine life.

A. Positional deformities.

1. **Metatarsus adductus.** In metatarsus adductus, the forefoot is deviated medially and is slightly supinated. In the normal foot, a line drawn through the hindfoot will pass between the second and third toe. With metatarsus adductus, this line will pass lateral to the third toe. The prognosis is excellent, with most cases of metatarsus adductus resolving spontaneously.

2. **Calcaneovalgus.** Calcaneovalgus deformity of the foot is commonly associated with lateral tibial torsion. The forefoot is abducted, and the ankle is severely dorsiflexed to where the foot folds against the anterolateral surface of the tibia. The deformity is usually flexible, and the foot can be passively placed in the normal position. Calcaneovalgus deformity of the foot usually resolves spontaneously.

3. **Talipes equinovarus.** Talipes equinovarus, or club foot, has an incidence of approximately 1.5 in 1,000. Fifty percent of the time, the condition is bilateral. It can be associated with other conditions such as spina bifida and arthrogryposis. The foot turns inward and downward and remains tight in this position. Talipes equinovarus requires immediate evaluation since the timing of corrective casting, if necessary, can affect optimal outcome.

XVII. **Hips.** The hips require special attention in the newborn period. Early detection of developmental dysplasia of the hip (DDH) is associated with better outcome. In general, developmental dysplasia of the hip refers to an abnormal relationship between the femoral head and the acetabulum. This encompasses instability, subluxation, acetabular dysplasia, and frank dislocation. Risk factors include first-born, female, left side, breech delivery, and family history. DDH can be associated with torticollis, foot abnormalities, and other musculoskeletal disorders.

A complete exam of the hips is imperative. In the older infant, limited range of motion is a common presenting sign. However, in the newborn, examination of range of motion in the newborn is not adequate for checking stability of the hip. Two maneuvers are essential to the newborn exam, the Barlow and Ortolani maneuvers (Fig. 3-10A, B). The optimal method in examining the hips of the newborn is when the infant is relaxed. Always examine the infant with a released diaper. Each hip should be examined separately.

The Ortolani maneuver reduces a dislocated hip. With the infant lying supine, the Ortolani is performed with the index and third finger positioned on the greater trochanter and the thumb positioned on the inner thigh. The other hand should be used to stabilize the pelvis. While the hip is flexed at a 90-degree angle and the leg is kept in a neutral position, abduct the hip and raise the leg anteriorly. With a positive Ortolani sign, this maneuver reduces an already dislocated hip and will produce a "clunk" sensation. This sign is produced by the head of the femur sliding over the edge of the acetabulum and into the socket. The term "click" should not be used and is not a diagnostic term.

The Barlow maneuver is a provocative test to detect those hips that are unstable, that is, able to be displaced from the acetabulum to a dislocated position. As with the Ortolani, one hand performs the maneuver and the other stabilizes the pelvis. The hand positioning is also similar to the Ortolani. Gently adduct the hip while applying a posterior pressure with the weight of the hand. The normal hip will not dislocate but the dislocatable hips will move very smoothly and subtly out of the socket. The second part of the Barlow maneuver is the classical Ortolani test, that is, abducting the hip and lifting the dislocated femoral head over the rim of the socket.

A positive Ortolani or Barlow requires immediate referral for further evaluation and correction. More subtle findings (i.e., asymmetric gluteal creases, unequal leg length,

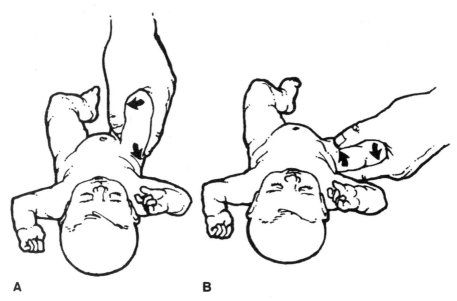

A **B**

Figure 3-10. Barlow **(A)** and Ortolani maneuvers **(B)**.

etc.) should be combined with presence of risk factors to determine further evaluation, including pediatric orthopedic referral and ultrasonography.

XVIII. **Neurologic system.** The neurologic examination of the newborn serves many purposes. It is a useful tool in helping to assess the maturity of a newborn; it can aid in the detection of acute disorders such as sepsis, cerebral edema, or nerve palsy; and it can assist in the detection of abnormalities that will affect subsequent development. The timing of the exam is important because after the first hours of life the newborn may experience a so-called "physiologic depression." Intrapartum medications received by the mother can also affect the examination. Both of these issues are usually resolved by 24 hours of age. Serial exams may be necessary. The neurologic examination of the newborn is thoroughly outlined in Chapter 16.

XIX. **Clinical pearls.**
- Perform exam with baby undressed, preferably under the warmer.
- Plot all anthropometric measurements versus gestational age on chart.
- Skin findings include petechiae (don't blanch with pressure) that are common on the face; erythema toxicum will appear after birth (generally after 24 hours); the pustules of pustular melanosis may be present at birth.
- Caput succedaneum is a collection of subcutaneous edema and can cross suture lines, whereas a cephalohematoma is a subperiostal hemorrhage, and because it is under the periosteum will not cross suture lines.
- Heart murmurs, while common, should be carefully evaluated, including repeating the examination prior to discharge.
- Genitalia: examine the penis for hypospadias (if present would be a contraindication for circumcision); a whitish vaginal discharge and some bleeding can normally occur in the newborn period.
- Extremity examination includes careful performance and documentation of the hip examination.
- The timing of the examination will influence the general tone and appearance of the newborn, with an initial period of alertness after birth followed by a variable period of "physiologic depression."

BIBLIOGRAPHY

American Academy of Pediatrics and American College of Obstetricians and Gynecologists. *Guidelines for perinatal care,* 5th ed. Elk Grove Village, IL: American Academy of Pediatrics, 2002.

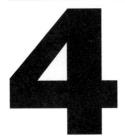

Assessment of Gestational Age

Julia Foster

I. **Rationale for assessment.** An essential part of every newborn assessment is the gestational age/birth weight classification. A newborn's behavior is a function of age as well as size. By knowing gestational age and growth patterns, clinicians can identify infants at risk for postnatal complications and develop care plans accordingly.

II. **Assessment tools.** The focus of this chapter is the physician's assessment of gestational age using the expanded New Ballard Score (Fig. 4-1). This universally accepted tool estimates the maturation of neonates from 20 to 44 weeks gestational age based on six

New Ballard Score

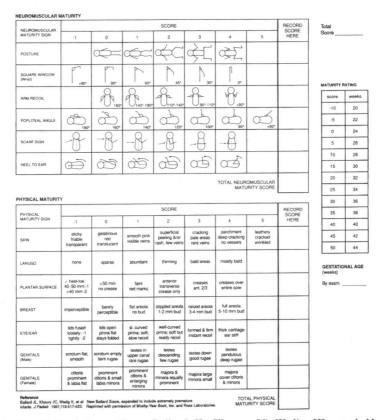

Figure 4-1. New Ballard Score. (From Ballard JL, Khoury JC, Wedig, KL, et al. New Ballard Score, expanded to include extremely premature infants. *J Pediatr* 1991;119:417–423; Mosby-Year Book, Inc. and Ross Laboratories, with permission.)

neuromuscular criteria and six physical criteria. It is accurate to within 2 weeks. Reliability is highest if the examination is completed within 12 hours after birth for infants less than 26 weeks gestational age, and within 2 to 3 days after birth for infants greater than 26 weeks gestational age.

On the basis of the examination, scores are assigned for each of the neuromuscular and physical criteria. The individual scores are totaled for the final maturity rating score and corresponding gestational age assessment in weeks. With experience, the assessment can easily be completed in just a few minutes.

A. Neuromuscular criteria.
   1. **Position.** The infant is observed resting quietly in the supine position. The score is determined by the degree of flexion. Flexion increases with advancing gestational age and proceeds from foot to head. Ankles flex first, then knees with wrists, followed by hips with elbows, and so on (Fig. 4-2).
   2. **Square window.** The hand is flexed at the wrist. The score is determined by the angle formed between the palm and the forearm. Flexion angle decreases with advancing gestational age.
   3. **Arm recoil.** The infant is placed in the supine position. Arms are flexed and then extended and released. The score is determined by the degree of flexion and the strength of recoil. Flexion and strength increase with advancing gestational age.
   4. **Popliteal angle.** The infant is placed in the supine position, flexed at the hip and knee with the thigh resting on the abdomen. The leg is gently extended until resistance is met. The score is determined by the angle formed at the knee. This angle decreases with advancing gestational age.

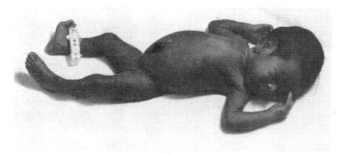

A

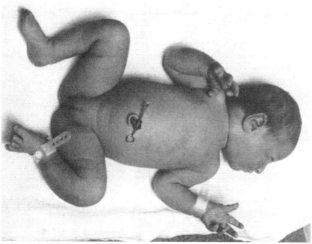

B

Figure 4-2. Resting posture in a premature **(A)** and full-term **(B)** infant.

5. **Scarf sign.** The infant is placed in the supine position. The arm is pulled across the chest and posteriorly around the neck until resistance is met. The score is determined by the position of the elbow on the chest: contralateral axillary line (score = 0), contralateral nipple line (score = 1), xyphoid process (score = 2), ipsilateral nipple line (score = 3), and ipsilateral axillary line (score = 4). Resistance increases with advancing gestational age.

6. **Heel to ear.** The infant is placed in the supine position with the hips flat on the examining table. The foot is gently pulled toward the ear until resistance is met. The score is determined by the location of the heel to the ear (score = -1), nose (score = 0), chin (score = 1), nipple line (score = 2), umbilicus (score = 3), and femoral crease (score = 4). Resistance increases with advancing gestational age.

B. Physical criteria.

1. **Skin.** The skin of the very premature infant is fragile and transparent. It becomes thicker with fewer visible blood vessels with increasing gestational age.

2. **Lanugo.** Lanugo is the soft, fine hair abundant over the body from 20 to 28 weeks gestation. It begins to thin after 28 weeks gestation and has essentially disappeared at term.

3. **Plantar surface.** The score for the extremely premature infant is determined by heel-to-toe measurements. The sole of the foot is smooth until approximately 30 weeks gestation, when the first anterior crease appears. Sole creases increase in number and depth with advancing gestational age. Creases extend to the heel at term (Fig. 4-3).

4. **Breast.** Before 34 weeks gestation, the nipple and areola are barely visible and there is no palpable breast tissue. The areola becomes raised by 34 weeks gestation and a small breast bud is palpable by 36 weeks gestation. Breast tissue increases with advancing gestational age and is approximately 5 to 6 mm in diameter at term (Fig. 4-4).

5. **Eyes and ears.** The score for the extremely premature infant is determined by fusion of the eyelids. Eyelids are fused in the extremely premature infant. Loosely fused eyelids open at least partially with gentle traction. Tightly fused eyelids remain fused with gentle traction.

   There is little cartilage formation prior to 34 weeks gestation; therefore, prior to this time, the pinna of the ear is essentially flat and shapeless and will remain

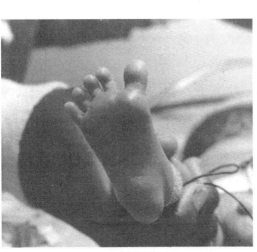
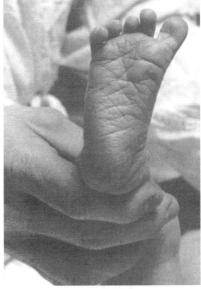

A   **B**

Figure 4-3. Sole of a premature **(A)** and full-term **(B)** infant.

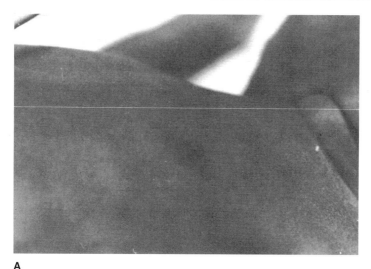

A

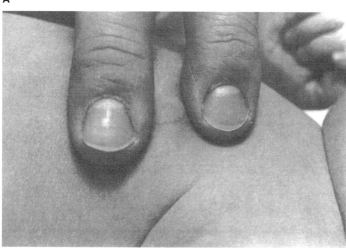

B

Figure 4-4. Breast tissue in a premature **(A)** and full-term **(B)** infant.

folded on itself. At approximately 34 weeks, gestation incurvature begins superiorly and progresses to the ear lobe with advancing gestational age (Fig. 4-5).

6. **Genitalia.** In the male, descent of the testes from the abdomen to the scrotum begins at 28 to 30 weeks gestation. At 34 weeks gestation, the testes are palpable in the inguinal canal and the scrotal skin begins to thicken and develop rugae (Fig. 4-6).

In the female, the clitoris is prominent and the labia majora are small and widely separated in the premature female infant. At term, the labia minora and the clitoris are completely covered by the labia majora (Fig. 4-7).

III. **Understanding the result of examination.** The result of the examination is compared with the obstetric best estimate (using factors such as menstrual dates, uterine size, auscultation of fetal heart tones, ultrasound examination, and amniotic fluid studies), and any discrepancy is documented in the medical record. Newborns are classified as premature (less than 37 weeks), term (37 weeks to 41 weeks and 6 days) or postterm (42 weeks or greater).

Premature infants may develop respiratory distress syndrome, apnea, temperature instability, hypoglycemia, hypocalcemia, feeding difficulties, infection, and/or jaundice.

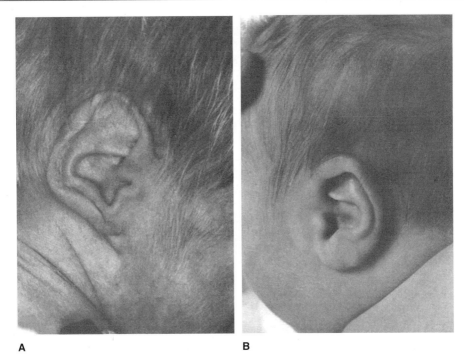

A   **B**

Figure 4-5. Premature **(A)** and full-term **(B)** ear.

Postterm infants may develop hypoglycemia, fetal distress, asphyxia, and/or meconium aspiration pneumonia, or may be small for gestational age.

The determined gestational age is plotted against birth weight using standard growth charts (Fig. 4-8). The gestational age is plotted along the horizontal axis, with weight

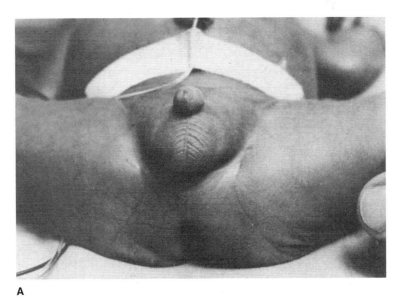

A

Figure 4-6. Male genitalia in a premature **(A)** and full-term **(B)** infant.   (*continued*)

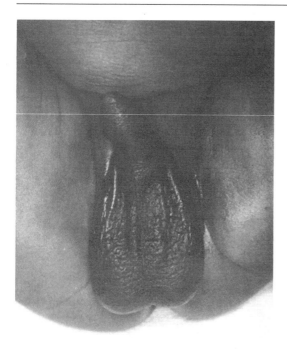

B

Figure 4-6. *(Continued)*

plotted along the vertical axis. Newborns are classified as large, appropriate, or small for gestational age. An infant is large for gestational age (LGA) if the weight is greater than the 90th percentile for gestational age or is two standard deviations above the mean weight for gestational age. Problems associated with LGA infants include birth trauma (cephalohematoma, fractured clavicle, and peripheral nerve injuries), asphyxia, and hypoglycemia. An infant is appropriate for gestational age (AGA) if the weight is between the 10th and 90th percentiles for gestational age. An infant is small for gestational age (SGA) if the weight is less than the 10th percentile for gestational age or is two standard deviations below the mean weight for gestational age. SGA infants are likely to develop hypoglycemia, hypocalcemia, temperature instability, and polycythemia. Congenital infection and chromosome disorders should be considered in SGA infants.

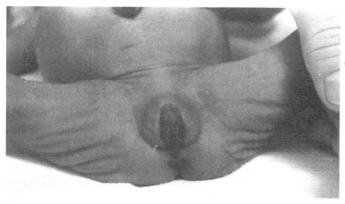

A

Figure 4-7. Female genitalia in a premature **(A)** and full-term **(B)** infant. *(continued)*

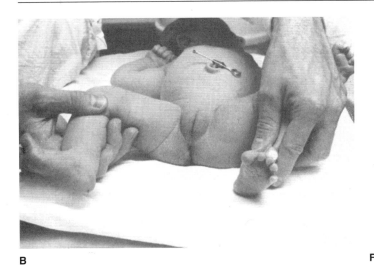

B

Figure 4-7. *(Continued)*

Colorado Intrauterine Growth Charts

Name

Birth date

Hospital number

Date

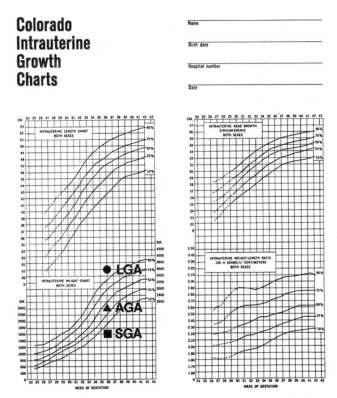

Figure 4-8. Plot of birth weight against gestational age. (From Lubchenco LO, Hansman C, Boyd E. Intrauterine growth in length and head circumference as estimated from live births at gestational ages from 26 to 42 weeks. *Pediatrics* 1966;37:403–408; copyright American Academy of Pediatrics, 1966, with permission.)

IV.   **Clinical pearls.**
- The New Ballard Score estimates the gestational age of infants delivered between 20 and 44 weeks gestation and is accurate to within 2 weeks.
- SGA infants are at risk for hypoglycemia, hypocalcemia, and temperature instability and should be monitored closely for these aberrations.
- LGA infants are at risk for trauma during delivery and should be carefully evaluated for this. These infants are also at risk of developing hypoglycemia and should be closely monitored for this.

BIBLIOGRAPHY

Ballard JL, Khoury JC, Wedig, KL, et al. New Ballard Score, expanded to include extremely premature infants. *J Pediatr* 1991;119:417–423.

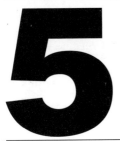

Thermoregulation

Vicki Powell-Tippit

I. **Description of the issue.** The provision of an optimal thermoneutral environment is of utmost importance in enhancing the survival of newborn infants, especially those born prematurely. In the early 1900s, Pierre Budin discovered a correlation between the maintenance of a euthermic environment and the increased survival rates of premature infants. The work of Budin and his followers established the foundation for neonatal care, and a thorough understanding of the concepts of thermoregulation is essential.

A. **Physiology.** Humans are naturally homeothermic and ordinarily maintain a steady body temperature via metabolic processes, despite changes in the environmental temperature. The regulation of body temperature is controlled by the hypothalamus and involves input from thermal receptors found on the skin's surface and deep within the body. The hypothalamus can readily influence heat production by altering vasomotor function, voluntary and involuntary muscle activity, metabolism, and nonshivering thermogenesis. Because of immaturity, newborn infants are susceptible to difficulty in maintaining optimal body temperature. Neonates are incapable of shivering and must rely on nonshivering thermogenesis, or brown fat metabolism, as a source of heat production. Unlike white fat, brown fat harbors a rich vascular supply with abundant sympathetic innervation. It begins to appear at approximately 26 to 28 weeks gestation and comprises 2% to 7% of total body weight at term. Brown fat is located around the great vessels, kidneys and adrenals, axillae, nape of the neck, and between the scapulae. Upon stimulation of the thermal receptors, a surge of norepinephrine stimulates the hydrolysis of brown fat triglycerides into nonesterified free fatty acids and glycerol. Heat generated from this process reaches the skin via transmission into body tissue and blood vessels. Although effective in heat generation, this metabolic process relies heavily upon oxygen and glucose. This increased demand for oxygen may result in hypoxia, metabolic acidosis, pulmonary vasoconstriction, and, if allowed to remain unchecked, death. Hypoglycemia may occur as well, secondary to the rapid consumption of carbohydrate stores. The amount of brown fat is reduced in the premature and very-low-birth-weight infant. Additionally, effective utilization of this process may be blunted in those infants with increased oxygen demands. Brown fat cannot be replenished once consumed. However, the ability to respond to cold stress is most limited during the first day of life and gradually increases thereafter.

B. **Risk factors for thermal instability.** Infants are at an increased risk for thermal instability secondary to a variety of factors. Premature and low-birth-weight infants harbor decreased stores of brown fat. Additionally, diminished subcutaneous fat fails to provide adequate insulation in this population. Infants have a large surface-area-to-body-mass ratio and will undergo heat loss through exposed surfaces. This is exacerbated in those with large open anomalies, such as abdominal wall and neural tube defects. Higher body water content and increased skin permeability promote evaporative heat and insensible water loss. Common issues such as the development of hypoxia and hypoglycemia directly impair the infant's ability to effectively metabolize brown fat. Infants suffering an insult to the central nervous system, such as hypoxic-ischemic encephalopathy, may suffer from blunted or absent thermoregulatory capabilities. The administration of sedation, analgesia, and anesthesia will decrease muscle tone and activity, thereby decreasing heat production.

C. **Heat transfer.** Heat transfer from the infant occurs along a thermal gradient. This gradient can be reflected internally (as heat transfers from the body's core to the skin surface) and externally (as heat transfers from the skin surface to the environment). Heat is transferred to the external environment via four pathways:

1. **Evaporation.** Evaporation is the transfer of heat through the conversion of liquid into a vapor. Evaporative heat transfer is most pronounced in the delivery setting where the neonate is covered in amniotic fluid and may result in a decrease in skin temperature of 0.5°F per minute. Additional examples of evaporative heat transfer include bathing, aerosol treatments, and the application of skin preparation solutions.

2. **Conduction.** Conduction can be defined as the transfer of heat between two surfaces lying in direct contact with one another. Conductive heat transfer may occur when the infant is placed upon a cold surface, such as an x-ray plate or a scale.

3. **Convection.** Convection refers to the transfer of heat from the body surface to cooler air currents that flow over the body. The amount of heat transfer is dependent upon the air temperature and velocity of flow.

4. **Radiation.** Radiation is defined as the transfer of heat from the body to cooler solid objects in the environment. This may occur when the infant's incubator is placed adjacent to a cold outside wall or window.

II. **Monitoring body temperature.** How often body temperature should be monitored is often based on the clinical status and individual needs of the infant. Body temperature should be assessed frequently during the first several hours following birth. Those infants deemed critically ill, premature, or low birth weight require frequent monitoring as well.

   A. **Measuring body temperature.** Body temperature can be measured by obtaining skin, axillary, rectal, or tympanic readings. Skin and axillary temperature readings are utilized most frequently in the neonatal population. Rectal temperature monitoring is no longer the preferred mode because of the risk of intestinal perforation. Additionally, the rectal temperature reading is reflective of the core body temperature and may initially be normal even though the infant is suffering from cold stress, because skin temperature falls before a change is noted in core readings. The reliability of tympanic temperature monitoring remains questionable in the neonatal population and is not recommended at this time.

   B. **Normal body temperature range.** The normal skin temperature for a newborn infant ranges between 36°C and 36.5°C (96.8°F to 97.7°F). The normal axillary and rectal temperature ranges between 36.5°C and 37°C (97.7°F to 98.6°F). The measurement of skin temperature is utilized most frequently because a decrease in skin temperature may indicate the first sign of cold stress.

III. **Hypothermia.** Hypothermia is often iatrogenic and nearly always preventable. Hypothermia is defined as a skin temperature less than 36°C (96.8°F) or an axillary temperature less than 36.5°C (97.7°F). The clinical manifestations of hypothermia are outlined in Table 5-1 and its consequences are listed in Table 5-2. Efforts to avert evaporative, conductive, convective, and radiant heat transfer should be initiated upon delivery of the infant and maintained thereafter. Interventions at the time of delivery include raising the environmental temperature, drying the infant quickly and thoroughly, and placing the infant on a prewarmed, covered surface. Additional measures may include using a chemical heat mattress and placing plastic wrap across the gap between the side rails of the radiant warmer bed. In the healthy, term infant, the initial

Table 5-1. Clinical manifestations of hypothermia

Body cool to touch
Acrocyanosis
Mottling
Bradycardia
Apnea,
   shallow, or irregular respirations
Decreased activity
Diminished or absent reflexes
Hypotonia
Central nervous system depression
Hypoglycemia
Metabolic acidosis

Table 5-2. Consequences of hypothermia

Hypoglycemia
Metabolic acidosis
Pulmonary vasoconstriction
Hypoxia
Altered surfactant production
Weight loss or poor weight gain

bath should be delayed until the body temperature has stabilized. The infant should be dressed and swaddled in prewarmed linens upon placement into an open crib.

A. Assessment of hypothermia. The infant's skin temperature can be assessed by utilizing the servo-control mode of the radiant warmer bed or incubator. The servo-control mode provides feedback from the infant, thus allowing the radiant warmer or incubator to titrate heat output dependent upon the skin temperature set point. The skin sensor probe must be covered with a reflective patch and it must be firmly applied to the infant's skin. Avoiding bony prominences and the extremities will ensure accurate temperature readings. The infant should not be laid directly on the probe as inadvertent cooling may occur. When the servo-control mode is employed, the use of temperature as a clinical sign may be lost. Therefore, it is important to record the radiant warmer or incubator temperature, in addition to the infant's axillary temperature, as the infant may experience relative hypo- or hyperthermia. When servo-control is no longer utilized, the incubator must be regulated manually to maintain a thermal neutral environment. This thermal neutral environment is dependent on weight, gestational age, and chronologic age (Table 5-3).

Additional measures to decrease heat loss include the provision of warmed, humidified inspired gases and the use of double-wall designed incubators. Incubator portholes should be opened only when necessary, and hands and equipment should be warmed prior to examining the infant.

B. Management of hypothermia. Rewarming the infant with severe hypothermia (less than 35°C or 95°F) requires special care to avoid raising the body temperature too rapidly, which could result in hypotension or apnea. The ambient temperature should be increased 1°C to 1.5°C above the infant's body temperature. The axillary temperature should be assessed every 15 to 30 minutes, and the ambient temperature should continue to be increased to maintain it 1°C to 1.5°C above the infant's body temperature until it reaches a normal range. The infant's cardiopulmonary and hemodynamic status must be monitored closely during rewarming.

IV. Hyperthermia. Hyperthermia may be iatrogenic or indicative of a disease process. Hyperthermia is defined as a skin temperature greater than 36.5°C (97.7°F) or an axillary temperature greater than 37°C (98.6°F).

A. Assessment of hyperthermia. Although hyperthermia frequently results from the presence of additional heat sources, such as phototherapy lamps, viral and bacterial infection must be considered. Maternal fever often results in neonatal hyperthermia in the first minutes of postnatal life, because a fetus's body temperature is normally greater than that of its maternal host. Those infants suffering from hypoxic ischemic encephalopathy may experience difficulty in heat regulation secondary to damage to the hypothalamus. Additionally, the administration of certain medications, such as prostaglandin E1, has been shown to increase the risk for hyperthermia.

Table 5-3. Neutral thermal environment

Age (d)	Birth weight (1 kg)	Birth weight (2 kg)
1	35.0–35.5	34.0–34.6
5	34.5–35.0	33.0–33.8
10	34.0–34.6	32.5–33.5
15	33.5–34.4	32.3–33.3
20	33.2–34.2	32.1–33.2

From Hey EN, Katz G. The optimal thermal environment for naked babies. *Arch Dis Child* 1970;45:328–334, with permission.

Table 5-4. Clinical manifestations of hyperthermia

Body warm to touch
Flushing
Diaphoresis
Tachycardia
Tachypnea
Apnea
Hypotension
Extended posturing

Table 5-5. Consequences of hyperthermia

Increased metabolic rate
Increased oxygen consumption
Dehydration secondary to increased insensible water loss
Peripheral vasodilatation that may lead to hypotension

The clinical manifestations of hyperthermia are outlined in Table 5-4 and its consequences in Table 5-5.

B. Management of hyperthermia. Management of hyperthermia should stem from identifying and preventing the risk factors involved. Ensuring proper bed temperature programming and servo-control probe placement is vital. Additional heat sources such as overhead phototherapy lamps should be positioned in accordance to the manufacturer's guidelines.

Upon encountering hyperthermia, a careful assessment of heat output equipment should be performed. External heat sources such as phototherapy lamps should be discontinued. Loosening and removing blankets and clothing will facilitate dissipation of heat. The infant's body temperature should be monitored every 15 to 30 minutes until it is stabilized, with the clinician taking care not to potentiate rebound hypothermia.

V. Clinical pearls.

- Neonates are incapable of shivering and must rely on nonshivering thermogenesis, or brown fat metabolism, as a source of heat production.
- Premature and low-birth-weight infants are at an increased risk for thermal instability secondary to a decreased supply of brown fat and subcutaneous tissue.
- A decrease in skin temperature is often the first sign of cold stress as the core body temperature strives to remain within a normal range.
- Correct placement of the skin sensor probe, utilized during the servo-control mode of the radiant warmer or incubator, is of utmost importance in the regulation and maintenance of a thermal neutral environment.

BIBLIOGRAPHY

Armstrong V. *Neonatal thermoregulation: guidelines for practice.* Petaluma, CA: National Association of Neonatal Nurses, 1998.

Infant Nutrition

Brenda B. Poindexter

I. **Description of the issue.** Adequate nutrition in the neonatal period is essential for normal growth and development. It is important to note that the nutrition needs of the preterm infant differ from those of the term infant.
  A. **Incidence of growth failure.** At birth, approximately 22% of very-low-birth-weight (501 to 1500 g) infants are small for gestational age when defined as less than the 10th percentile for gestational age using the Alexander reference fetal growth curve. At 36 weeks postmenstrual age, as many as 97% of these same infants have experienced in-hospital growth failure, that is, weight less than 10th percentile for anticipated weight. Of even greater concern, these infants also have a high incidence of poor head growth, which is particularly worrisome given the association between small head size and poor neurodevelopmental outcome.
  B. **Consequences of early nutrition inadequacies.** There is increasing evidence that early nutrition inadequacies may have long-term consequences, some persisting into adulthood. Lucas and colleagues have reported the results of a randomized trial of early diet (standard term formula versus a nutrient-enriched premature formula) in preterm infants. Receipt of standard term formula was associated with disadvantages in neurodevelopment at 18 months and in cognition at 7 to 8 years of age, despite the fact that these infants only received the nutrition intervention for an average of 1 month.

II. **Nutrient considerations.** Although current recommendations for nutrient intake in premature infants are designed to approximate the rate of growth and composition of weight gain for a normal fetus of the same postmenstrual age and to maintain normal concentrations of blood and tissue nutrients, there is not universal agreement that this is the appropriate standard for premature infants. In addition, most recommendations for the requirements of extremely low-birth-weight (<1000 g) infants have been extrapolated from studies in larger premature infants.
  A. **Estimated energy requirements—premature infants (see Table 6-1).**
    1. The basal metabolic rate (BMR) is the largest component of energy expenditure. In neonates, the resting metabolic rate (RMR) is used as a surrogate for BMR because BMR can be measured only after overnight fasting. The BMR also includes a "disease factor" and is increased with fever, sepsis, and hypoxia.
    2. On a per-kilogram basis, the RMR of a premature infant is higher than that of a term infant. Therefore, energy requirements of infants weighing <1000 g may exceed 120 kcal/kg/day for adequate growth. Key differences between premature and term infants with respect to energy metabolism include the following:
      • Premature infants have lower energy stores (less body fat and lower glycogen stores).
      • Factors such as temperature and activity may have a relatively greater effect on energy expenditure in premature infants.
      • Increased caloric intake is required to compensate for the energy expended in growth in premature infants.
    3. Energy requirements are considerably lower in infants exclusively receiving parenteral nutrition and are approximately 90 to 100 kcal/kg/day. This is primarily because of less energy excretion (see Table 6-1).
  B. **Carbohydrates.**
    1. Lactose is the primary carbohydrate in human milk.
    2. Despite lower activity of intestinal lactase in premature infants (approximately 30% activity at 34 weeks gestation compared with term infants), lactose digestion is relatively efficient.
    3. Glucose polymers are added to most premature formulas (approximately 50% to 60% of total carbohydrate content) because they are digested by $\propto$12-glucosidases (which approximate adult levels of activity sooner than does lactase).

Table 6-1. Estimate of total energy requirements in premature infants

Factor	kcal/kg/d
Energy expenditure	
Resting metabolic rate	40–60
Activity	0–5
Thermoregulation	0–5
Synthesis/energy cost of growth	15
Energy stored	20–30
Energy excreted	15
ESTIMATED TOTAL	90–130

C. Lipid.
1. Half of the calories in human milk are provided by fat (40% to 50% in commercial preterm formulas). The fat content of human milk varies throughout lactation and in response to maternal diet.
2. Cow's milk fat is predominantly saturated and is poorly absorbed by premature infants. Premature formulas contain medium-chain triglycerides (MCT) and vegetable oils (polyunsaturated, long-chain triglycerides) that are better absorbed.
3. Most formulas are now supplemented with docosahexanoic (DHA) and arachidonic (ARA) acids, which are long-chain polyunsaturated fatty acids found in breast milk and thought to be important for brain and retinal development.

D. Protein.
1. Protein requirements to mimic *in utero* growth are estimated to be 2.7 to 3.5 g/kg/day (may be higher for infants weighing <1000 g). Adequate total calories are necessary for efficient protein utilization.
2. The protein content of human milk from mothers who deliver prematurely is higher than that of mothers who deliver at term. This difference persists for the first several weeks of life and then the increased protein content decreases to that of term milk. The protein contents of premature and term human milk are as follows:
   - Premature human milk: 2.4 to 3.1 g protein/100 kcal
   - Term/mature human milk: 1.0 to 1.5 g protein/100 kcal
3. Infant formulas and human milk fortifiers contain higher protein content than does human milk. Premature infants receiving human milk require fortification to supply adequate protein. The protein contents of fortified human milk and of formulas are as follows:
   - Fortified human milk: 2.6 to 3.1 g protein/100 kcal
   - Premature formula: 2.5 to 3.0 g protein/100 kcal
   - Term formula: 2.0 to 2.1 g protein/100 kcal
4. Human milk supplies a 80:20 whey:casein ratio (55:45 in mature milk). Although bovine whey is added to premature formulas to maintain a whey-predominant ratio similar to that of human milk, the amino acid profiles are different.
5. Soy-based formulas are not routinely recommended for premature infants for the following reasons:
   - Optimal carbohydrate, protein, and mineral absorption from these formulas has not been documented.
   - Soy formulas result in significantly lower serum phosphorus levels compared with human milk or cow-milk based formula (those fed soy feedings because of feeding intolerance should be closely monitored for metabolic bone disease).
   - Phytates in soy formulas can interfere with iron absorption.

III. Parenteral nutrition for the hospitalized neonate.
  A. Indications. Parenteral nutrition should be considered for all very-low-birth-weight (<1500 g) neonates and any newborn who cannot sustain a minimum intake of 60 kcal/kg/day from enteral nutrition.
  B. Composition and administration of parenteral nutrition (see Table 6-2).
    1. Dextrose is provided to maintain normal plasma glucose concentrations and to meet rates of glucose production/utilization, which are as follows:
      a. Rates of glucose production:
        3 to 5 mg/kg/minute for term infants
        6 to 8 mg/kg/minute for premature infants

Table 6-2. Typical composition of parenteral nutrition

Component	Usual daily requirements
Neonatal amino acid solution	1.5–4.0 g/kg/d (for ELBW infants, start minimum of 1.5 g/kg/d ASAP after birth)
Cysteine hydrochloride	40 mg/g amino acids (120 mg/kg maximum)
Dextrose	6–8 mg/kg/min
Lipid (20% emulsion)	0.5–4.0 g/kg/d
Electrolytes and minerals	
Sodium	2–4 meq/kg/d
Potassium	2–3 meq/kg/d
Chloride	2–4 meq/kg/d
Calcium	1.5–4.5 meq/kg/d
Magnesium	0.25–1.0 meq/kg/d (start ELBW at lower end)
Phosphorus	1.3–2.0 mMol/kg/d
Zinc (as sulfate or in pediatric trace-metal solution)	
Preterm and with increased GI losses	400 μg/kg/d
Term <3 mo	250 μg/kg/d
Pediatric trace-metal solution (Zn, Cu, Mn, Cr)	1.5–2 μg/kg/d
Not indicated if on parenteral nutrition <2 wk	
May consider omission if cholestasis or renal dysfunction	
Vitamins (MVI-pediatric)	2 cc/kg/d, maximum 5 cc/d

ELBW, extremely low birth weight; ASAP, as soon as possible; GI, gastrointestinal.

    b. Glucose infusion rate (GIR); use the following formula to calculate the GIR:

$$\frac{\% \text{ dextrose (expressed as a whole number)} \times \text{infusion rate (cc/h)}}{\text{weight (kg)} \times 6}$$

    c. A dextrose concentration of 12.5% should not be exceeded with peripheral catheters and a concentration of 25% should not be exceeded with a central catheter.

  2. Lipid is supplied in the following components: neutral triglycerides derived from soybean or safflower oil; phospholipid emulsifier; and glycerin.
- A minimum of 0.5 g/kg/day is needed to prevent essential fatty acid (linoleic and linolenic) deficiency.
- Initially, lipid is provided at 0.5 to 1.0 g/kg/day and advanced by 0.5 g/kg/day as tolerated to a maximum of 4.0 g/kg/day.
- Monitor serum triglycerides with each advancement in dose and maintain <200 mg/dL.
- Use only 20% or greater intravenous lipid solutions because they contain a lower phospholipid to triglyceride ratio (10% emulsions contain excessive phospholipids and should not be used in neonates).

  3. Protein is provided as crystalline amino acids. Pediatric mixtures are used because these have been designed to match the amino acid pattern of term breast-feeding infants.
- Begin providing 3 g/kg/day on the first day of parenteral nutrition. To avoid excessive protein loss, intravenous amino acids should be initiated as soon as possible after birth in all infants weighing <1000 g.
- Add cysteine hydrochloride (40 mg/g amino acids; 120 mg/kg maximum). Cysteine is not supplied by standard amino acid solutions and is thought to be conditionally essential in premature infants. With the addition of cysteine, consider using acetate to buffer excess anions.

Table 6-3. Calculating caloric intake from parenteral nutrition

Component	kcal/g	kcal/cc
Dextrose	3.4	
5% dextrose		0.17
10% dextrose		0.34
20% Intralipid	10	2.0
10% amino acid solution	4	0.4

    C. Calculating caloric intake from parenteral nutrition (see Table 6-3).
       1. The usual caloric goal is 80 to 100 kcal/kg/day.
       2. Nonprotein calories from carbohydrate and lipid should be at a ratio of approximately 60:40 to maximize protein retention.
  IV. **Enteral nutrition for the hospitalized neonate.** Premature and critically ill neonates may have several complex medical and surgical problems, which may interfere with the provision of adequate nutrition. Each infant must be assessed individually to determine the best method and type of feeding for each clinical situation. When selecting the most appropriate feeding, clinicians must consider the following: gestational age, birth weight, coordination of sucking and swallowing reflexes, rate of respiration, and gastrointestinal pathology.
    A. Human milk (Table 6-4 and Table 6-5).
       1. Always use full strength human milk that supplies 20 kcal/oz.
       2. Premature infants require fortification of human milk to supply adequate calories, protein, vitamins, and minerals. Commercial human milk fortifiers are typically recommended for in-hospital use only.
          a. Powder—Similac or Enfamil Human Milk Fortifier (HMF): Add 1 packet to 25 cc human milk (supplies 24 kcal/oz).
          b. Liquid—Similac Natural Care (helpful when maternal milk supply is limited): Mix 1:1 with human milk (supplies 22 kcal/oz).
          c. Formula powder can be used on a temporary basis if HMF is not tolerated. Add 1 tsp Pregestimil powder to 60 cc human milk (supplies 24 kcal/oz).

Table 6-4. Nutrient composition of human milk (HM) and human milk fortifiers (HMF)

Nutrient (per 100 kcal)	Human milk		Similac HMF (1 packet: 25 cc HM)	Enfamil HMF (1 packet: 25 cc HM)	Similac Natural Care (50:50 HM)
	Term	Preterm			
Protein, g	1.5	2.1	2.97	3.12	2.6
Calcium, mg	45	37	175	145	132
Phosphorus, mg	22.6	19	98	77	72
Iron, mg	0.06	0.18	0.58	1.93	0.28
Zinc, mg	0.38	0.51	1.7	1.3	1.1
Vitamin A, IU	319	581	1246	1652	949
Vitamin D, IU	3	3	151	187	84
Folic acid, μg	12	5	32	35	23
Osmolality	286	290	385	350	280

Table 6-5. Increasing caloric density of human milk

Caloric density	Human milk	Human milk fortifier	Pregestimil powder	MCT oil
22 kcal/oz	50 cc	1 packet	—	—
24 kcal/oz	25 cc	1 packet	—	—
27 kcal/oz	25 cc	1 packet	1/4 tsp	—
30 kcal/oz	25 cc	1 packet	1/4 tsp	0.3 cc

MCT, medium-chain triglycerides.

Table 6-6. Nutrient composition of standard preterm formula, follow-up formula, and standard term formula

Nutrient (per 100 kcal)	Premature formula		Follow-up formula		Term formula	
	Similac Special Care 24 kcal/oz	Enfamil Premature 24 kcal/oz	NeoSure 22 kcal/oz	Enfacare 22 kcal/oz	Similac 20 kcal/oz	Enfamil 20 kcal/oz
Protein, g	3.0	3.0	2.6	2.8	2.07	2.1
Fat, g	5.43	5.1	5.5	5.3	5.4	5.3
Carbohydrate, g	10.6	11.1	10.3	10.7	10.8	10.9
Calcium, mg	180	165	105	120	78	78
Phosphorus, mg	100	83	62	66	42	53
Iron, mg	1.8	1.8	1.8	1.8	1.8	1.8
Zinc, mg	1.5	1.5	1.2	1.25	0.75	1
Vitamin A, IU	1250	1250	460	450	300	300
Vitamin D, IU	150	270	70	80	60	60
Folic acid, μg	37	35	25	26	15	16
Osmolality	280	310	250	260	300	300

  B. **Premature formulas (Table 6-6).**
    1. Similac Special Care Advance and Enfamil Premature Lipil (available as 20 or 24 kcal/oz) are standard formulas for hospitalized premature infants. Pregestimil powder, vegetable oil, MCT oil, or polycose powder can be added to increase caloric density.
    2. Similac NeoSure Advance and Enfamil EnfaCare Lipil (standard 22 kcal/oz) are designed to provide more calories and higher levels of protein, vitamins, and minerals than term formulas. Fat blend is with medium-chain triglycerides (MCT oil) to enhance absorption in premature infants. These formulas can be used in growing premature infants once they begin to feed orally, or as discharge formulas for premature infants. They can also be used to fortify human milk postdischarge. These formulas can be considered for use as the initial formula for healthy premature infants with birth weight >1800 g.
 V. **Postdischarge nutrition.**
  A. **Fortification of human milk for home use.** Maintaining optimal infant growth following discharge often requires continued fortification of expressed breast milk to a higher caloric density. Recipes to achieve this are outlined in Table 6-7.
  B. **Follow-up formulas for premature infants.** The use of preterm discharge formulas to 9 months corrected age results in greater linear growth, weight gain, and bone mineral content compared with the use of term infant formula. Recipes to increase the caloric density of these formulas are outlined in Table 6-8.
  C. **Vitamins.** Pediatric multivitamin supplementation is needed to supply vitamin D, ascorbic acid, thiamine, riboflavin, pyridoxine, and niacin to preterm infants who receive unfortified human milk or formula not specifically designed for the premature infant. Indications for vitamin and iron supplementation are outlined in Table 6-9.
  D. **Iron.**
    1. Premature infants have lower iron stores on a per-kilogram basis at birth. In addition, the frequent blood sampling premature infants often undergo further depletes iron stores.

Table 6-7. Fortification of human milk for home use

Caloric density	Formula powder*	Human milk
24 kcal/oz	1 level teaspoon	60 cc
24 kcal/oz	1 level scoop	300 cc
27 kcal/oz	1 level scoop	160 cc
30 kcal/oz	1 level scoop	120 cc

*Formula powders for use with this recipe include Similac Neosure, Enfamil Enfacare, Similac Advance, and Enfamil Lipil; use unpacked scoops and use only the scoop that comes in the original can.

Table 6-8. Formula to reconstitute Similac Neosure Advance or Enfamil Enfacare Lipil

Caloric density	Formula powder*	Water
20 kcal/oz	2 scoops	135 cc
22 kcal/oz (standard)	1 scoop	60 cc
24 kcal/oz	3 scoops	165 cc
27 kcal/oz	5 scoops	240 cc

*Use level scoops for these recipes.

2. Recommended intake is a total of 2 to 4 mg/kg/day of elemental iron by 4 weeks of age. Some infants requiring catch-up growth may need as much as 4 to 6 mg/kg/day (inclusive of feedings). Premature formulas with iron (Similac Special Care, Premature Enfamil) and preterm follow-up formulas (NeoSure, Enfacare) provide 2 mg/kg/day elemental iron (per 120 kcal/kg).
3. Use of "low-iron" formulas is not warranted. In its Pediatric Nutrition Guidelines, the American Academy of Pediatrics (AAP) makes the following statement: "The AAP sees no role for the use of low-iron formulas in infant feeding and recommends that all formulas fed to infants be fortified with iron." Additional iron supplementation is recommended for infants <1500 g at birth and is to be continued through 6 months corrected age. Premature infants fed human milk need 2 to 4 mg/kg/day elemental iron supplementation, which should be started by 4 weeks of age. Available iron supplements are listed in Table 6-10.
   E. **Fluoride.** Fluoride is not recommended until 6 months of age and only if fluoride concentration in community drinking water is <0.3 ppm.
VI. **Breastfeeding.**
   A. **Current statistics.** The World Health Organization (WHO) Healthy People 2010 initiative includes a goal of achieving a 75% rate of breastfeeding in the early postpartum period, 50% at 6 months, and 25% at 1 year.
   B. **Supplemental nutrient requirements for the breastfed infant.**
      1. **Vitamin K.** All infants should receive intramuscular vitamin K at the time of birth.
      2. **Vitamin D.** The AAP recommends that all breastfed infants receive 200 IU of vitamin D beginning during the first 2 months of life to prevent rickets and vitamin D deficiency.
      3. **Fluoride.** Supplementation is only required after 6 months of age if water supply is fluoride deficient (see section on postdischarge nutrition).
      4. **Complementary foods.** Exclusive breastfeeding provides adequate, optimal nutrition for the first 6 months of life. Iron-enriched solid foods are introduced during the second 6 months of life.

Table 6-9. Vitamin and iron supplementation

Feeding type	Multivitamin	Iron supplement
Unfortified human milk	Yes	Yes
Human milk + HMF*	No	Similac HMF powder supplies 0.58 mg iron/100 kcal fortified human milk. Enfamil HMF powder supplies 1.93 mg iron/100 kcal fortified human milk.
Similac Natural Care	Yes	Yes
Premature formula	No	Yes
Other formula (term, specialized)	Yes	Yes
Follow-up formula	Yes (until taking 24 oz/d)	Yes

*Infants who take volumes >360 cc/d (15 fortifier packets) will receive intakes of some vitamins 200% of amounts recommended for preterm infants; for these infants, fortification with infant formula powder should be considered.

Table 6-10. Available iron supplements

Preparation	Elemental iron
FerInSol drops	15 mg/0.6 cc
FerInSol liquid	18 mg/5.0 cc
Generic ferrous sulfate liquid	60 mg/5.0 cc
Pediatric multivitamin with iron (PolyViSol with iron)	10 mg/1.0 cc

C. **Special circumstances.**
   1. **Early discharge.** All infants who are breastfeeding at the time of hospital discharge should be seen for a follow-up visit and weight check within 48 hours.
   2. **Hyperbilirubinemia.** Early jaundice in a breastfeeding infant is commonly a function of milk production. It is not necessary to interrupt breastfeeding in this situation but rather to increase milk production and intake with more frequent nursing and the use of supplementation following nursing sessions.
   3. **Prematurity.** Promote early skin-to-skin contact whenever feasible. Encourage use of human milk as a medication, as some mothers who would otherwise choose not to nurse their infant are often willing to provide expressed breast milk for their premature or hospitalized infant if they understand the health benefits that breast milk provides. The age at which the ability to suck, swallow, and breathe in a coordinated fashion is attained varies among premature infants, but most infants can safely begin breastfeeding attempts by 34 weeks corrected gestational age.
   4. **Breastfeeding failure-to-thrive.** Breastfeeding failure can result from unrecognized inadequacy of milk production. Infants typically present at 1 to 3 weeks of age with severe hypernatremic dehydration (serum sodium often >180 meq/L). Complications include venous thrombosis, cerebral infarcts, and seizures (with rehydration therapy).

D. **Contraindications to breastfeeding.**
   1. **Maternal**
     • Illicit drug use (e.g., cocaine)
     • Certain infectious diseases (e.g., HIV, tuberculosis)
   2. **Infant**
     • Metabolic contraindications (e.g., galactosemia)
   3. **Drugs**
     • Bromocriptine
     • Cyclophosphamide
     • Cyclosporin
     • Doxorubicin
     • Ergotamine
     • Lithium
     • Methotrexate
     • Phencyclidine

E. **Advising and advocating for breastfeeding mothers.**
   1. **Hospital support**
     • Recommend lactation consultation and private areas for breastpumping.
     • Begin breastfeeding as soon as possible after birth.
     • Mother and infant should room in together.
     • Discourage use of unjustified supplements.
   2. **Parenting programs.** Physicians caring for infants should be aware of programs in their community that erroneously teach rigid scheduling rather than on-demand feeding for the nursing infant. Parents should be educated regarding the need to nurse newborns whenever they show any signs of hunger and that crying is a very late indicator of hunger.
   3. **Maternal employment.** Mothers returning to the workplace should be educated of their right to appropriate time and facilities for breastpumping.
   4. **Duration of breastfeeding.** The AAP recommends that "breastfeeding continue as long as is mutually desired." Reasonable evidence, rather than personal opinion, should direct recommendations regarding weaning.

VII.   Clinical pearls.

- Premature infants receiving breast milk require fortification to supply adequate protein, calcium, vitamins, and minerals.
- The ability to suck, swallow, and breathe in a coordinated fashion appears between 32 and 34 weeks gestation and most infants can safely begin oral feeding attempts at 34 weeks corrected gestational age.
- Preterm discharge formulas (22 cal/oz) are recommended to a postnatal age of 9 months.
- Evaluation of the breastfeeding newborn by a health care professional 48 to 72 hours after release from the hospital will minimize the risk of breastfeeding failure.
- Vitamin D supplementation should be initiated in the first 2 months of life in all breastfed infants to prevent rickets and vitamin D deficiency.

BIBLIOGRAPHY

Hay WW, Lucas A, Heird WC, et al. Workshop summary: nutrition of the extremely low birth weight infant. *Pediatrics* 1999;104(6):136–138.

Kleinman RE, ed. *Pediatric nutrition handbook*, 5th ed. Elk Grove Village, IL: American Academy of Pediatrics, 2004.

Lucas A, Morley R, Cole T. Randomised trial of early diet in preterm babies and later intelligence quotient. *British Medical Journal* 1998;317(7171):1481–1487.

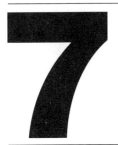

Common Metabolic Problems: Hypoglycemia, Hyperglycemia, and Hypocalcemia

Scott C. Denne

Disorders of glucose and calcium homeostasis in the neonate are quite common, although usually transient. With appropriate monitoring of neonates that are most at risk for these disorders, some of these problems can be prevented, and when present, effectively treated.

HYPOGLYCEMIA

I. **Description of the issue.** Glucose is the major metabolic fuel of the fetus. It is transported across the placenta, and the fetal serum glucose concentration is about two-thirds of the maternal concentration. Insulin, on the other hand, is not transported across the placenta. The fetal pancreas synthesizes insulin early in gestation and is an important regulator of fetal glucose concentration. Upon delivery of the infant, the maternal supply of glucose stops and the neonate must provide glucose from glycogenolysis and gluconeogenesis. Usually, the newborn serum glucose concentration decreases after birth. After 1 to 2 hours of age, it normally rises slowly and reaches adult values by 1 week of age. Because glucose is the preferred fuel for brain metabolism and the newborn brain is relatively large for body size, the neonate's basal rate of glucose utilization (4 to 6 mg/kg/minute for term neonates, 5 to 8 mg/kg/minute for preterm infants) is greater than that of the adult. Limited glycogen stores and the potential for decreased glucose intake make neonatal hypoglycemia a relatively common clinical problem.

A. **Epidemiology.** Estimates of the incidence of hypoglycemia vary and depend upon the risk group. Symptomatic hypoglycemia occurs in <1% of normal term newborns, in approximately 5% of small-for-gestational-age infants, and in 15% of infants of diabetic mothers.

B. **Etiology/contributing factors.**

1. **Limited glycogen stores/increased metabolic rate.** Premature neonates and small-for-gestational-age infants are at risk for hypoglycemia because of limited glycogen stores and high glucose utilization. Without sufficient intake, glycogen stores are rapidly depleted and hypoglycemia can occur. Infants with sepsis, respiratory distress, and other critical illness can also have increased glucose needs and are also at risk for hypoglycemia. Cold stress and hypothermia can also increase metabolic rate and glucose utilization.

2. **Hyperinsulinism.** Infants of diabetic mothers are at risk for hypoglycemia because of hyperinsulinism. Maternal hyperglycemia results in fetal hyperglycemia, which in turn results in pancreatic β-cell hyperplasia and hyperinsulinism. Better glucose control in the mother reduces the risk of complications for the neonate, including hypoglycemia. Other problems associated with infants of diabetic mothers are shown in Table 7-1. Hyperinsulinism is also present in some other uncommon

Table 7-1. Problems of infants of diabetic mothers

Hypoglycemia
Hypocalcemia
Hyperbilirubinemia
Respiratory distress
Polycythemia
Macrosomia/birth injuries
Congenital anomalies
Congestive heart failure (hypertrophic cardiomyopathy, congenital heart defects)
Small left colon syndrome
Renal vein thrombosis

conditions, particularly Beckwith-Wiedemann syndrome and congenital hyperinsulinism (previously known as nesidioblastosis). Congenital hyperinsulinism can be a genetic disorder, with both recessive and dominant forms.

3. **Inborn errors of metabolism.** Hypoglycemia can result from a wide variety of inborn errors of metabolism; however, these are very uncommon. Inborn errors of metabolism produce hypoglycemia by limiting or blocking normal gluconeogenic pathways or by preventing normal glycogenolysis. Hypopituitarism results in hypoglycemia because of counter-regulatory hormone deficiency, particularly growth hormone and adrenocorticotropic hormone (ACTH). Deficiency of these hormones permits unopposed insulin action resulting in hypoglycemia. Adrenal insufficiency can result in hypoglycemia by the same mechanism. A list of common and uncommon causes of hypoglycemia is provided in Table 7-2.

II. **Making the diagnosis.**

A. **Definition.** Controversy remains about the precise definition of hypoglycemia in the neonate. At present, a glucose concentration of <40 mg/dL is a reasonable practical threshold for neonatal hypoglycemia. There is no justification to use a different definition for preterm infants.

B. **Signs and symptoms.** Clinical manifestations of hypoglycemia (Table 7-3) include apnea, cyanosis, jitteriness, lethargy, abnormal cry, hypotonia, hypothermia, poor feeding, seizures, coma, sweating, and tachypnea. None of these symptoms are specific for hypoglycemia and all are seen commonly in other serious neonatal disorders. Therefore, it is important to consider hypoglycemia in the evaluation of any sick neonate.

C. **Tests.** Glucose concentrations can be accurately determined in plasma with standard laboratory techniques. The blood should be handled expeditiously and in a manner so that glucose concentrations are not altered by *in vitro* glycolysis from red cells. Screening for hypoglycemia is often done using glucose test strips, but there are significant limitations to this method. Glucose test strips are optimized to detect hyperglycemia rather than hypoglycemia and their ability to accurately reflect low glucose concentrations may be limited. The glucose strip method also measures whole blood glucose, which is significantly affected by hematocrit. Whole blood has a lower concentration of glucose than that of plasma (typically measured by standard laboratory techniques). In the presence of polycythemia, the differences between whole blood and plasma glucose concentrations can be quite large. If an abnormal glucose concentration is obtained using a glucose strip method, samples should be sent for standard laboratory analysis at the same time therapy is initiated.

III. **Management.**

A. **Screening/preventive measures.** At-risk neonates, in particular, infants of diabetic mothers, small-for-gestational-age infants, and premature neonates, should be screened for hypoglycemia. For these high-risk neonates, routine screening should be begun on admission and before the first 2 to 4 feedings, or at 2 to 4 hour intervals for the first 24 to 48 hours. Glucose concentration should also be measured if any clinical symptoms consistent with hypoglycemia are observed. Early feedings should be initiated in these high-risk neonates if they are clinically stable. If infants are unable to be fed, an intravenous glucose infusion should be begun as early as possible.

Table 7-2. Causes of hypoglycemia

Common causes

Infants of diabetic mothers
Large-for-gestational-age infants
Small-for-gestational-age infants
Prematurity
Respiratory distress
Sepsis
Other critical illness
Hypothermia

Less common causes

Inborn errors of metabolism (galactosemia, amino acid disorders)
Beckwith–Wiedemann syndrome (macroglossia, macrosomia, omphalocele)
Congenital hyperinsulinism
Hypopituitarism/adrenal insufficiency

Table 7-3. Clinical manifestations of hypoglycemia

Jitteriness
Lethargy
Apnea
Cyanosis
Seizures
Poor feeding
Tachypnea
Hypothermia
Abnormal cry
Sweating
Hypotonia

    B. Treatment. Infants with asymptomatic hypoglycemia may be fed if they are able to tolerate enteral feeds (Table 7-4). In symptomatic infants with a screening blood sugar <40 mg/dL, a blood sample for laboratory glucose determination should be obtained and a bolus of 2 to 4 mL/kg of D10W should be given by intravenous push followed by constant intravenous infusion of D10W to deliver 5 to 6 mg/kg/minute (3.5 mL/kg/hour D10W) of glucose. Hypoglycemia may persist despite a constant intravenous glucose infusion, so glucose levels should continue to be frequently monitored. For infants of diabetic mothers (and other conditions with hyperinsulinemia), higher glucose infusion rates may be necessary. This will often require a catheter in the inferior vena cava or other large vessel so that glucose concentrations of >12.5% can be delivered. Infants with congenital hyperinsulinism may require glucose infusion rates in excess of 20 mg/kg/minute and yet still remain hypoglycemic. These infants require subspecialty consultation and may need treatment with diazoxide, somatostatin, or steroids. In infants who respond to an intravenous glucose concentration with normal blood sugars, it is important to decrease the rate and/or concentration of intravenous glucose gradually while increasing enteral intake. Frequent monitoring of blood glucose is required during this time.

IV.   **Clinical pearls and pitfalls.**
- In the first few hours after birth, asymptomatic hypoglycemia is common in term newborns (approximately 20% of infants). In addition, term newborns that are breastfed often have lower glucose concentrations. Asymptomatic hypoglycemia in term neonates is transient and without clinical consequences. Routine screening of term neonates for hypoglycemia is not recommended.
- For all conditions resulting in hypoglycemia, other than hyperinsulinism, a glucose infusion rate of 4 to 8 mg/kg/minute is usually effective in achieving glucose concentrations in the normal range (60 to 90 mg/dL).
- If glucose infusions of >8 mg/kg/minute are required, the mechanism of hypoglycemia is almost certainly hyperinsulinism. Gradual increases in glucose infusions are particularly important in these infants to avoid reactive insulin release.

HYPERGLYCEMIA

I.   **Description of the issue.** Hyperglycemia is a common problem within the neonatal intensive care unit, most often occurring in premature and sick neonates receiving intravenous glucose.

Table 7-4. Treatment of hypoglycemia

Preventative measures	In infants at risk for hypoglycemia, feed early if clinically stable.
Asymptomatic infants	Feed with breast milk or formula and recheck glucose after 30 min.
Symptomatic infants	Give 2 cc/kg of D10W by IV push followed by IV infusion of D10 W at 75–150 mL/kg/d. Adjust glucose infusion on the basis of frequent blood glucose determinations.
Intractable hypoglycemia	Diazoxide, somatostatin, steroids. Subspecialty consultation required.

A. Epidemiology. Estimates of the incidence of hyperglycemia in premature infants vary widely, with some reported rates as high as 70%. It is clear, however, that the smallest, most immature neonates have the highest incidence of hyperglycemia.

Neonatal diabetes is a very rare cause of hyperglycemia, with an estimated incidence of 1 in 500,000. There is a genetic component to some cases of neonatal diabetes.

B. Etiology/contributing factors.

1. **Prematurity.** Premature infants are at risk for hyperglycemia, especially the most immature (<27 weeks gestational age, <1,000 g birth weight). The mechanisms of hyperglycemia in this population are not entirely clear, but may include decreased insulin response to a glucose load, as well as elevated levels of cortisol, glucagon, and catecholamines associated with illness and stress.

2. **Sepsis/stress/critical illness.** Sick and septic neonates are also at high risk for hyperglycemia, probably as a result of elevated stress hormones as described above. Interestingly, critically ill and septic children and adults are at similar risk for hyperglycemia.

3. **High glucose infusion rates.** In order to provide sufficient fluid intake to premature neonates, high glucose infusion rates are sometimes inadvertently administered. Glucose infusion rates in excess of 8 mg/kg/minute can result in hyperglycemia, especially in the extremely premature neonate.

4. **Neonatal diabetes mellitus.** Neonatal diabetes mellitus is an extremely rare condition, with affected infants usually born small for gestational age. This condition usually presents within the first 1 to 3 months of life, and affected infants have low insulin levels in the face of hyperglycemia.

II. **Making the diagnosis.**

A. Definition. Definitions of hyperglycemia vary among authorities. A typical definition of hyperglycemia in neonates is a glucose concentration >150 mg/dL. However, clinical intervention is usually more often required in neonates with glucose concentrations exceeding 180 mg/dL.

B. Signs and symptoms. Clinical manifestations of hyperglycemia are primarily polyuria, dehydration, and weight loss. Acidosis (lactic acidosis rather than ketosis) is also sometimes observed.

III. **Management.**

A. Screening/prevention. Because premature infants in the neonatal intensive care unit are at relatively high risk for hyperglycemia, glucose concentration should be frequently monitored in the first 24 hours until the infant is stable, and periodically thereafter, especially when glucose infusion rates are changed. Glucose infusions should be delivered at rates providing at most 8 mg/kg/minute of glucose during the first 24 hours.

B. Treatment. The treatment for hyperglycemia primarily involves decreasing the amount of glucose being administered by lowering either the rate or glucose concentration of the infused solution. In rare instances when glucose concentrations exceed 200 mg/dL despite minimal glucose infusion rates, insulin might be required. A continuous intravenous insulin infusion can be used beginning at 0.01 units/kg/hour and increasing gradually as necessary up to 0.05 to 0.1 units/kg/hour. Frequent monitoring of glucose concentrations is required during an insulin infusion.

IV. **Clinical pearls.**

- Early amino acid administration to premature neonates improves glucose tolerance and reduces hyperglycemia, possibly by increasing insulin secretion.

HYPOCALCEMIA

I. **Description of the issue.** Hypocalcemia is common among sick and premature neonates in the neonatal intensive care unit. The fetus receives active calcium transfer from the mother, which reaches a peak of 150 mg/kg/day during the third trimester. After birth, this calcium supply ceases, and serum calcium concentration is maintained either by exogenous intake or by calcium from bone. During this transition phase, early neonatal hypocalcemia (<2 days of age) is common and is often asymptomatic. Late hypocalcemia, on the other hand, is often symptomatic and is the result of unusual and uncommon conditions.

A. Epidemiology. Approximately 20% of premature infants will develop early neonatal hypocalcemia. The incidence of hypocalcemia in infants of diabetic mothers is approximately 17%. However, with poor maternal glucose control, the risk of hypocalcemia in infants of diabetic mothers is substantially higher.

    B. Etiology/contributing factors.

        1. Prematurity. Hypocalcemia of prematurity is related to decreased calcium intake, increased serum calcitonin, and transient functional hypoparathyroidism. Hypocalcemia is usually temporary and resolves in 1 to 3 days.

        2. Infants of diabetic mothers. Hypocalcemia in infants of diabetic mothers appears to be related to maternal and neonatal hypomagnesemia and secondary functional hypoparathyroidism. Hypocalcemia is observed early in neonatal life and often resolves in 1 to 3 days.

        3. Perinatal asphyxia. Several factors are likely responsible for hypocalcemia in infants with perinatal asphyxia, such as increased endogenous phosphorus load, increased serum calcitonin concentration, and decreased calcium intake. Hypocalcemia in these infants presents in early neonatal life.

        4. Congenital hypoparathyroidism. This grouping of disorders includes congenital hypoparathyroidism secondary to agenesis of the parathyroid gland, DiGeorge syndrome with parathyroid hypoplasia, and transient hypoparathyroidism in offspring of hypoparathyroid mothers. Hypocalcemia in these infants tends to present after the first 2 days of life. These disorders are uncommon.

II.   **Making the diagnosis.**

    A. Definition. Hypocalcemia is usually defined as a serum calcium level of <7 mg/dL or an ionized calcium level of 3 to 4 mg/dL. Ionized calcium is the physiologically relevant fraction and may not correlate well with total serum calcium under pathologic conditions. Therefore, measuring ionized calcium in sick and potentially symptomatic infants is desirable.

    B. Signs and symptoms. Clinical manifestations of hypocalcemia include jitteriness, hypotonicity, laryngospasm with inspiratory stridor, and focal and generalized seizures. These signs are not specific for hypocalcemia. Many infants with hypocalcemia are asymptomatic.

III. **Management.**

    A. Screening. Sick premature infants and neonates who have experienced perinatal asphyxia should be screened for hypocalcemia for at least the first 2 days of life. In infants with potential symptoms, ionized calcium should be measured. Sick infants of diabetic mothers should also be screened; however, asymptomatic infants of diabetic mothers who are able to begin normal enteral feedings on the first day do not require routine calcium monitoring.

    B. Treatment. Symptomatic hypocalcemia can be treated with a low intravenous infusion of 100 to 200 mg/kg of calcium gluconate (1 to 2 mL/kg of 10% calcium gluconate) given over 10 minutes with heart rate monitoring. If bradycardia occurs, the infusion must be stopped. This can be followed by continuous intravenous calcium supplementation at the rate of 500 to 800 mg/kg of calcium gluconate over a 24-hour period. The complications of intravenous calcium include skin slough, tissue necrosis, and bradycardia. Alternatively, if infants can tolerate oral feedings, the same dose of calcium gluconate can be provided orally after the initial correction of hypocalcemia. The approach to asymptomatic hypocalcemia varies widely among clinicians. Owing to the potential complications of intravenous calcium, it may be reasonable to treat preterm infants only when their total serum calcium is <6 mg/dL or ionized calcium <3.0 mg/dL.

IV. **Clinical pearls and pitfalls.**

    • Serum magnesium should be measured in all infants with hypocalcemia, especially infants of diabetic mothers. Hypomagnesemia (<1.6 mg/dL) often accompanies hypocalcemia, and it may not be possible to resolve hypocalcemia until magnesium levels are normalized. Treatment consists of 0.1 to 0.2 mg/kg of 50% magnesium sulfate IM or IV.

BIBLIOGRAPHY

Cornblath M, Hawdon J, Williams AF, et al. Controversies regarding definition of neonatal hypoglycemia: suggested operational thresholds. *Pediatrics* 2000;105:1141–1145.

Cornblath M, Ichord R. Hypoglycemia in the neonate. *Semin Perinatol* 2000;24:136–149.

Cowett RM, Loughead JL. Neonatal glucose metabolism: differential diagnoses, evaluation, and treatment of hypoglycemia. *Neonatal Netw* 2002;21:9–19.

Farrag HM, Cowett RM. Glucose homeostasis in the micropremie. *Clin Perinatol* 2000;27:22.

Hsu SC, Levine MA. Perinatal calcium metabolism: physiology and pathophysiology. *Semin Neonatol* 2004;9:23–26.

Kalhan S, Peter-Wohl S. Hypoglycemia: what is it for the neonate? *Am J Perinatol* 2000;17:11–18.

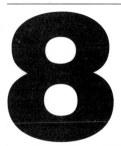

Jaundice

Jo Ann E. Matory

I. **Description of the issue.** Jaundice, the clinical manifestation of hyperbilirubinemia, occurs in many term and most premature infants.
   A. **Epidemiology.** The overall incidence of jaundice in the newborn is 65%. It affects 50% of term newborns and 80% of premature newborns. Elevated bilirubin levels have been associated with several factors during the newborn period, including the following:
   - low birth weight
   - breastfeeding
   - prematurity
   - sepsis
   - delivery requiring instrumentation
   - history of maternal diabetes
   - Asian descent

   Other factors have been inconsistently identified, such as epidural anesthesia and oxytocin during labor.
   B. **Bilirubin metabolism.** Bilirubin results from the breakdown of heme-containing proteins such as hemoglobin in red blood cells. This process is initiated in the reticuloendothelial system and is responsible for 75% of the body's production of bilirubin. The remaining 25% of bilirubin production results from the breakdown of other heme sources. These include the breakdown of immature red cell precursors in the bone marrow, known as "ineffective erythropoiesis," and the breakdown of other heme-containing proteins such as myoglobin and free hemoglobin. For bilirubin metabolism to proceed (Fig. 8-1), heme is presented to the reticuloendothelial system. The heme ring is oxidized to biliverdin by the microsomal enzyme heme oxygenase with subsequent release of carbon monoxide (excreted from the lungs) and iron (reutilized). Biliverdin is reduced by biliverdin reductase to bilirubin and is transported to the liver in the plasma bound to albumin. When the bilirubin-albumin complex reaches the hepatocyte, the bilirubin crosses into the hepatocyte without the simultaneous uptake of albumin. In the hepatocyte, the bilirubin is bound to ligandin, also known as Y protein, and to a lesser extent Z protein, for transport into the smooth endoplasmic reticulum and eventual conjugation prior to excretion into bile. Conjugation results when bilirubin uridine diphosphate glucuronyl transferase (UDPG-T) transfers the glucuronyl group from UDP-glucoronic acid to bilirubin, rendering the bilirubin water soluble. This conjugated bilirubin can then be actively transported across the canalicular membrane and excreted into bile for elimination in stool. In the newborn, however, much of this conjugated bilirubin is deconjugated by β-glucoronidase, an intestinal enzyme with increased activity in the neonatal period. The resultant unconjugated bilirubin is reabsorbed and again presented to the liver for conjugation. This is referred to as "enterohepatic circulation." Further increasing the bilirubin load in the neonate is the fact that the newborn produces between 8 and 9 mg bilirubin/kg/day (136 to 153 μm/kg/day), which is two to three times the rate of normal adult production.

II. **Making the diagnosis.**
   A. **Recognizing jaundice.** The newborn period is unique in that it is the only time of life when jaundice is extremely common and when an elevated serum bilirubin concentration may cause significant morbidity. Therefore, the ability to identify infants at risk for hyperbilirubinemia and subsequently provide appropriate management for these infants is extremely important. Jaundice can be detected by visual assessment of skin color following digital pressure and release. The serum bilirubin concentration must reach 4 to 6 mg/dL (68 to 102 μm/L) before jaundice is detectable in this fashion. Devices that provide transcutaneous bilirubin measurements to identify jaundice in newborns are available. These measurements are based on the assumption that

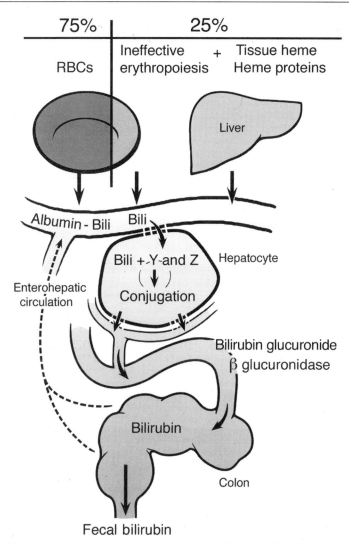

Figure 8-1. Bilirubin metabolism in the newborn. (From Maisels MJ, *Pediatric clinics of North America*, 19:452,1972, with permission.)

the "yellowness" of the skin is in a constant and consistent equilibrium with serum bilirubin. Certain clinical factors may alter this equilibrium, including changes in serum albumin concentration, use of phototherapy, or exchange transfusions. Skin color, gestational age, and ethnic background have all been shown to affect the correlation of the transcutaneous reading with the serum bilirubin concentration, and these factors must be taken into account when interpreting these measurements. Laboratory measurement of the serum bilirubin level will aid in the interpretation of questionable values.

B. **Etiology.** Jaundice is the clinical manifestation of hyperbilirubinemia and results from an imbalance between bilirubin production and removal. It can be classified according to whether the major bilirubin identified is unconjugated (indirect reacting) or conjugated (direct reacting). Indirect reacting and direct reacting reflect the ways the two forms of bilirubin react to certain dyes during laboratory analysis. Indirect bilirubin usually comprises 90% of bilirubin in newborn infants. Figure 8-2 identifies some common causes of clinical jaundice in newborns using Coombs antibody testing (described below), direct bilirubin levels, and the reticulocyte count.

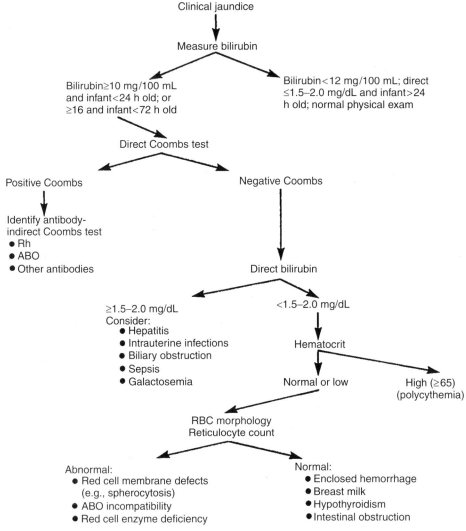

Figure 8-2. Diagnosis of the etiology of jaundice. (From Cloherty JP, Stark AR. *Manual of neonatal care.* Boston: Little, Brown,1980;202, with permission.)

   C. Differential diagnosis. Newborn jaundice can be further identified as physiologic, implying no underlying pathologic process, or nonphysiologic, implying underlying pathology. Common clinical conditions in the newborn that can potentially cause jaundice are listed in Table 8-1.
   Most cases of unconjugated or indirect hyperbilirubinemia in the newborn period are due to *physiologic jaundice,* which is defined as an elevation of unconjugated bilirubin during the first week of life with no other demonstrable cause. In the newborn period, physiologic jaundice can result from the following:
   · increased bilirubin production
   · increased enterohepatic circulation
   · defective uptake of bilirubin from plasma
   · decreased hepatic excretion of conjugated bilirubin
   In the full-term newborn with physiologic jaundice, the bilirubin level peaks by day 3 to 4 of life with a level of 6 to 8 mg/dL (102 to 136 µm/L); in the premature newborn, peak levels of 10 to 12 mg/dL (170 to 204 µm/L) are seen by day 5 or 6 of life

Table 8-1. Clinical conditions associated with jaundice

Physiologic jaundice
Nonphysiologic (pathologic) jaundice
  Hemolytic disease (usually Rh or ABO incompatibility)
  Infection
  Hematomas and bruising
  Polycythemia
  Breastfeeding
  Liver disease (neonatal hepatitis, bile obstruction)
  Metabolic disease (hypothyroidism, hypoglycemia, galactosemia)
  Diabetic mother
  Bowel obstruction

(Fig. 8-3). Of note, the existence of a bilirubin level within the "physiologic" range does not exclude a pathologic process and in every infant with clinical jaundice, physiologic jaundice should remain a diagnosis of exclusion. Direct hyperbilirubinemia with levels greater than 10% of the total or 1.5 to 2 mg/dL (25 to 34 μm/L) is never physiologic.

Nonphysiologic or pathologic jaundice can result in the following: jaundice within the first 24 hours of life; a rise in bilirubin level >0.5 mg/dL (8.5 μm/L) per hour; a change in clinical status unrelated to some other diagnosis; and/or prolonged jaundice lasting longer than 1 week in the term infant or 2 weeks in the preterm infant.

1. **Fetomaternal blood group incompatibility.** Isoimmunization develops in newborns as a result of blood group incompatibility secondary to red blood cell antigens. Although more than 100 antigens have been described, only a few have been associated with increased bilirubin levels and subsequent jaundice, namely, Rh blood group antigens (particularly the D antigen), A and B blood group antigens, and minor blood group antigens such as Kell and Kidd. In fetomaternal

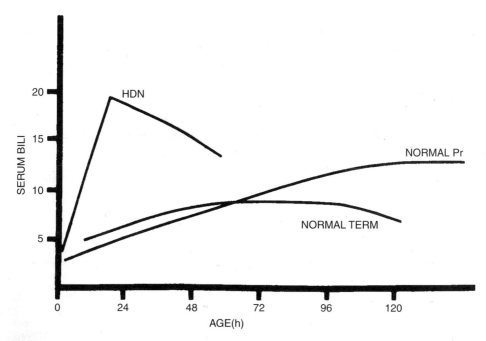

Figure 8-3. Physiologic jaundice peaks at an older age in premature (Pr) than in term infants. Hemolytic disease of the newborn (HDN) usually presents with jaundice in the first 24 hours of life.

blood group incompatibility secondary to Rh blood group antigens, red blood cells possessing an antigen lacking in the mother enter into the maternal circulation, where they stimulate maternal antibody production resulting in *Rh isoimmunization*. These immunoglobulin G (IgG) antibodies may then transplacentally enter the fetal circulation, attach to the surface of the Rh-positive fetal red cell, and lead to destruction of the cell. With Rh incompatibility, an Rh-negative mother may be sensitized by exposure to Rh-positive cells in several ways, including:

- previous undetected or forgotten Rh-positive pregnancies
- past transfusion with Rh-positive cells
- previous inadequate RhoGam* administration following a large fetomaternal hemorrhage
- Rh isoimmunization during pregnancy

Exposure to as little as 0.1 to 0.2 mL of fetal red blood cells can result in maternal sensitization. The management of a pregnancy complicated by Rh sensitization is extremely complex and is ideally supervised by a perinatal obstetrician in a center that has an obstetric intensive care unit as well as a neonatal intensive care unit. Antepartum RhoGam should be administered to nonimmunized pregnant women who are Rh-negative at 28 to 29 weeks of gestation. Additionally, RhoGam can be given to the Rh-negative mother within 72 hours of delivery after the first Rh-positive pregnancy or abortion to provide a further protective effect. If a large fetomaternal hemorrhage occurs, as with a traumatic delivery or manipulation of the placenta, a larger dose of RhoGam may be needed. The recommended amount of RhoGam may be determined by evaluating the quantity of fetal blood in the maternal circulation after delivery utilizing the Kleihauer-Betke assay. At the time of delivery, 15% to 20% of mothers who received antepartum prophylaxis will have anti-D antibody detected in their serum. These titers are usually low and dependent on the time between the injection of the RhoGam and delivery. This low, passively acquired anti-D antibody titer is not a contraindication to postpartum RhoGam.

Since the introduction of RhoGam and the resultant decrease in incidence of sensitization to the D antigen, *ABO incompatibility* is now the most common cause of isoimmune hemolytic disease in the newborn. Naturally occurring anti-A and anti-B antibodies in the serum of mothers with blood type O are of the IgG class and can therefore cross the placenta. Once in the fetal circulation, these antibodies attach to the A or B antigens on the fetal red cells and cause hemolysis. The cord blood direct Coombs test is positive in approximately one-third of these pregnancies. In contrast to Rh-sensitized pregnancies, the disease does not necessarily become worse with subsequent pregnancies.

2. **Red blood cell membrane defects and enzyme deficiencies.** Defects in the red blood cell membrane can predispose red cells to hemolysis to a degree that can result in jaundice. Examples of such defects include spherocytosis and elliptocytosis, both of which are autosomal dominant. Of note, jaundice due to the latter is rare in the newborn period.

 The most frequently encountered red blood cell enzyme deficiencies that can result in jaundice in the newborn are glucose-6-phosphate dehydrogenase (G6PD) deficiency and pyruvate kinase deficiency. G6PD is X-linked and responsible for variable disease in the newborn period. Pyruvate kinase deficiency with autosomal recessive inheritance can result in significant jaundice in a newborn infant. Both of these enzymes are important for efficient glycolysis in the red blood cell. Disruptions in this glycolytic pathway occur in infants with deficiencies of these enzymes with resultant red cell hemolysis and subsequent jaundice. Acidosis, infection, and some medications (i.e., sulfonamides and salicylates) are known to trigger this hemolytic process in G6PD-deficient infants.

3. **Polycythemia.** Polycythemia, associated with a venous hematocrit greater than 65%, is often seen in infants of diabetic mothers, intrauterine growth restricted infants, recipients of a twin-to-twin transfusion, and in cases of delayed cord clamping. With the increase in red blood cell mass, there is associated hyperviscosity. As a result of sluggish blood flow, there is impaired delivery of oxygen to tissues and the potential development of microthrombi. Due to these changes and the increased red cell mass, hyperbilirubinemia results as the red cells break down.

4. **Congenital hypothyroidism.** Jaundice, especially if persistent, may be a presenting symptom of hypothyroidism. Although the exact mechanism of action is not

*RhoGam = high titer anti-D immunoglobulin G

completely understood, it is believed to be because of deficient uridine diphosphate glucoronyl transferase activity. Once treatment is initiated for hypothyroidism, elevated bilirubin levels will decrease. Treatment for hypothyroidism should be initiated as early as possible to ensure the most favorable response for appropriate growth and neurologic development.

5. **Metabolic disorders.** Although less common, several metabolic disorders can present with jaundice in the newborn. Examples of these include Crigler-Najjar syndrome and galactosemia. In infants with Crigler-Najjar syndrome, types I and II, uridine diphosphate glucuronyl transferase activity is absent. Hyperbilirubinemia develops during the first days of life in these infants. Type I is the most severe form and is inherited as an autosomal recessive trait. Aggressive treatment with phototherapy for infants with type I is recommended during the newborn period and beyond to attempt to prevent the development of kernicterus. Type II is more common and less severe, and is an autosomal dominant trait with variable penetrance. Type II will respond to administration of phenobarbital.

   Infants with galactosemia may develop, in addition to jaundice, sepsis (particularly, due to gram negative organisms such as *E. coli*), urinary tract infections, hepatomegaly, vomiting, and hypoglycemia. It is crucial that these infants be identified early in the newborn period as cataracts, renal disease, and mental retardation can develop in untreated cases. Although three inborn errors of metabolism can cause galactosemia, the deficient enzyme is most commonly galactose-1-phosphate uridyl transferase, which can be measured in erythrocytes. Many states now require screening of newborns for several disorders that may present with jaundice, including hypothyroidism and galactosemia.

6. **Breast milk.** *Breastfeeding jaundice,* due primarily to decreased intake, inadequate hydration, and delayed passage of meconium, usually presents in the first week of life. Breastfed infants require close monitoring of their bilirubin levels and hydration status, while their mothers need ongoing support. Timely recognition of the need for treatment is important both in the inpatient and outpatient setting.

   In contrast, *breast milk jaundice* seems to be related to some alteration in breast milk composition possibly resulting in an increase in the bilirubin load presented to the liver in some infants. These infants appear healthy and without evidence of hemolysis; jaundice develops during the second week of life and usually resolves by 12 weeks. If the bilirubin level approaches a level that would require intervention, some would advocate the interruption of breastfeeding for 24 to 48 hours with supplementation of formula as such an interruption usually results in a prompt decline in bilirubin levels.

7. **Prematurity.** Premature newborns are more susceptible to the toxic effects of elevated bilirubin levels due to immaturity of the blood-brain barrier. These infants require close monitoring so that treatment may be initiated at the appropriate time. Sick premature newborns are particularly vulnerable to the development of jaundice as a result of respiratory distress and acidosis, delayed feedings, and impaired immune systems with resultant increased incidence of infections.

8. **Infections.** Jaundice in the newborn period can be associated with infection due to both bacteria and viruses. The pathogenesis is believed to be increased hemolysis secondary to bacterial endotoxin (e.g., *E. coli*) or to viremia with subsequent depression of hepatic function and hepatitis. Infants with intrauterine viral infections, including toxoplasmosis, rubella, cytomegalovirus, herpes simplex, and syphilis, may have pronounced hepatomegaly, hepatitis, and obstruction of bile flow. Of note, cholestasis due to these infections may also result in an elevated level of conjugated (direct) bilirubin.

9. **Additional entities.** Other diagnoses in the newborn period associated with jaundice include the following: any delay in the passage of meconium, as with intestinal atresias, meconium plugs, or meconium ileus, which result in increased enterohepatic circulation; swallowed blood with subsequent breakdown of hemoglobin by heme oxygenase located in the intestinal epithelium; and extravasated blood, which occurs with cephalohematomas, bruising, or occult abdominal hemorrhage resulting from a traumatic delivery. It should be noted that because meconium ileus is the most common presentation of cystic fibrosis in the newborn, family history and monitoring for pulmonary symptoms and evidence of cholestasis should be considered for infants with this diagnosis.

D. **History.** Establishing the appropriate diagnosis and subsequent management of a newborn with jaundice requires that the physician obtain a detailed history of the mother's pregnancy and the infant's delivery and initial status in the nursery. The maternal record should be reviewed for the following: illnesses during the prenatal period that may suggest a viral exposure; evidence of maternal diabetes mellitus; maternal screening labs, including blood type and serologies; and obstetric managements during the current and prior pregnancies. Additionally, any family history of jaundice or anemia should be noted. A history of hemolytic disease in siblings requiring treatment or extended hospital stay in the newborn period may suggest a potential blood group incompatibility or hemolytic process such as a red blood cell membrane or enzyme defect. Deliveries requiring instrumentation should be assessed for possible birth trauma and subsequent bruising or hematoma formation. Possible sepsis should be considered if maternal risk factors exist or if low Apgar scores and/or decreased activity are noted. Both the age of the infant at onset of jaundice or a history of prolonged jaundice may prompt the need for further investigations.

E. **Physical exam.** A complete physical examination of all newborns with jaundice should be performed regardless of the initial suspected diagnosis. If jaundice is noted during a visual examination, a decision must be made as to whether this represents physiologic or pathologic jaundice and what forms of treatment should be instituted. Particular concern exists for newborns with microcephaly, petechiae, and growth restriction as these conditions may be indicative of an associated intrauterine viral infection. Hepatosplenomegaly is significant as it may be the result of a hemolytic process, liver disease, or hepatic involvement due to infection. Any evidence of pallor or bruising may suggest extravascular blood and will require close monitoring of vital signs.

F. **Laboratory evaluation.** In addition to a complete history and thorough physical examination, laboratory testing is a key component in the evaluation of the jaundiced infant. A basic laboratory evaluation is indicated for all infants and an expanded evaluation for selected infants (Table 8-2). The basic evaluation should include the following: a fractionated bilirubin level that includes direct (conjugated) and indirect (unconjugated) bilirubin measurements; a complete blood count with peripheral smear and differential noting any nucleated red blood cells; a reticulocyte count; maternal blood type, Rh status, and antibody screen; and, if ABO incompatibility is suspected, the infant's blood type, Rh status, and direct and indirect Coombs should be assessed. The direct Coombs test, also known as the Direct Antiglobulin Test or "DAT," determines if IgG antibodies are attached to red blood cells (Fig. 8-4). A positive direct Coombs does not identify the type of antibody or specific antigen; therefore, it is impossible to determine if it is against the Rh, ABO, or some other red blood cell antigen group. The indirect Coombs tests for specific plasma antibodies that are not attached to red blood cells (Fig. 8-5). For example, an indirect Coombs test with A cells tests specifically for anti-A antibody in the patient's plasma. Further, established newborn metabolic screening tests (particularly to detect hypothyroidism and galactosemia) should be sent as a part of basic laboratory studies.

Additional studies may be indicated on the basis of the history (both maternal and perinatal) and physical examination of the infant. To test for possible sepsis, blood, urine, and perhaps cerebrospinal fluid should be collected for culture. If intrauterine viral infection is suspected, appropriate specimens should be sent, such as blood for total immunoglobulin M (IgM) and urine for cytomegalovirus (CMV)

Table 8-2. Laboratory evaluation of jaundice

Basic evaluation
Fractionated bilirubin level
Complete blood count including reticulocyte count
Blood type and Rh of mother
Blood type, Rh, direct Coombs of infant (indirect Coombs if ABO incompatibility)
Newborn screen

Additional studies (as indicated)
Blood, urine, and cerebrospinal fluid cultures
Titers and/or cultures for congenital infections
Further hemolytic evaluation
Further hepatic evaluation

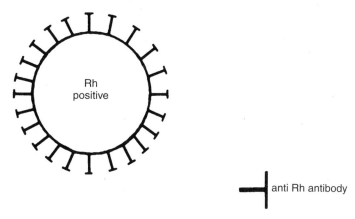

Figure 8-4. The direct Coombs test for antibodies attached to the red blood cell.

culture. Additional studies to investigate hepatic dysfunction or a more extensive hemolytic process may be necessary following preliminary laboratory results (for example, a reticulocyte count greater than 8% indicating excessive hemolysis). Persistence of elevated bilirubin levels may be associated with hypothyroidism or inborn errors of metabolism, which may need to be screened for as well.

III. Management.

    A. Goals of therapy. The recognition that neurotoxicity can result from exposure of the central nervous system to elevated bilirubin levels during the newborn period is the primary impetus to establish guidelines for the management of jaundiced newborns. Although controversy exists as to the specific bilirubin levels responsible for neurologic injury, agreement does exist as to the need for guidelines for the institution of therapies, supportive management regimens, and close follow-up of neonates requiring treatment for, or at risk for, hyperbilirubinemia. Neurotoxicity is associated with the passage of unconjugated bilirubin into the central nervous system. Unconjugated bilirubin not bound to albumin can pass through the blood-brain barrier and this passage may occur to a greater extent if the barrier is immature or if it is disrupted, for example, secondary to infection or anoxia. Evidence of neuronal injury

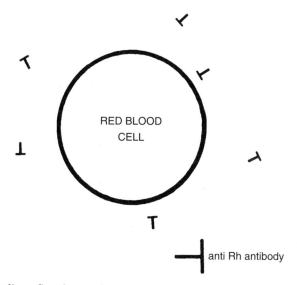

Figure 8-5. The indirect Coombs test for antibodies in the plasma not attached to red blood cells.

may be variable. It includes acute bilirubin encephalopathy with periods of hypotonia and hypertonia and, eventually, marked decreased tone and activity if chronic
bilirubin encephalopathy develops. Infants who die following severe injury may
demonstrate the pathologic finding of kernicterus, which refers to the yellow staining of the brain (most notably in the basal ganglia and cerebellum). This deposition
of bilirubin is associated with neuronal injury. The primary goal of therapeutic interventions ordered for jaundiced newborns is to prevent these neurologic injuries
and their long-term sequelae.

B. **Management strategies.**

   1. **General guidelines.** In accordance with current standard of care recommenda-
      tions from the American Academy of Pediatrics (AAP), the following guidelines
      should be considered for the management of hyperbilirubinemia:
      - Establish guidelines appropriate for individual institutions to identify and
        treat elevated bilirubin levels.
      - Ensure adequate monitoring of vital signs, hydration, bilirubin levels, and
        other appropriate laboratory evaluations.
      - Monitor for underlying illnesses requiring specific therapies.
      - Provide appropriate follow-up for identified at-risk newborns.

   a. **Term- and near-term infants.** Normograms have been established to identify
      potential risk for the development of significant hyperbilirubinemia in term-
      and near-term newborns. Utilizing predischarge bilirubin levels, four risk
      zones have been determined as shown in Fig. 8-6. These zones—low, interme-
      diate (low and high), and high—can be used to assess the likelihood that the
      bilirubin level will increase to a degree that intervention will be necessary. This
      is very useful in planning follow-up monitoring. Guidelines for the institution
      of phototherapy in term- and near-term infants are identified in Fig. 8-7.

   b. **Premature infants.** The decision of when to initiate therapy for premature
      newborns is controversial and is less well defined because of the lack of defini-
      tive evidence as to specific levels of bilirubin associated with neurologic injury
      in these infants. Because premature neonates have a fragile blood-brain bar-
      rier and are at greater risk of disruption of this barrier from acidosis, sepsis,
      and anoxia, a much lower threshold to initiate interventions for hyperbiliru-
      binemia should exist. These decisions must consider gestational age, associ-
      ated illnesses, current clinical status, and any coexisting neurologic injury. A
      conservative guideline for initiating phototherapy in "healthy" premature
      newborns is outlined in Table 8-3.

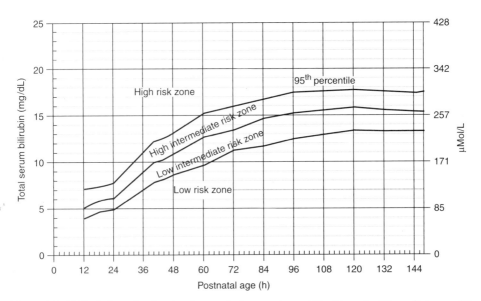

Figure 8-6. Risk designation for development of severe hyperbilirubinemia. [From Subcommittee
on Hyperbilirubinemia. Management of hyperbilirubinemia in the newborn infant 35 or more
weeks of gestation. *Pediatrics* 2004;114(1):297–316, with permission.]

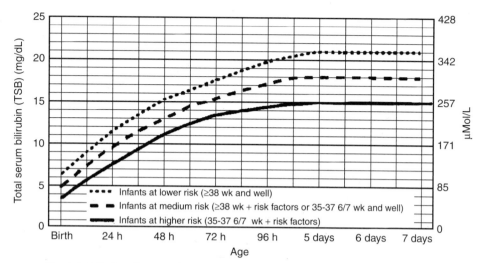

- Use total bilirubin. Do not subtract direct reacting or conjugated bilirubin.
- Risk factors = isoimmune hemolytic disease, G6PD deficiency, asphyxia, significant lethargy, temperature instability, sepsis, acidosis, or albumin <3.0g/dL (if measured)
- For well infants 35-37 6/7 wk can adjust TSB levels for intervention around the medium risk line. It is an option to intervene at lower TSB levels for infants closer to 35 wks and at higher TSB levels for those closer to 37 6/7 wk.
- It is an option to provide conventional phototherapy in hospital or at home at TSB levels 2-3 mg/dL (35-50 µMol/L) below those shown but home phototherapy should not be used in any infant with risk factors.

Figure 8-7. Guidelines for phototherapy use in term- and near-term newborns. [From Subcommittee on Hyperbilirubinemia. Management of hyperbilirubinemia in the newborn infant 35 or more weeks of gestation. *Pediatrics* 2004;114(1):297–316, with permission.]

2. **Specific managements.** Three basic modes of therapy are utilized to treat hyperbilirubinemia: phototherapy, exchange transfusion, and drugs that induce acceleration of normal metabolic pathways.
   a. **Phototherapy.** Phototherapy has been shown to be an effective means of preventing, treating, and modifying the course of significant hyperbilirubinemia. Phototherapy units act by converting bilirubin to photochemical products that are water soluble and can therefore be excreted in urine and bile without need for conjugation. The most effective forms of phototherapy lights provide wavelengths in the range of 425 to 475 nm with absorption in the blue region of the visible spectrum. In addition to standard phototherapy lights, high-intensity spotlights and fiberoptic phototherapy "bili-blankets" are also available. These "bili-blankets" are useful alternatives for outpatient management of infants with nonhemolytic jaundice secondary to breastfeeding. Infants treated in this manner require close monitoring of their bilirubin levels, hydration, and intake. In any infant receiving phototherapy, the serum bilirubin level must be followed, as clinical assessment of skin color is not adequate.
      It is important to remember that phototherapy may obscure a serious diagnosis for which other treatment is needed. For example, jaundice in infants

Table 8-3. Guidelines for initiating phototherapy in premature newborns

Weight (g)	Bilirubin level (mg/dL)
<1,000	5–7
1,001–1,500	7–10
1,501–2,000	10–12
2,001–2,500	12–15
>2,500	15–18

with sepsis or hypothyroidism may respond to phototherapy with a decrease in bilirubin level; however, failing to diagnose the underlying etiology may compromise treatment and outcome.

Potential side effects of phototherapy include the following:

- "bronze baby syndrome," in which the skin and urine of infants who have elevated direct bilirubin levels become "bronze" colored with the use of phototherapy, probably due to retention of bile pigments
- increased insensible water loss
- temperature instability
- loose stools due to increased gastrointestinal transit time
- skin rashes

Owing to increased insensible water loss, infants treated with phototherapy lights may need 15 to 20 mL/kg/day of additional fluids. Phototherapy is usually discontinued in infants who develop a conjugated (direct) hyperbilriubinemia in order to avoid "bronze baby syndrome." Also, in view of laboratory evidence of retinal damage in animals exposed to phototherapy and DNA breaks in cell culture, it is recommended that during phototherapy the infant's eyes and genitalia be covered.

b. Exchange transfusions. Exchange transfusions are high-risk procedures and, thus, should be performed only by experienced health care practitioners. The decision to do an exchange transfusion is often a difficult one and the bilirubin level is usually the main determinant. However, the bilirubin level chosen will vary depending on several factors: gestational age, chronologic age, underlying diagnosis, rate of rise of the bilirubin level, and the infant's current

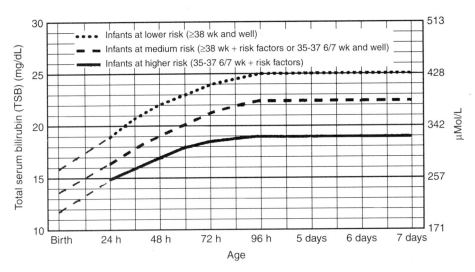

- The dashed lines for the first 24 hours indicate uncertainty owing to a wide range of clinical circumstances and a range of responses to phototherapy.
- Immediate exchange transfusion is recommended if infant shows signs of acute bilirubin encephalopathy (hypertonia, arching, retrocollis, opisthotonos, fever, high pitched cry) or TSB is ≥5 mg/L (85 μMol/L) above these lines.
- Risk factors = isoimmune hemolytic disease, G6PD deficiency asphyxia, significant lethargy, temeperature instability, sepsis, acidosis.
- Measure serum albumin and calculate B/A ratio.
- Use total bilirubin. Do not subtract direct-reacting or conjugated bilirubin.
- If infant is well and 35-37 6/7 wk (median risk), individualize TSB levels for exchange based on actual gestational age.

Figure 8-8. Guidelines for exchange transfusion in term- and near-term newborns. [From Subcommittee on Hyperbilirubinemia. Management of hyperbilirubinemia in the newborn infant 35 or more weeks of gestation. *Pediatrics* 2004;114(1):297–316, with permission.]

clinical status. Figure 8-8 provides recommendations from the American Academy of Pediatrics for performing an exchange transfusion in term and near-term infants. For premature infants, as described previously for the initiation of phototherapy, the criteria to perform an exchange transfusion are less well defined. Because lower levels of hyperbilirubinemia are thought to put these infants at risk for adverse sequelae, the threshold for treatment is lower.

Once the decision is made to do an exchange transfusion, several parameters of the newborn's status must be monitored closely. These include temperature, hydration, oxygenation, acid-base balance, and serum glucose and electrolyte levels. For a double-volume exchange transfusion, fresh (<72-hour old), heparinized or citrate-phosphate-dextrose-anticoagulated blood is used. If the blood bank does not have access to fresh blood, then a unit of packed red blood cells of the proper type and Rh compatibility can be resuspended in fresh frozen plasma to a hematocrit of approximately 50%. The blood should have a serum potassium concentration <10 meq/L and should be appropriately screened for hepatitis, HIV, and CMV. A double-volume exchange transfusion, assuming a neonate's blood volume to be 80 to 100 mL/kg, should remove 87% of the infant's original blood. Because of equilibration between extravascular and plasma bilirubin, the serum bilirubin concentration several hours after a double-volume exchange will be about 65% of the pre-exchange bilirubin level. Continued production of bilirubin from red blood cell hemolysis and the degradation of other heme proteins may further increase the serum bilirubin concentration, thus necessitating additional exchange transfusions.

A double-volume exchange transfusion is usually performed via an umbilical venous catheter using a push–pull method. Continuous exchange transfusion by infusing donor blood into a venous line while extracting infant blood from an arterial line is also a safe and efficacious method. On occasion, venous access may be necessary via the antecubital fossa or femoral vein if the umbilical vessels cannot be used.

During an exchange transfusion, appropriate monitoring of the infant's heart rate, temperature, oxygenation, and serum glucose must be performed. If an infant is requiring supplemental oxygen, the concentration of oxygen may need to be increased 5% to 10% during the procedure. Immediately prior to performing an exchange transfusion, the infant's hematocrit, fractionated bilirubin, and electrolytes including calcium should be measured. The serum glucose should be monitored throughout the procedure and for 4 hours following completion of the procedure.

The blood to be used should be warmed to 37°C using a heating coil. An umbilical venous catheter should be placed under sterile technique with the infant adequately restrained. Optimally, the umbilical venous catheter is inserted until the tip is in the inferior vena cava and below the right atrium or proximal to the portal sinus as detailed in Chapter 11. The catheter is almost always in the inferior vena cava if it can be introduced beyond 8 cm in a premature infant or 11 cm in a term infant without meeting resistance. If resistance is encountered, the catheter can be withdrawn to approximately 3 cm in premature infant or 5 cm in a term infant and, once secured, the procedure can be completed from these depths of catheter insertion.

The exchange transfusion is then performed by exchanging aliquots of the infant's blood for aliquots of donor blood. The volume of each aliquot is based on the infant's weight: <1500 g—5 mL aliquots; 1500 to 2500 g—10 mL aliquots; 2500 to 3500 g—15 mL aliquots; and >3500 g—20 mL aliquots. The ideal duration of time to complete a double-volume exchange is approximately 50 to 70 minutes.

At completion of the exchange transfusion, blood is obtained from the last aliquot of blood removed and sent for laboratory testing to include hematocrit, fractionated bilirubin, electrolytes including calcium, pH, platelet count, and glucose. Potential risks of exchange transfusions are listed in Table 8-4. The mortality rate from this procedure is directly related to the severity of illness in the baby and the experience of the personnel performing the procedure and should be less than 1%.

c. **Drugs.** Several drugs have been used experimentally to facilitate bilirubin metabolism and decrease elevated levels. Phenobarbital, which increases bilirubin excretion, uptake, and conjugation, is effective for the management

Table 8-4. Potential complications of exchange transfusions

Vascular
Embolization (air, clots)
Thrombosis
Infarction of organs
Perforation of vessels, bowel
Cardiac
Arrhythmias
Volume overload
Arrest
Hematologic
Bleeding
Hemolysis
Metabolic
Hyperkalemia
Hypernatremia
Hypocalcemia/hypomagnesemia
Hypoglycemia (postexchange)
Thrombocytopenia
NEC
Infection

NEC, necrotizing enterocolitis.

of indirect hyperbilirubinemia in Crigler-Najjar Type II and the direct hyperbilirubinemia associated with hyperalimentation. Intravenous immune globulin (IVIG), believed to decrease the rate of red cell hemolysis in infants with isoimmune hemolytic anemia, has been employed in addition to phototherapy and exchange transfusions in the management of these infants. Although metalloporphyrins, which are competitive inhibitors of heme oxygenase, have been used experimentally to treat infants with ABO incompatibility and Crigler-Najjar type I, they are not recommended for routine clinical use.

IV.　**Clinical pearls.**
- The overall incidence of jaundice in newborns is 65%, which includes 50% of term and 80% of premature infants.
- Jaundice in the first 24 hours of life is pathologic until proven otherwise.
- One gram of hemoglobin yields 35 mg of bilirubin.
- Serum bilirubin levels must reach 4 to 6 mg/dL (68 to 102 μm/L) to be visually detected.
- If resistance is met with placement of an umbilical venous catheter for an exchange transfusion, it should be withdrawn to 3 cm for premature infants and 5 cm for term infants where it can be secured and used to accomplish the exchange transfusion.
- In infants with hemolytic disease, ongoing hemolysis may continue for many weeks owing to the persistence of antibodies in the infant's blood. This can result in significant anemia and therefore the hematocrit of these infants should be followed closely after discharge from the hospital.

BIBLIOGRAPHY

American Academy of Pediatrics, Subcommittee on Hyperbilirubinemia. Management of hyperbilirubinemia in the newborn infant 35 or more weeks of gestation. *Pediatrics* 2004;114:297–301.

Bhutani VK, Johnson L, Siveri EM. Predictive ability of a predischarge hour-specific serum bilirubin for subsequent significant hyperbilirubinemia in healthy term and near-term newborns. *Pediatrics* 1999;103:1–4.

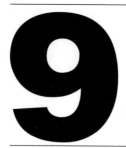

Nonsurgical Causes of Respiratory Distress

William A. Engle,
Michael Stone Trautman, and
Kimberly E. Applegate

I. **Description of the issue.** Respiratory distress is a common presenting sign for many illnesses during the neonatal period. Approximately 3% of neonates suffer from respiratory distress during the first days of life. The most common etiologies include the following:
   - respiratory distress syndrome (i.e., surfactant deficiency)
   - transient tachypnea
   - pneumothorax
   - pneumonia
   - meconium aspiration syndrome
   - persistent pulmonary hypertension of the newborn
   - miscellaneous group of surgical and nonsurgical disorders

   Of those newborns suffering from respiratory distress during the neonatal period, 10% to 16% will succumb, especially those at lower gestational ages, and many others will require prolonged hospitalizations and intensive care (Table 9-1).

II. **Making the diagnosis.** This chapter will discuss the following common respiratory disorders that present during the immediate neonatal period: respiratory distress syndrome, transient tachypnea, meconium aspiration, persistent pulmonary hypertension, pneumothorax, and pneumonia. Other, less common problems, such as congenital heart disease, sepsis, congenital diaphragmatic hernia, metabolic/thermoregulatory disorders, and congenital anomalies of the pulmonary, thoracic, and cardiac systems, are beyond the scope of this chapter; however, these conditions will be included during discussions of differential diagnosis and treatment. Historical risk factors, signs and symptoms, radiographic findings, treatments, and outcomes for the most common respiratory disorders will be presented.

   A. **Historical clues.** History is very helpful when a clinician is presented with a newborn infant suffering from respiratory distress. Although often nonspecific, historical information combined with prenatal diagnostic studies, clinical pattern of respiratory distress, chest radiographs, time course, and response to specific therapies will lead to specific diagnoses (Table 9-2). Significant risk factors for respiratory distress presenting during the immediate perinatal period include the following:
      - prematurity
      - emergency cesarean delivery
      - elective cesarean delivery
      - male gender (1.3:1 male:female ratio)
      - fetal distress
      - prenatally identified congenital anomalies

      Premature infants account for 60% of respiratory distress cases. The incidence in premature infants is 50% compared with a 0.8% incidence in term neonates. Following emergency cesarean birth, the incidence of respiratory distress is 12%; this is nearly four times the incidence following elective cesarean birth (3.1%) and eight times the incidence following vaginal delivery (1.6%). Any of these risk factors is an alert to clinicians that respiratory compromise may occur and, if known before delivery, preparations for illness-specific interventions can be arranged (i.e., surfactant for respiratory distress syndrome prophylaxis in extremely preterm infants, immediate intubation for congenital diaphragmatic hernia, prostaglandin infusion for ductal-dependent congenital heart disease, etc.).

      1. **Surfactant deficiency.** Specific risk factors associated with respiratory distress syndrome, or surfactant deficiency respiratory distress, include prematurity, pregnancy-induced hypertension, abruptio placenta, intrauterine growth retardation, emergency cesarean section, and an Apgar score at 5 minutes ≤3. Other risk factors for respiratory distress syndrome include previous preterm

infant with respiratory distress syndrome, maternal diabetes (especially if insulin dependent), and blood group isoimmunization.

2. **Transient tachypnea.** Transient tachypnea of the newborn is caused by delayed resorption of intrapulmonary fluid following birth. Historical clues for development of transient tachypnea in newborns include emergency cesarean section, elective cesarean section, male gender, forceps application, pregnancy-induced hypertension, prolonged rupture of membranes, and precipitous delivery. Infants with hypotonia (asphyxia, neuromuscular disorders, hypermagnesemia) or depressed respiratory efforts (maternal narcotics, asphyxia, hypermagnesemia) may also have delayed absorption of intrapulmonary fluid and respiratory distress.

Table 9-1. Causes of respiratory distress in neonates

<u>Pulmonary</u> Respiratory pump (lungs, chest wall, diaphragm, intercostals and accessory muscles)

Acute parenchymal disease:
Respiratory distress syndrome
Transient tachypnea
Pneumonia/sepsis
Meconium aspiration
Persistent pulmonary hypertension
Pneumothorax
Pulmonary edema
Pleural effusions

Subacute/chronic parenchymal disease:
Bronchopulmonary dysplasia
Mikity-Wilson disease
Chronic pulmonary insufficiency of prematurity

Congenital parenchymal disease:
Cystic malformations (e.g., cystic adenomatoid malformation, lobar emphysema)
Other malformations (e.g., sequestration, hypoplasia)

Diaphragm and chest wall:
Diaphragmatic hernia
Eventration, thoracic cage anomalies

<u>Upper airway</u>

Nose, mouth, and pharynx:
Choanal atresia
Cleft lip/cleft palate
Micrognathia
Macroglossia
Pharyngomalacia

Larynx:
Laryngomalacia
Vocal cord paralysis
Subglottic stenosis

Trachea and bronchi:
Tracheal stenosis
Tracheal ring/web
Tracheomalacia
Bronchomalacia
Tracheoesophageal fistula
Laryngotracheal cleft

<u>Nonpulmonary</u>

Cardiovascular:
Congenital heart disease
Congestive heart failure

(continued)

Table 9-1. Causes of respiratory distress in neonates (*continued*)

Metabolic/endocrine:
Asphyxia
Hypothermia
Hyperthermia
Hypoglycemia

Hematologic:
Polycythemia
Anemia
Leukemoid reaction
Thrombocytosis

Neurologic:
Apnea of prematurity
Central nervous system malformation
Hydrocephalus
Arnold-Chiari malformation

Table 9-2. Historical clues and causes of neonatal respiratory distress

Any respiratory distress	Prematurity, emergent or elective cesarean birth, male gender, fetal distress, prenatally diagnosed congenital anomaly
Respiratory distress syndrome	Prematurity, pregnancy-induced hypertension, abruptio placenta, intrauterine growth restriction, five minute Apgar ≤3, previous preterm birth, second of twins, insulin-dependent diabetic mother, blood group isoimmunization, emergent cesarean section
Transient tachypnea	Emergent or elective cesarean birth, male gender, forceps delivery, pregnancy-induced hypertension, prolonged rupture of membranes, prematurity, fetal distress, maternal diabetes, delayed cord clamping, maternal narcotics or hypermagnesemia, precipitous delivery
Pneumonia	Maternal group B streptococcal colonization, chorioamnionitis, maternal urinary tract or other infection
Meconium aspiration syndrome/ persistent pulmonary hypertension	Meconium-stained amniotic fluid, fetal distress, cesarean birth, meconium aspiration, sepsis/pneumonia, transient tachypnea, respiratory distress syndrome, congenital diaphragmatic hernia, congenital heart disease

3. **Pneumonia.** Pneumonia often occurs without known prenatal or perinatal risk factors. However, maternal colonization with group B streptococcus and maternal chorioamnionitis increase risk.
4. **Meconium aspiration.** Meconium aspiration as a cause for respiratory distress is considered when respiratory distress occurs in the presence of meconium-stained amniotic fluid or following perinatal depression.
5. **Persistent pulmonary hypertension.** Persistent pulmonary hypertension may occur following cesarean birth, perinatal depression, meconium aspiration, pneumonia, transient tachypnea, and respiratory distress syndrome, or it may be a primary process. It often accompanies congenital diaphragmatic hernia and, occasionally, congenital heart disease, both of which are often diagnosed on prenatal ultrasound.

B. **Clinical presentation of respiratory distress: signs, symptoms, and physiologic responses.** Clinical presentation of respiratory distress varies with the underlying etiology and severity of illness. Some newly born infants with common respiratory disorders may be clinically asymptomatic. However, most infants with respiratory disorders show one or more signs, such as tachypnea, nasal flaring, retractions, grunting, see-saw respirations, apnea, and cyanosis. In general, the number and severity of these signs is proportional to the severity of illness.

1. **Tachypnea.** The normal respiratory rate during the neonatal period is 20 to 60 breaths per minute. Tachypnea, therefore, is a respiratory rate greater than 60 breaths per minute. Tachypnea is the most sensitive sign of respiratory distress. With rapid respiratory rates, expiratory time is decreased; this allows the volume of gas within the lung, especially functional residual capacity, to be maintained and oxygenation stabilized. This is especially important for neonates who are at high risk for diffuse atelectasis because of immature respiratory controls, highly compliant chest walls, and low lung volumes. Illnesses that alter respiratory control or decrease lung volume are complicated by loss of lung volume (i.e., atelectasis) when functional residual capacity is decreased. Tachypnea also increases minute ventilation to acutely reduce partial pressure of carbon dioxide and raise pH; this compensatory response occurs in many illnesses that cause respiratory and metabolic acidosis, hypoxemia, hypercarbia, or hyperthermia (Table 9-3).

   Although sustained tachypnea is a sign of respiratory distress, intermittent or brief periods of tachypnea occur in healthy neonates. Respiratory patterns in newborn infants are notably irregular. This is especially apparent during the rapid eye movement phase of sleep, when increased respiratory rates are common. Caregivers examining an infant during the tachypneic phase of rapid eye movement sleep may mistakenly interpret this as a sign of an underlying pathologic process. Brief periods of tachypnea following the respiratory pause during periodic breathing may similarly be misinterpreted. Therefore, it is important to evaluate for sustained tachypnea, other signs of respiratory distress, and improvement after awakening or transitioning to quiet sleep.

   Sustained tachypnea or tachypnea associated with other signs of respiratory distress require evaluation and treatment. Neonates with parenchymal lung disease often present with tachypnea, cyanosis, and other signs of respiratory distress such as nasal flaring, retractions, and grunting respirations. In contrast, neonates with respiratory distress but without parenchymal lung involvement often present with unlabored tachypnea and cyanosis (e.g., those with cyanotic congenital heart disease, primary persistent pulmonary hypertension, or sepsis without pneumonia).
2. **Nasal flaring.** Nasal flaring is one of the first physiologic compensations for illnesses that impair oxygenation or ventilation. Flaring of the nares decreases airway resistance and improves gas flow through the upper airway. This is especially important in neonates who are obligate nose breathers. If nasal flaring cannot increase gas flow sufficiently due to severe disease, additional physiologic responses such as tachypnea, retractions, and/or cyanosis will be present.
3. **Retractions.** Retractions are active contractions of intercostal, subcostal, and suprasternal chest wall muscles, which function to stabilize the relatively compliant chest wall of the neonate. This occurs in neonates with parenchymal lung disorders that cause an increase in respiratory effort (i.e., generation of a more negative pleural pressure than normal) needed to move air into and out of the lung. As the negative pleural pressure needed to move air increases, the diaphragm contracts downward pulling the chest wall muscles inward and pushing the abdomen outward; this is called "see-saw" breathing. "See-saw" respirations indicate severe respiratory distress.
4. **Grunting.** Grunting respirations describe another physiologic compensation for low lung volume or parenchymal lung disease. When an infant exhales against a partially closed glottis, which increases functional residual capacity,

Table 9-3. Respiratory distress and physiologic actions

Tachypnea	Shorten expiratory time
	Increase functional residual capacity
	Increase minute ventilation
Nasal flaring	Decrease airway resistance
Retractions	Stabilize chest wall
Grunting	Increase end expiratory pressure
	Increase functional residual capacity
Apnea and periodic breathing	Decrease lung volume and minute ventilation
Cyanosis	Decreased oxygen delivery

an expiratory grunt or moan may be audible. The loudness of the grunt is proportional to the severity of lung disease. The presence of tachypnea, nasal flaring, retractions, and/or grunting respirations is described as increased "work of breathing."

5. **Apnea and periodic breathing.** Irregular respiratory efforts characterize the neonate, especially premature neonates, and may manifest as periodic breathing or apnea. Irregular respiration is associated with immature chemoreceptor, mechanoreceptor, thermal, and neural controls; preponderance of rapid eye movement sleep; low respiratory muscle tone; and a compliant chest wall. Conditions or illnesses that affect central respiratory drive, airway patency, and proper functioning of the respiratory pump (lungs, chest wall, diaphragm, intercostal muscles, and accessory respiratory muscles) can cause periodic breathing and apnea. Many illnesses, airway anomalies, conditions, and medications impair respiratory drive, airway patency, and respiratory pump function and may cause central and/or obstructive apnea (Table 9-4).

   Short pauses in breathing occur in normal newborns, children, and adults following large sigh breaths, crying, or hyperventilation. This physiologic response to hypocarbia is normal but should be brief (<5 seconds). Periodic breathing is a gradual decrease in frequency and depth of breathing efforts until a short pause occurs; no fall in oxygenation or heart rate occurs. The pause in breathing is followed by a brief (approximately 15 seconds) period of tachypnea. The term apnea is used to describe a pause in breathing that lasts greater than 20 seconds or a pause of any duration that is associated with bradycardia (heart rate <80 beats per minute), oxygen desaturation (saturation <88%), cyanosis, or hypotonia. Although periodic breathing is common in preterm and term neonates, apnea occurs predominantly in preterm infants (apnea of prematurity). Apnea in term neonates, or preterm neonates with additional signs of illness, is usually pathologic and additional evaluation and intervention is warranted. "Apnea of prematurity" is a diagnosis of exclusion and other pathologic causes should be ruled out, especially if the onset is in the first days of life. The presence of apnea or periodic breathing is not predictive of sudden infant death syndrome.

6. **Cyanosis.** Cyanosis is subdivided into two categories, central and peripheral (acrocyanosis). Central cyanosis (cyanosis of the mucous membranes of the mouth and tongue) is visibly apparent when greater than 5 grams of unsaturated hemoglobin/100 mL of blood is present; this occurs when pulmonary disorders

Table 9-4. Causes of central and/or obstructive apnea

Illness	Sepsis
	Pneumonia
	Necrotizing enterocolitis
	Atelectasis
	Central nervous system hemorrhage
	Hypoxia/ischemia
	Metabolic abnormalities
Airway anomalies	Choanal atresia
	Micrognathia
	Macroglossia
Conditions	Prematurity
	Hypoxemia
	Acidosis
	Hypo/hyperthermia
	Anemia
Medications	Antepartum magnesium sulfate
	General anesthesia during delivery
	Prostaglandins
	Sedatives
	Analgesics
	Paralytics

prevent oxygenation of arterial blood due to ventilation:perfusion mismatching, hypoventilation, or impaired respiratory membrane diffusion. Cyanosis is also present in congenital cardiovascular disorders, owing to mixing of unsaturated venous blood with oxygenated pulmonary venous blood (single ventricle), insufficient pulmonary blood flow, or perfusion of the systemic circulation with unsaturated venous blood (transposition of the great vessels).

Because it is the absolute amount of unsaturated hemoglobin in the blood that is visible as cyanosis, neonates with low hemoglobin concentrations (anemia) may not be visibly cyanotic because the physiologic compensation is to maximize binding of oxygen to hemoglobin to maintain oxygen delivery to tissues. On the other hand, neonates with high concentrations of hemoglobin (polycythemia) may look cyanotic because they have excess hemoglobin to supply oxygen needs of the tissues; therefore, they may circulate greater than 5 grams of unsaturated hemoglobin/100 mL of blood. Central cyanosis is particularly visible in the mucous membranes of the mouth and tongue because the thin epidermis in highly vascular tissues allows the blue color of the unsaturated hemoglobin in capillary blood to be easily seen.

Central cyanosis is difficult to detect in neonates until a partial pressure of oxygen reaches as low as 30 to 40 mm Hg (oxygen saturation 75% to 85%) because fetal hemoglobin binds oxygen more avidly than adult hemoglobin. Therefore, by the time cyanosis becomes visible during an illness, the neonate has little physiologic margin to compensate. Noninvasive transcutaneous oxygen saturation measurement in the delivery room and nursery is useful to detect hypoxemia before cyanosis becomes clinically apparent in neonates with respiratory distress. Because cyanosis is often a presenting sign of illness in neonates (especially cyanotic congenital heart disease), some clinicians advocate that oxygen saturation become one of the routine vital signs measured prior to discharge in all neonates.

Acrocyanosis, or peripheral cyanosis of the hands and feet, is common in healthy neonates. Unless associated with central cyanosis or symptoms of diminished cardiac output, no investigation is needed. Acrocyanosis is apparent in the hands and feet because of relatively sluggish blood flow, especially when cold stress exists. The slow rate of blood flow through the capillaries allows enough time for the capillary blood to lose most of its oxygen to the tissues and therefore appear blue even though the hemoglobin is fully oxygenated in the arterial blood.

C. Evaluation of the neonate with respiratory distress.

    1. Physical findings. Antenatal testing (serum screening, sonography, magnetic resonance imaging, karyotype, etc.) and intrapartum findings may detect fetal anomalies or conditions that predispose to respiratory distress (e.g., congenital diaphragmatic hernia, meconium staining, fetal distress). Knowledge of these findings helps alert the clinician so that specific preparations for delivery room and nursery management can be anticipated. When antenatal diagnoses have been determined, the clinician is responsible to stabilize the neonate, confirm the antenatal diagnoses, search for associated findings that may not be apparent with antenatal studies, and begin diagnostic and therapeutic interventions. Signs of respiratory distress, physical findings in other body systems, and severity of illness in the delivery room guide the urgency for evaluation and treatment.

    For neonates that present with respiratory distress without antenatal risk factors or diagnoses, physical findings in all body systems and age at onset of symptoms provide clues to determine diagnosis and guide stabilization and treatment. Physical findings and commonly associated causes or conditions are found in Table 9-5.

    2. Age at onset of respiratory distress. Age at onset of respiratory illness tends to be either immediately after birth or within hours to days of birth depending on the cause of respiratory distress. Because some illnesses that present at birth may have minimal symptoms initially, they may go undetected for hours. Those entities that often present immediately after birth include transient tachypnea, respiratory distress syndrome, meconium aspiration, spontaneous pneumothorax, pulmonary hypoplasia, congenital pneumonia, sepsis, persistent pulmonary hypertension of the newborn, congenital diaphragmatic hernia, large lung masses, and nonductal-dependent cyanotic congenital heart disease. Respiratory distress that presents after the first hours or days of life is often due to sepsis and pneumonia acquired during birth, ductal-dependent congenital heart disease, or progression or recognition of illnesses that were present immediately after birth.

Table 9-5. Physical findings and selected causes for respiratory distress

Stridor	Upper airway obstruction
	Laryngomalacia
	Vocal cord paresis/paralysis
Nares not patent	Choanal atresia or stenosis
Noisy breathing	Nasal edema from suctioning
	Meconium in trachea
Neck mass	Cystic hygroma
	Goiter
	Thyroglossal duct or branchial cleft cyst
Absent breath sounds	Obstructive or central apnea
	Pneumothorax
	Diaphragmatic hernia
	Cystic lung disease
	Pleural effusion
Asymmetric breath sounds	Pneumothorax (unilateral)
	Pulmonary hypoplasia (unilateral)
	Atelectasis
	Diaphragmatic hernia
	Endotracheal tube malposition
Coarse crackles	Pneumothorax
	Pneumonia
	Meconium aspiration
	Transient tachypnea
Increased anterior-posterior diameter	Pneumothorax
	Diaphragmatic hernia
	Atelectasis (unilateral with contralateral hyperexpansion)
	Cystic lung disease
Bell-shaped chest	Hypotonia
	Pulmonary hypoplasia

Illnesses that present as respiratory distress after the first days of life include sepsis, congenital heart disease, pneumonia, apnea of prematurity, metabolic abnormalities, endocrine disorders, and some neurologic disorders.

The peak in severity of respiratory distress syndrome (surfactant deficiency) occurs at about 3 days of age in premature infants. Although this peak in severity of the disease process itself has been reduced considerably with antenatal steroids and postnatal surfactant therapy, the timing of peak illness continues to be at about 3 days. The peak severity for persistent pulmonary hypertension, either primary or complicating other respiratory disorders, occurs during the first 3 days of life. Meconium aspiration is often most severe at 24 to 48 hours of age, which correlates with progression of chemical pneumonitis. Transient tachypnea, uncomplicated by air leak or pulmonary hypertension, often peaks within the first 12 to 24 hours of life.

3. **Laboratory studies.** Arterial blood gases, transcutaneous oxygen saturation measurements, and transcutaneous arterial oxygen and carbon dioxide recordings provide evidence for severity of respiratory compromise. White blood cell and differential counts, hematocrit, glucose, ionized calcium, and electrolytes screen for infection, anemia, and common metabolic disorders that lead to respiratory distress. Cultures of blood and other normally sterile body fluids help determine the presence of infectious etiologies for respiratory distress.

4. **Radiography.** Chest radiography adds valuable diagnostic information to the evaluation of respiratory distress. Although some radiographic findings are characteristic of specific disorders, most are adjunctive only to history and physical findings. Assessment of lung volume, interstitial markings, pulmonary vascularity, cardiothymic silhouette, diaphragm position, and soft tissue or bony anomalies is particularly useful (Table 9-6).

Table 9-6. Chest radiographic findings and neonatal respiratory distress

Reticulogranular lung fields with air bronchograms	Respiratory distress syndrome
	Group B streptococcal pneumonia
Low lung volume	Respiratory distress syndrome
	Pulmonary hypoplasia
High lung volume	Transient tachypnea
	Meconium aspiration
	Persistent pulmonary hypertension
	Cystic lung diseases
	Excessive positive pressure ventilation
Diffusely hazy lung fields	Transient tachypnea
	Respiratory distress syndrome
	Meconium aspiration
	Pneumonia
Patchy infiltrates	Meconium and other aspiration syndromes
	Pneumonia
	Transient tachypnea
Diminished pulmonary vascularity	Persistent pulmonary hypertension
	Pneumothorax
	Pneumomediastinum
	Pulmonary outflow obstruction (pulmonary atresia)
	Cystic lung diseases
Increased pulmonary vascularity	Transient tachypnea
	Congenital heart disease with increased pulmonary blood flow or obstruction of pulmonary venous drainage
	Pulmonary edema
	Interstitial pneumonia
	Pulmonary lymphangiectasia
Pleural effusion	Transient tachypnea
	Pneumonia
	Chylothorax
	Hydrops fetalis
	Leakage from central venous catheters

A radiographic pattern with reticulogranular lung fields, air bronchograms, and low lung volumes most often represents respiratory distress syndrome. This pattern may also be found with group B streptococcal pneumonia and pulmonary hypoplasia (Figs. 9-1 and 9-2). History of maternal group B streptococcus status, prematurity, white blood cell count, differential white cell count, and clinical course help determine the specific diagnosis.

Diffuse patchy infiltrates with normal to high lung volume is consistent with meconium aspiration, congenital pneumonia, and transient tachypnea of the newborn (Figs. 9-3 to 9-5). Presence of meconium-stained amniotic fluid, history of maternal chorioamnionitis, and history of cesarean delivery help differentiate these diagnoses.

Pleural effusion can be found with pneumonia, transient tachypnea, chylothorax, hydrops fetalis, and inadvertent drainage of intravenous solutions into the pleural space. Persistent radiographic infiltrates, history of cesarean delivery, chylous fluid, anasarca, or recent placement of a central venous catheter can aid in the determination of the diagnosis. Normal chest radiographs may be found with primary pulmonary hypertension of the newborn, transient tachypnea, sepsis, and some forms of congenital heart disease.

Pneumothorax characteristically shows dark, lucent lung fields without lung markings with the atelectatic lung outlined; however, medial pneumothorax and pneumomediastinum may appear similar as hyperlucency in one or both perihilar

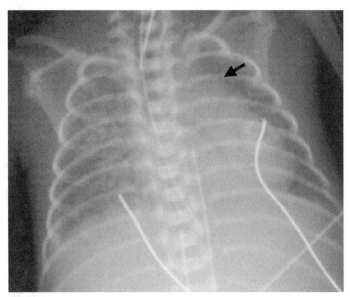

Figure 9-1. Respiratory distress syndrome. Diffuse reticulogranular pattern with air bronchogram (arrow) and low lung volume.

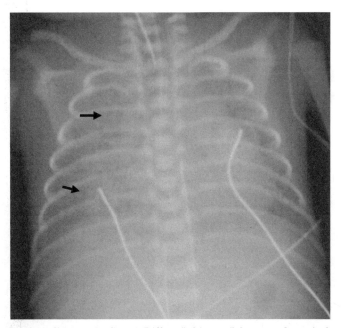

Figure 9-2. Respiratory distress syndrome. Diffuse "white out" due to atelectasis, low lung volume, and air bronchograms (arrows).

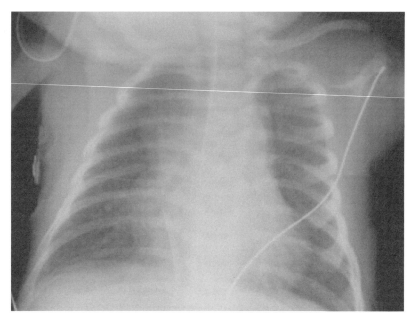

Figure 9-3. Transient tachypnea of the newborn. Perihilar prominence of vasculature, normal lung volume, fluid in the minor fissure.

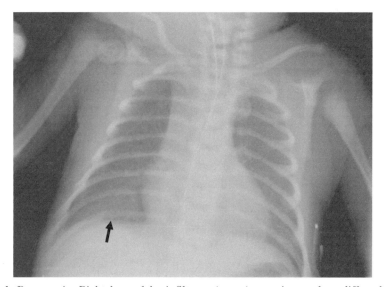

Figure 9-4. Pneumonia. Right lower lobe infiltrate (arrow) superimposed on diffuse hazy lung fields with normal lung volume.

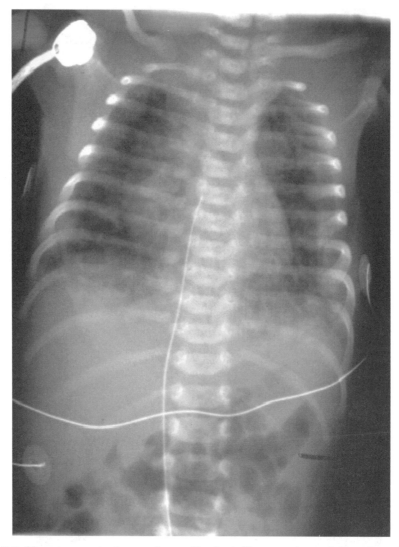

Figure 9-5. Meconium aspiration syndrome. Patchy infiltrates scattered throughout the lung fields with hyperexpansion.

locations (Figs. 9-6 and 9-9). Superior layering of air on decubitus chest radiograph, transillumination of the hemithorax, or return of air on thoracentesis confirms pneumothorax. The absence of these findings with persistent perihilar hyperlucency, air dissecting within the neck, and thymic elevation (sail sign) suggests pneumomediastinum.

III.   **Supportive care.** Neonates with respiratory distress require rapid assessment and quick intervention, especially if clinical deterioration or moderate to severe distress is complicated by hypoxemia, respiratory acidosis, and/or cardiopulmonary insufficiency. General supportive care measures such as supplemental oxygen, mechanical ventilation, volume expansion, vasopressor agents, and antibiotics may be required until history, laboratory findings, and radiographic interpretations can be gathered. For example, if extreme prematurity is present by history and on physical examination, prophylactic surfactant administration in the delivery room may be warranted. When congenital diaphragmatic hernia has been diagnosed antenatally, immediate intubation,

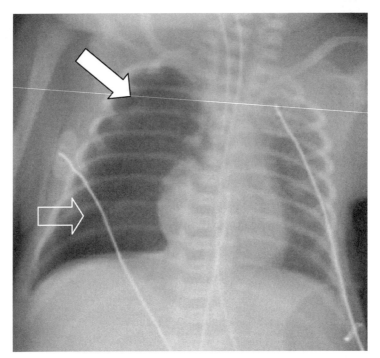

Figure 9-6. Right pneumothorax. Collapsed right lung (white arrow) and right middle lobe lung segment (transparent arrow) surrounded by pneumothorax.

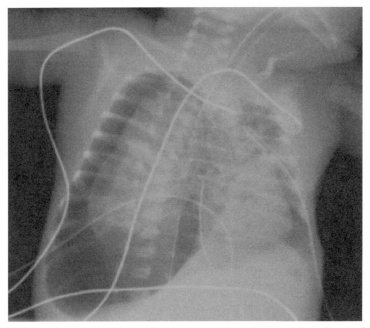

Figure 9-7. Right tension pneumothorax. Large right pneumothorax with mediastinal shift to left causing contralateral atelectasis.

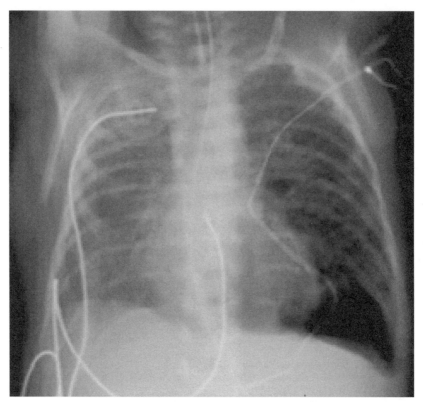

Figure 9-8. Left subpulmonic pneumothorax, left pulmonary interstitial emphysema, and right respiratory distress syndrome.

mechanical ventilation, and pediatric surgery consultation is often required. Lastly, in a neonate several days to weeks old with acute onset respiratory distress, poor perfusion, and absent pulses, the immediate institution of antimicrobials and prostaglandin E1 is indicated while the possible diagnoses of sepsis, ductal-dependent congenital heart disease, or metabolic disorder can be sorted out.

IV.   **Frequently encountered disorders, diagnostic clues, and therapies.**

A. **Respiratory distress syndrome (hyaline membrane disease).** Respiratory distress syndrome, or hyaline membrane disease, is a primary surfactant deficiency complicated by anatomic pulmonary immaturity, especially at low gestational ages (Figs. 9-1 and 9-2). Postnatal signs and symptoms result from the loss of functional residual capacity and lung volume; however, reduced compliance, pulmonary hypertension, and apnea may also complicate the pathophysiology.

Respiratory distress syndrome primarily affects premature infants. However, term infants, especially infants of diabetic mothers, asphyxiated infants, and infants with congenital diaphragmatic hernia, can be affected as well. Secondary surfactant deficiency may complicate many disorders that result in surfactant-inactivating substances or conditions within alveolar sacs, such as meconium, blood, albumin, hyperoxia, hyperexpansion, high airway pressure, atelectasis, pneumonia, and pulmonary edema.

The course of respiratory distress syndrome peaks at 3 days of age, often associated temporally with a marked urinary diuresis. With exogenously administered surfactant and antenatal maternal steroids, the severity of illness and frequency of complications such as pneumothorax and pulmonary interstitial emphysema have decreased during these first days of life (Figs. 9-6–9-9). However, the incidence of chronic lung disease has not decreased despite these advances. Although the incidence of chronic lung disease (approximately 20%) has not changed significantly

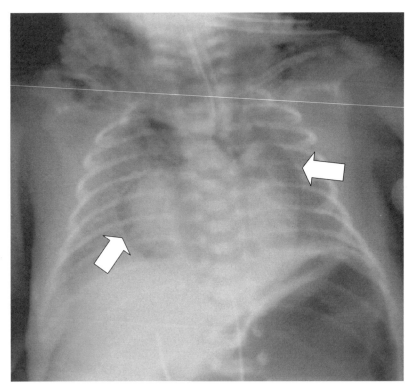

Figure 9-9. Respiratory distress syndrome, pneumomediastinum (arrows), subcutaneous air in neck.

since surfactant became available, this may be a reflection of the survival of more extremely premature infants who formerly would not have survived. It appears that the severity of chronic lung disease is less in comparable gestational age infants. In addition to antenatal steroids and surfactant, other management refinements have contributed to reduction in air leaks and chronic lung disease. These include the avoidance of lung over-distension, the avoidance of high airway pressures, and the avoidance of high concentrations of supplemental oxygen beginning with the first breaths in the delivery room. Early use of continuous positive airway pressure beginning in the delivery room and reducing the use and duration of mechanical ventilation may also decrease the risk for complications. Minimizing endotracheal tube suction pressure and consequent loss of lung volume during suctioning may reduce the contribution of atelectasis to development of chronic lung disease.

Exogenous surfactant is given through an endotracheal tube directly into the lungs. This is often initiated within the first minutes to hours of life. If the gestational age is less than approximately 30 weeks, prophylactic surfactant administration within the first minutes of life may be considered. Rescue administration is given to infants greater than or equal to 30 weeks a gestation who have signs of respiratory distress severe enough to require respiratory intervention with continuous positive airway pressure or mechanical ventilation. For this group of infants, if the diagnosis is confirmed by physical examination, chest radiographs, and high amount of continuous positive airway pressure (CPAP >4 cm H_2O), mean airway pressure (MAP >7 cm H_2O), or supplemental oxygen (FIO_2 >0.3), surfactant is recommended. When using a surfactant rescue approach for low-birthweight neonates with respiratory distress, keep in mind that about 60% of neonates less than 1500 grams birth weight have respiratory distress syndrome (i.e., qualify to receive surfactant) and approximately 40% have transient tachypnea, mild respiratory distress syndrome, or persistent pulmonary hypertension.

Postnatal surfactant and antenatal maternal steroids have dramatically improved survival in premature infants, especially those suffering from respiratory distress syndrome. Respiratory distress syndrome now ranks below congenital anomalies and short gestation/low birth weight as the most frequent cause for death during the neonatal period. Survival of neonates born at 23 to 27 weeks gestation is 30% to 80%, respectively. For neonates born at 28 to 32 weeks, survival rates of 90% to 98% are anticipated. Neonates with gestational ages greater than 32 weeks have a survival rate greater than 98%.

B. **Transient tachypnea of the newborn.** Transient tachypnea of the newborn is one of the most common respiratory illnesses that affect newly born infants, especially those born at term. Perinatal history of cesarean delivery, forceps-assisted delivery, preeclampsia, hypotonia, and rapid labor alert clinicians to the possibility of transient tachypnea. The primary pathophysiology is delayed resorption of alveolar and interstitial fluid into the pulmonary interstitial vessels and lymphatics after birth. Lack of vaginal delivery and chest "squeeze" followed by rebound expansion of the lung has been proposed to explain the association of delayed resorption of lung fluid with cesarean birth and hypotonia. The hypothesis is that lung expansion triggers rapid resorption of lung fluid and establishes adequate functional residual capacity.

All of the signs of respiratory distress may be present with transient tachypnea, although tachypnea is the predominant finding. Chest radiographs characteristically show perihilar streaking (engorgement of perivascular lymphatics and interstitial vessels) with normal lung volume and heart size (Fig. 9-3). A diffuse hazy background due to alveolar and interstitial fluid collections, or lakes, is commonly found during the first hours after birth with transient tachypnea. Patchy infiltrates and pleural effusions are occasionally present with transient tachypnea and make differentiation from congenital pneumonia, sepsis, and meconium aspiration syndrome difficult. Historical clues help to establish the diagnosis. Without meconium-stained amniotic fluid, meconium aspiration can be excluded. More difficult to exclude is the possibility of mild persistent pulmonary hypertension, congenital pneumonia, and early onset sepsis. A retrospective diagnosis of transient tachypnea may be determined if the clinical symptoms and radiographic findings resolve and blood cultures are negative at 48 hours of age. Supportive care with oxygen, antibiotics, and occasionally continuous positive airway pressure or mechanical ventilation is often initiated while awaiting the evolution or resolution of clinical symptoms and laboratory investigations.

The time course of transient tachypnea is variable, lasting minutes to several days. Severity is also variable although most neonates require only supplemental oxygen and close cardiopulmonary monitoring. Antibiotics are often initiated until infection is excluded. The course of neonates with more severe disease may be complicated by persistent pulmonary hypertension and pneumothorax. Although neonates with severe transient tachypnea may have large pleural effusions and numerous infiltrates, the respiratory distress and radiographic findings resolve remarkably quickly, often within 24 to 48 hours. If infiltrates persist after 48 hours of age, many clinicians will consider congenital pneumonia a more likely diagnosis and continue antibiotics for up to 7 days. If respiratory distress is associated with hypotonia complicating maternal narcotics, hypermagnesemia, perinatal asphyxia, or neuromuscular syndrome, these underlying problems will need to be evaluated and a treatment plan developed.

The outcome of transient tachypnea of the newborn without complication or predisposing conditions is very optimistic. Survival is expected and long-term morbidities are infrequent. Complications or underlying illnesses increase the risk for mortality and long-term neurologic and developmental sequelae.

C. **Pneumothorax and other air leak syndromes.** Pneumothorax is the most frequently encountered air leak syndrome in neonates with an incidence of 0.5% to 2% of babies, although symptomatic pneumothorax is found in only 0.05% to 0.07% of live births. Pneumothorax is the presence of air in the pleural space between the lung and chest wall. Like other air leak syndromes, high intraalveolar pressure may cause rupture of air into the perivascular sheath surrounding intraalveolar capillaries. This air dissects into the lymphatic tree but does not usually collect in peribronchial spaces. Air then dissects along the perivascular sheath toward the hilum of the lung where blebs collect at the reflection of the visceral pleura onto the parietal pleura. Air may also dissect to form blebs in the subpleural surface of the lung.

These blebs of air may be reabsorbed or dissect into the pleural space to cause pneumothorax (Figs. 9-6 and 9-8). If the blebs of air at the hilum are large or if they drain into the mediastinum, pneumomediastinum results (Fig. 9-9). When perivascular and lymphatic air accumulates within the interstitium of the lung, pulmonary interstitial emphysema results. This is most common in premature infants with fragile pulmonary tissues receiving mechanical ventilation (Fig. 9-8). Air may dissect into the peritoneal space (pneumoperitoneum) along the pulmonary ligament and the intravascular space (air emboli); both of these problems only occur with severe air leak conditions.

Pneumothorax and pneumomediastinum may occur spontaneously during the initial breaths following birth. Tachypnea, retractions, grunting, see-saw respirations, and/or cyanosis may occur. Many infants are asymptomatic and pneumothorax is discovered as an incidental finding on chest radiographs that were obtained for other reasons. Some clinicians suggest evaluation of the genitourinary system when spontaneous pneumothorax is present because of case series reporting an association between these entities. Pneumothorax may also occur as a complication of aspiration syndromes, positive pressure ventilation, or continuous positive airway pressure when susceptible lung segments become hyperinflated and air ruptures into the perivascular space of pulmonary arterioles.

The time course for resolution of pneumothoraces and other air leaks is variable. With many air leaks, spontaneous resolution occurs without intervention. Some air leaks, especially those under tension, may compromise pulmonary and cardiac function. In these situations, immediate diagnosis based on absent or reduced breath sounds, coarse crackles, positive transillumination, and, if time permits, radiographic evidence is imperative and immediate intervention may be lifesaving. Emergent thoracentesis and/or thoracostomy tube placement and conventional mechanical or high frequency ventilation may be helpful to resolve the air leak and stabilize the neonate.

Term and near-term neonates with respiratory signs and symptoms of distress due to air leaks without cardiovascular compromise are managed expectantly or treated with a nitrogen washout maneuver. Nitrogen washout is accomplished by administering 100% oxygen, usually by oxyhood, for 6 to 24 hours. The concentrated oxygen within the lung sets up a gradient for nitrogen to move from the pneumothorax into the airways and from there it is exhaled. No controlled trials of the nitrogen washout technique have been performed. If a neonate is receiving positive pressure ventilation, resolution of pneumothorax or pulmonary interstitial emphysema may require thoracostomy tube placement or high frequency ventilation.

Pneumomediastinum may be difficult to differentiate from medial pneumothorax on chest radiographs. Layering of air superiorly in cross table lateral radiographs and positive transillumination of the hemithorax is most consistent with medial pneumothorax. With large pneumomediastinum, peripheral lung fields appear hazy due to atelectasis, whereas with pneumothorax, peripheral lung fields appear dark without lung markings. If air dissects into the neck or elevates the thymus (the sail sign), pneumomediastinum is present.

Pneumothorax and pulmonary interstitial emphysema are risk factors for the subsequent development of chronic lung disease, especially in extremely premature infants. Pneumomediastinum may resolve spontaneously and is often asymptomatic. Pneumoperitoneum caused by dissection of air through the pulmonary ligaments of the diaphragm and intravascular air generally accompany other severe air leak phenomena and are, therefore, additional indicators of severe air leak syndrome.

D. **Meconium aspiration and other aspiration syndromes.** Meconium aspiration is the most frequently identified aspiration syndrome in neonates. Meconium-stained amniotic fluid is present in 10% to 20% of pregnancies and is often a normal maturational occurrence during late fetal life. However, passage of meconium *in utero* may be a response to hypoxic or ischemic stresses. When this occurs, fetal distress may cause fetal gasping respirations and *in utero* aspiration. Postnatal aspiration of meconium also occurs in neonates who have labored respirations, apnea, bradycardia, or hypotonia (i.e., perinatal depression). However, postnatal meconium aspiration in vigorous, healthy neonates is unusual and likely due to the normal protective reflexes of the upper airway. Aspiration of blood, amniotic fluid, and vaginal fluid also may present as respiratory distress, although these are infrequently identified as causes for neonatal respiratory illness.

All of the signs of respiratory distress occur with the aspiration syndromes. Meconium, amniotic fluid, and blood aspiration most often present immediately after delivery. Chest radiographs are variable. Classic findings of the aspiration syndromes include diffuse patchy infiltrates, hyperexpansion, and barrel chest (Fig. 9-5). Bacterial and fungal pneumonia present clinically and radiographically the same; therefore, antibiotic administration and evaluation for infection is indicated. Chest radiographs may also show perihilar streakiness similar to transient tachypnea. When secondary surfactant inactivation develops, low lung volume, reticulogranular lung fields, and air bronchograms may be seen.

The presence of respiratory distress and meconium-stained amniotic fluid are prerequisite for making a diagnosis of meconium aspiration syndrome. This syndrome occurs in about 1% of pregnancies in which meconium-stained amniotic fluid is present. The classic clinical and radiographic syndrome results from thick tenacious meconium particles causing physical obstruction of large airways. During exhalation, airways normally narrow. If meconium is aspirated into the large airways, particles of meconium may be lodged in the airways as they narrow during exhalation. This results in gas being trapped distal to the obstruction and possible air leak due to elevated airway and alveolar saccular pressure and volume.

Meconium also causes inflammation that may progress during the first days of life, thereby causing obstruction of small airways; destruction of alveolar saccules and interstitium; proteinaceous exudates; and interstitial edema. For the next hours and days, progression in illness severity may occur. Surfactant inactivation by meconium and intraalveolar proteinaceous debris further compromises pulmonary function. Pulmonary hypertension may additionally complicate hypoxic respiratory failure associated with severe meconium aspiration, owing to ventilation–perfusion mismatch, hypoxic pulmonary constriction, generation of pulmonary vasoconstrictor mediators, and platelet aggregation within pulmonary capillaries.

Treatment of meconium aspiration begins with prevention. Obstetric interventions include amnioinfusion in selected pregnancies complicated by meconium-stained amniotic fluid, delivery before 41 weeks gestation, and suctioning of the oropharynx following delivery of the head but before delivery of the torso. Postnatal intubation and suctioning of the trachea in neonates who are hypotonic, apneic, bradycardic, or gasping is recommended to prevent postnatal aspiration. General supportive care including oxygen, mechanical ventilation, and fluid maintenance is indicated. Exogenous surfactant, inhaled nitric oxide, and extracorporeal membrane oxygenation may be required in the most severe cases. Survival is expected in more than 90% of cases.

E. **Persistent pulmonary hypertension of the newborn.** Persistent pulmonary hypertension of the newborn most often complicates the course of hypoxic respiratory failure in neonates suffering from pneumonia, sepsis, aspiration syndromes, congenital diaphragmatic hernia, respiratory distress syndrome, air leaks, and transient tachypnea. Other risk factors for persistent pulmonary hypertension include maternal aspirin, maternal indomethacin, or other prostaglandin inhibitors, polycythemia, hypothermia, and hypoglycemia. It may also present as a primary condition. Approximately 0.2% of live births are complicated by persistent pulmonary hypertension of the newborn.

Fetal oxygenation and ventilation are managed by the placenta and maternal circulations. Therefore, the volume of blood flow through fetal lungs is normally low (approximately 10%) during pregnancy. Active pulmonary vasoconstriction *in utero* causes elevation in pulmonary vascular resistance and diversion of umbilical venous blood (Po_2 approximately 30 torr) across the ductus venosus and foramen ovale to supply the fetal brain with relatively well oxygenated blood. Venous blood returning to the fetal heart is directed across the patent ductus arteriosus into the descending aorta for return back to the low resistance placental vascular bed. At birth, lung inflation; improved oxygenation, ventilation, and acid-base balance; and release of endogenous vasodilators (e.g., nitric oxide, prostacyclin, histamine, etc.) cause pulmonary vascular resistance to fall. This initiates a cascade of events that increases pulmonary blood flow that includes closure of the ductus venosus, foramen ovale, and ductus arteriosus and separation of the systemic and pulmonary circulations.

Excessive pulmonary blood flow through the fetal lung causes increased muscularization of the peripheral and alveolar pulmonary vasculature. These hypermuscular arterioles are vasoreactive and increase pulmonary vascular resistance because of small intraluminal diameters resulting from vasoconstriction. Fetal conditions that increase pulmonary blood flow include maternal aspirin or ibuprofen (fetal ductus arteriosus closure), systemic hypertension due to fetal hypoxic-ischemic stress, pulmonary hypoplasia, and congenital heart lesions that preferentially perfuse the pulmonary circulation. Increased pulmonary blood flow induces this muscularization of intraacinar vessels. Although pulmonary arteriole and capillary muscularization may occur in preterm infants, it is presumed that this remodeling takes a number of days to weeks to occur. Therefore, term and near-term neonates who are stressed, often undetectably, *in utero* are at highest risk for severe pulmonary hypertensive crises. In contrast, many preterm infants are born before *in utero* stressors have induced medial smooth muscular remodeling.

Pulmonary vasoconstriction in the postnatal neonate causes venous blood with low oxygen saturation to shunt from the venous, or right sided, circulation across a patent foramen ovale, patent ductus arteriosus, and/or diseased lung parenchyma into the systemic, or left-sided, circulation (right-to-left shunting). If this right-to-left shunt carries a high volume of venous blood into the systemic circulation, systemic hypoxemia occurs. Pulmonary vasoconstriction may be induced by hypoxia, acidosis, insufficient lung volume, vasoconstrictive mediators (e.g., endothelin and thromboxane), pneumonia, intraalveolar protein and debris, cold stress, polycythemia, and hypoglycemia. When cardiorespiratory or metabolic dysfunction precipitates pulmonary hypertension, cyanosis and tachypnea occur. If severe pulmonary hypertension and hypoxemia occur, grunting respirations, retractions, and see-saw respirations appear.

Neonates with pulmonary vasoconstriction without pulmonary vascular muscularization (maldevelopment) may have hypoxemia that recovers spontaneously or with limited interventions, such as supplemental oxygen and/or fluid resuscitation. This transient pulmonary hypertension accounts for arterial oxygen saturations during the first hours after birth in the 85% to 95% range. With the anticipated decline in pulmonary vascular resistance during this time, arterial oxygen saturation normally increases to greater than 95%. This transient pulmonary hypertension presents with cyanosis and tachypnea similar to those infants with transient tachypnea. If the chest radiograph is clear and no evidence of ductal shunting is present, an echocardiogram is necessary to differentiate these diagnoses.

Severe cyanosis and hypoxemia are presenting signs for severe persistent pulmonary hypertension of the newborn, cyanotic congenital heart disease, and severe hypoxemic respiratory failure from many causes. Patients with cyanotic congenital heart disease often present with cyanosis and unlabored tachypnea, whereas those with persistent pulmonary hypertension and severe hypoxemic respiratory failure present with cyanosis, tachypnea, and labored respiratory efforts (retractions, grunting, see-saw respirations).

Hypoxemic respiratory failure and persistent pulmonary hypertension often respond to a trial of 100% inspired oxygen or hyperventilation with an increase in oxygen saturation, whereas cyanotic congenital heart disease does not respond to these maneuvers. If right-to-left shunting occurs at the level of a patent ductus arteriosus, differential oxygen saturation will occur between the preductal and postductal circulation, and this can be demonstrated by the presence of transcutaneous oxygen saturation on the right hand (preductal) being greater than that on a foot (postductal). This difference in pre- and postductal oxygen saturations can be noninvasively monitored during therapy using transcutaneous probes to continuously assess the presence of ductal level shunting. If ductal level shunting is not present (i.e., right-to-left shunting is through a patent foramen ovale or across diseased lung parenchyma) or if cyanotic heart disease is present, diffuse cyanosis and absence of a difference between preductal and postductal oxygen saturations will be present. Unfortunately, chest radiographs may not definitively differentiate between these causes for cyanosis and an echocardiogram may be required to establish the diagnosis.

It is important to establish a diagnosis in the cyanotic neonate because therapy differs among those with severe persistent pulmonary hypertension, cyanotic congenital heart disease, and severe hypoxemic respiratory failure. Severe persistent pulmonary hypertension is treated with potentially high oxygen concentrations, mechanical ventilation including high frequency devices, surfactant, volume expansion, vasopressor agents, inhaled nitric oxide, and extracorporeal membrane oxygenation. Infants with severe hypoxemic respiratory failure may receive similar treatments. However, cyanotic congenital heart disease is usually treated with lower oxygen concentrations, prostaglandins, vasopressors, judicious volume expansion, and mechanical ventilation if apnea, congestive heart failure, or severe acidosis develop. Operative intervention may be necessary. Oxygen saturation greater than 70% is generally acceptable in the cyanotic heart patient in contrast to a goal of greater than 90% in those with persistent pulmonary hypertension or hypoxemic respiratory failure.

Survival for neonates with transient persistent pulmonary hypertension is greater than 95%. Neurologic and developmental morbidities are infrequent. However, survival for severe persistent pulmonary hypertension requiring extracorporeal membrane oxygenation is about 80%. Additionally, these infants are at risk for complications such as air leaks, intracranial hemorrhage, infection, disseminated intravascular coagulation, hypoxic–ischemic encephalopathy, multisystem organ dysfunction, metabolic imbalances, and electrolyte abnormalities. Severe disabilities including hearing loss, seizures, developmental delay, and cerebral palsy may occur in 10% of these neonates, while lesser disabilities can be seen in as many as 40%.

F. Congenital pneumonia. Pneumonia during the first days of life may be acquired *in utero*, during delivery, or postnatally. Aspiration of infected amniotic fluid or vaginal secretions is the most frequent route for infection, although transplacental and postnatal nosocomial acquisition does occur. Infants who experience aspiration of bacteria, viruses, fungi, spirochetes, and protozoa may be asymptomatic for hours after birth. However, during the following hours and days, respiratory distress occurs with severity dependent on the amount of intrapulmonary exudate, airway and pulmonary inflammation, and alveolar necrosis that develops.

Most organisms that infect humans can affect the fetus and newborn. Several bacteria are especially prevalent during the perinatal period including group B streptococcus and *E. coli*. The clinical signs of respiratory distress owing to pneumonia are similar to many of the illnesses that present during the neonatal period; therefore, symptoms alone are inadequate to establish a diagnosis of pneumonia. Additional information such as history, physical findings, age at onset, laboratory evaluation, radiographic evidence, and clinical course are necessary to make a definitive diagnosis. Because of similar presentation and potential for rapid progression and deterioration with pneumonia, most neonates with respiratory distress will be treated with antibiotics until a diagnosis is established.

Clues for pneumonia or sepsis as the cause for respiratory distress in the neonate include a history of maternal infection, maternal colonization with group B streptococcus, prolonged rupture of membranes (>18 hours), temperature instability, elevated white blood cell count with more immature white blood cells in the differential, positive cultures of blood or tracheal aspirate, and infiltrates or effusions on chest radiographs. Pneumonia may appear on chest radiographs as diffuse haziness (similar to respiratory distress syndrome and pulmonary edema), perihilar streakiness (similar to transient tachypnea), patchy infiltrates (similar to meconium aspiration), or as focal infiltrates (similar to atelectasis, Fig. 9-2). Pleural effusions can be seen as well and suggest group B streptococcus as an etiologic agent.

The course of pneumonia varies with the organism and host response. The neonate may be asymptomatic, tachypneic, apneic, hypothermic, hypotensive, or severely compromised with multisystem organ dysfunction. Supportive care, antibiotics, supplemental oxygen, and mechanical ventilation provide the bulk of support usually required in the sicker neonate. For more severe disease, high frequency ventilation, vasopressors, inhaled nitric oxide, and extracorporeal membrane oxygenation may be needed. Prophylactic intrapartum antibiotics have been successful in reducing the number of neonatal infections caused by group B streptococci.

Most neonates with congenital pneumonia survive. Those who succumb usually have underlying pathophysiology that predisposes to infection. Examples include extreme prematurity, maternal infectious illness or colonization, and congenital anomalies, especially of the heart, nervous, gastrointestinal, and genitourinary systems.

IV. Clinical pearls and pitfalls.
- Respiratory distress is a common problem during the neonatal period.
- The most common causes for respiratory distress in neonates are respiratory distress syndrome, transient tachypnea, pneumothorax, pneumonia/sepsis, meconium aspiration syndrome, and persistent pulmonary hypertension of the newborn.
- Historical details about the pregnancy, labor, delivery, and family provide important clues to alert the neonate's caregivers about potential medical or surgical illnesses that may require resuscitation and intervention at birth.
- The signs and symptoms of respiratory distress in neonates reflect physiologic compensations to improve oxygenation, ventilation, and acid-base balance.
- Key physical findings and historical clues guide clinical assessment, establishment of differential diagnoses, and preparations for resuscitation and stabilization of the sick neonate.

- Radiographic findings in neonates with respiratory distress are often nonspecific and should be interpreted along with clinical and laboratory information to best determine specific diagnoses.

BIBLIOGRAPHY

Donnelly LF. Chapter 3: Chest. *Fundamentals of pediatric radiology*. Philadelphia, PA: WB Saunders, 2001.
Fanaroff AA, Martin RJ. *Neonatal-perinatal medicine*, 7th ed. St. Louis: Mosby, 2002.
Hansen TH, Cooper TR, Weisman LE. *Neonatal respiratory disease*, 2nd ed. Newtown, PA: Handbooks in Health Care Company, 1998.
Kuhn JP, Slovis TL, Haller JO. Chapter 3: Neonatal lung and thorax. *Caffey's pediatric diagnostic imaging*, 10th ed., Vol. 1. St. Louis: Mosby, 2004.

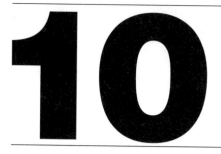

Surgically Correctable Causes of Respiratory Distress

Alan P. Ladd and
Jay L. Grosfeld

I. **Description of the issue.** The newborn infant with respiratory distress represents a challenge to the family practitioner, pediatrician, neonatologist, and pediatric surgeon alike. While the majority of causes of neonatal respiratory distress are nonsurgical in nature (e.g., hyaline membrane disease, meconium aspiration, sepsis, etc.), a much smaller percentage are related to disorders amenable to surgical intervention.

The signs and symptoms of surgical respiratory distress do not differ significantly from those of a medical etiology. Cyanosis and pallor, tachypnea, and poor feeding are classic signs of respiratory insufficiency and should alert the clinician. Stridor and chest wall retractions are suggestive of upper respiratory obstruction in the pharyngeal or subglottic regions. Respiratory arrest is unusual without at least a brief period of distress but does occur in babies who become exhausted from the increased work of breathing associated with obstructive or parenchymal lesions. An appearance unique to diaphragmatic hernias is a "barrel" chest with scaphoid abdomen resulting from translocation of the intraabdominal viscera into the chest.

Prompt physical examination of the infant in respiratory distress is mandatory and often unenlightening. Breath sounds are freely transmitted throughout the thorax in the neonate. Mediastinal shift may produce confusing breath sounds bilaterally, and dullness to percussion is difficult to judge in the infant chest. The most important diagnostic test in an infant with respiratory distress remains the chest radiograph. Prompt decisions on therapy can usually be made on the basis of the initial chest x-ray. The evolution of changes in serial chest radiographs can be helpful in making a definitive diagnosis.

II. **Pneumothorax.** Pneumothorax is a common cause of respiratory distress in newborn infants. It has been estimated that spontaneous pneumothorax occurs in 0.5% to 2% of all newborn infants and this disorder occurs even more frequently in infants with hyaline membrane disease, aspiration pneumonia, or after resuscitation. The use of positive-pressure ventilators and continuous positive airway pressure (CPAP) may further increase the incidence (Table 10-1). An association between spontaneous pneumothorax and renal malformations has been made. In infants with spontaneous pneumothoraces, an evaluation of renal structure and function may be indicated and accomplished by measuring urine output and serum creatinine and by obtaining a renal ultrasound.

The pathophysiology of pneumothorax (Table 10-2), pneumomediastinum, and pneumopericardium begins with hyperinflation of alveoli. In spontaneous pneumothoraces, this alveolar hyperinflation may result from the high intrathoracic pressures generated during the first extrauterine breaths. At the time of birth, a combination of factors, including uneven ventilation, poor lung compliance, high viscosity of lung fluid, and high surface tension, may result in intraalveolar pressures over 40 cm H_2O with the first gasp by the infant. This can result in alveolar rupture, allowing air to escape under a pressure gradient into the interstitium and advance along the perivascular spaces in the lung. The air continues to dissect along the perivascular spaces toward the hilum and may rupture into the mediastinum, producing a pneumomediastinum; through the visceral pleura, resulting in a pneumothorax (Fig. 10-1); into the pericardial space, resulting in a pneumopericardium (Fig. 10-2); or into the peritoneal cavity, causing a pneumoperitoneum.

A. **Diagnosis.** The symptoms of a pneumothorax in the newborn include tachypnea, retractions, cyanosis, grunting, and tachycardia or bradycardia (Table 10-3). Breath sounds may be decreased on the ipsilateral side, although the absence of this sign does not rule out a pneumothorax. The heart sounds may be shifted to the contralateral side, and there may be enlargement of the hemithorax. Elevated intrathoracic pressure from an expanding pneumothorax may cause mediastinal shift and reduce venous return to the heart. Subsequent impairment of cardiac output

Table 10-1. Predisposing factors to a pneumothorax

Resuscitation
Aspiration (blood, mucus, meconium)
Continuous positive airway pressure (CPAP)
Ventilator therapy
Endotracheal tube down right mainstem bronchus
Hyaline membrane disease
Pneumonia
Congenital lobar emphysema
Hypoplastic lungs (e.g., Potter syndrome, diaphragmatic hernia)

Table 10-2. Pneumothorax pathophysiology

Increased intraalveolar pressure
↓
Alveolar rupture
↓
Interstitial air
↓
Dissection of air along perivascular spaces toward root of lung
↓
Rupture into pleural space, mediastinum, pericardial space

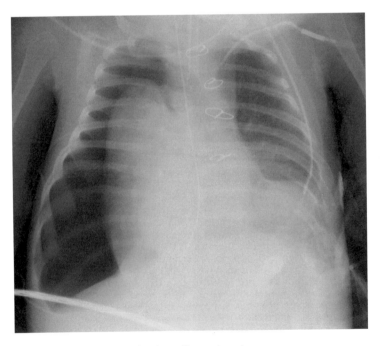

Figure 10-1. Pneumothorax as a result of ventilatory barotrauma.

may result in hypotension and metabolic acidosis. Arterial blood gases may show hypoxia and hypercapnia.

It is impossible to rule out a pneumothorax by clinical examination; therefore, a chest radiograph is mandatory in any infant with respiratory distress. Transillumination of the chest with a high-intensity fiberoptic light provides an additional means of prompt diagnosis of a pneumothorax. Appropriate application and interpretation of this technique requires extensive experience, as subcutaneous edema,

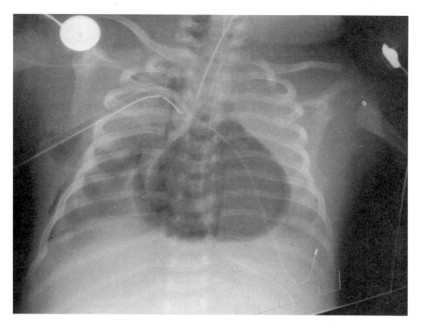

Figure 10-2. Pneumopericardium secondary to pulmonary barotrauma.

Table 10-3. Signs of a pneumothorax

Tachypnea
Retractions
Grunting
Cyanosis
Tachycardia, bradycardia
Decreased Pa_{O_2}
Increased Pa_{CO_2}
Hypotension
Metabolic acidosis
Decreased breath sounds
Shift of heart sounds
Chest bulge
Fighting the ventilator
Increased ventilator support

pneumomediastinum, lobar emphysema, or pulmonary interstitial emphysema may easily be confused with a pneumothorax. Transillumination should be used in conjunction with radiographs and not as a replacement for them. Intervention based on transillumination alone should only be done when the infant's deteriorating condition precludes waiting for the chest radiograph.

When the infant is in the supine position the pneumothorax may accumulate anteriorly. In these situations, it may be difficult to diagnose the pneumothorax by an anterior-posterior chest radiograph since lung markings may still be visible extending to the lateral chest wall. Increased lucency of one hemithorax should suggest the possibility of an anterior pneumothorax (Fig. 10-3A). A lateral decubitus or cross-table lateral film can confirm the diagnosis with the hyperlucent hemithorax in the superior position (Fig. 10-3B).

Air in the subpulmonic space or over the apex of the lung may be the earliest sign of a pneumothorax. An often confusing radiographic finding is the medial stripe sign, which may be associated with a pneumothorax or pneumomediastinum. Skin folds and the border of the scapula may mistakenly suggest a pneumothorax. The best method of confirming a pneumothorax is to obtain a lateral decubitus film.

B. Treatment. There are several treatment modalities for a pneumothorax. In the term infant with mild respiratory distress, 100% inspired oxygen may be provided for a few hours; the pneumothorax may resolve by nitrogen washout. A follow-up chest radiograph can be obtained to monitor the response of this treatment. This treatment should not be used in premature infants or infants requiring mechanical ventilatory assistance, or as the sole means of therapy for infants in moderate to severe distress.

In an infant who is critically ill and a pneumothorax is suspected clinically, diagnostic and therapeutic thoracentesis should be performed immediately. A size 20- or 22-gauge angiocatheter may be used to aspirate the pneumothorax in such emergencies. The angiocatheter and stylet are attached to a syringe and passed into the third or fourth interspace. Because the intercostal blood supply runs along the inferior margin of the rib, the needle is passed along the superior aspect of the rib to avoid hemorrhage from this vascular area. While the needle is advanced into the chest, negative pressure is applied to the plunger of the syringe. With aspiration of air, the catheter may be advanced into the chest and the stylet removed. The catheter can then be directly aspirated by a syringe and stopcock to relieve the pressure of the pneumothorax. A 23-gauge scalp vein needle may be used similarly to aspirate the pneumothorax in such emergencies (Fig. 10-4). This technique may be used to relieve a pneumothorax until support personnel arrive. If an error in diagnosis is made and there is, in fact, no pneumothorax present, this technique rarely induces one.

The angiocatheter may be used as a temporary chest tube. After removal of the needle, the catheter may be connected to a stopcock and syringe for aspiration of the pneumothorax or may be connected to intravenous tubing, which in turn is connected to an underwater drainage system. This procedure may serve as a temporizing measure to relieve a pneumothorax until a thoracostomy tube can be placed.

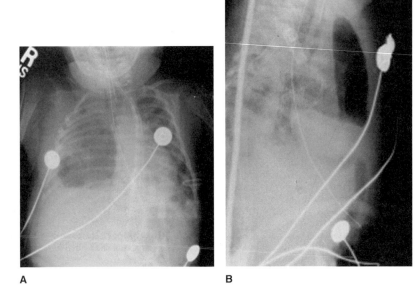

A   **B**

Figure 10-3. (A) Hyperlucency overlying right anterior hemithorax. **(B)** Occult anterior pneumothorax identified on cross-table lateral chest radiograph in patient from Figure 10-3A.

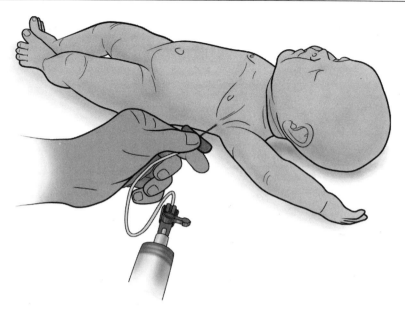

Figure 10-4. Needle aspiration technique for pneumothorax utilizing stopcock. (Courtesy of Office of Visual Media, Indiana University School of Medicine, 2004.)

1. **Chest tubes.** A size 8 French chest tube is usually used for a simple pneumothorax; however, a larger tube such as a size 10 or 12 French may be necessary if draining purulent material or blood. Additional equipment includes sterile instruments, an infant-sized underwater seal drainage system, a sterile connector, suture with a curved needle, suction tubing, tape, chest tube clamp, and surgical light.

   Sterile technique is necessary. The person performing the procedure and an assistant wear a sterile gown, cap, mask, and gloves. Adequate lighting is essential. The infant's heart rate must be monitored. Maintenance of oxygenation, ventilation, and warmth is essential.

   The infant's extremities are restrained with the arms positioned away from the chest (Fig. 10-5). The anterior chest wall on the side in which the tube is to be inserted should be carefully prepared as for any surgical procedure.

   After infiltration with a local anesthetic, an incision of approximately 0.3 to 0.4 cm is made lateral to the nipple in the anterior axillary line. Extreme care should be taken not to traumatize the areola or surrounding breast tissue.

   The tip of the tube (size 8 to 12 French) should be grasped with a small curved hemostat. The hemostat is then placed through the incision, point down, perpendicular to the plane of the chest, and advanced with a rotary "screwing"-type motion into the pleural cavity through the interspace superior to the level at which skin incision was made (Fig. 10-6). A fair amount of force is required to accomplish this, even in small premature babies.

   Once the pleural cavity is entered, the hemostat is rotated so that the tip is pointing in the direction desired for tube placement. The tube is then advanced into the chest for a length of about 5 cm, with the clinician being certain that all holes of the tube are within the thoracic cavity. After the hemostat is removed, a purse-string suture is tightened and tied. This prevents leakage of air around the incision. The ends of the suture are tied around the chest tube itself to prevent slippage (Fig. 10-7). An antibiotic ointment is applied to the incision area, and the tube is carefully secured with tape.

   The tube is then connected to the underwater drainage system, and the water level is observed for fluctuation with respiration. If this is absent, the chest tube is probably obstructed or improperly placed. A common error is placement of the tube in the subcutaneous tissue rather than in the intrapleural space.

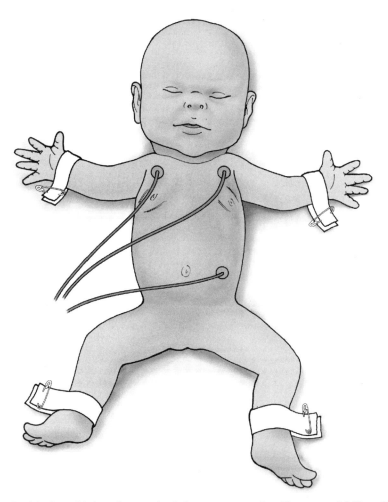

Figure 10-5. Positioning of infant for standard thoracostomy tube. (Courtesy of Office of Visual Media, Indiana University School of Medicine, 2004.)

A chest radiograph is obtained to determine placement and the effectiveness of lung reinflation. In addition, a cross-table lateral chest x-ray can be performed to determine whether the tube is placed anteriorly or posteriorly.

If the infant is on a ventilator or if the pneumothorax persists and proper placement is assured, the chest tube is connected to a continuous suction of 10 to 12 cm H_2O. If negative pressure is applied to the chest tube and continuous bubbling results, one of two problems may be present: (1) there may be a large rent in the visceral pleura (i.e. the pneumothorax is so large that the chest tube continuously drains air); or (2) more likely, there is a leak in the system (e.g. one hole of the chest tube may be outside of the chest), or there may be a loose connection within the chest tube system (Fig. 10-8).

2. **Complications of chest tubes.** One of the most serious complications of chest tube placement is perforation of the lung. The diagnosis of a perforated lung should be suspected when a pneumothorax does not resolve over a prolonged time despite apparent proper placement of the chest tube. These infants usually show continuous bubbling in the drainage system. When placement of a chest tube results in this complication, surgical closure of the lung injury may be indicated.

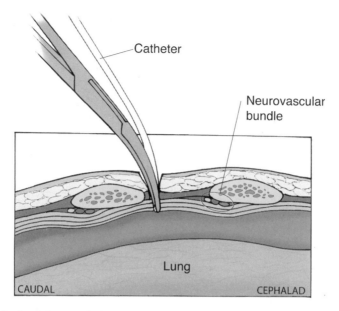

Figure 10-6. Path of chest wall dissection for thoracostomy tube. (Courtesy of Office of Visual Media, Indiana University School of Medicine, 2004.)

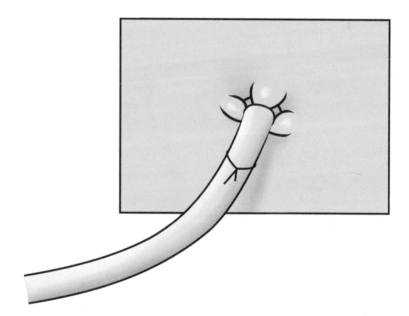

Figure 10-7. Securing of thoracostomy tube with purse-string closure.

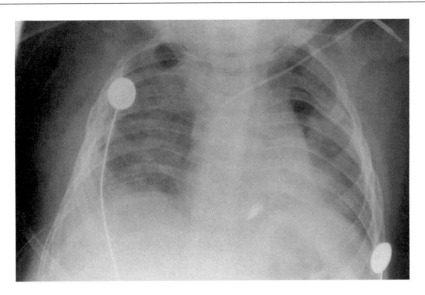

Figure 10-8. Malpositioned chest tube with extrathoracic side port.

3. **Care and maintenance of chest tubes.** Generally, a chest tube placed for a pneumothorax drains very little fluid, whereas a chest tube placed postoperatively has more drainage. The presence of fluctuation or bubbling in the drainage system should be monitored and recorded. Pleur-evac or other drainage systems are frequently used in the newborn intensive care unit. These devices control the amount of actual suction through either a column of water set to a desired height or through suction control settings on the device itself. The "water seal chamber" in each type of system is connected toward the baby. Bubbling in this area reflects drainage of air from the chest. Fluctuation of water in the water seal chamber signifies a patent chest tube within the intrapleural space.

A chest tube placed for treatment of a pneumothorax should not be clamped if the chest tube is still draining air from the intrapleural space. Clamping the chest tube results in reaccumulation of air within the intrapleural space and typical symptoms and signs of a pneumothorax.

4. **Chest tube removal.** The chest tube is usually left to suction until bubbling has not been observed for 24 hours. The tube is then placed to water seal only, the baby's clinical condition is closely monitored, and a chest radiograph is obtained to identify a possible reaccumulation of air. If a pneumothorax reaccumulates, the tube is returned to suction for at least another 24 hours. If the lung remains inflated with no identifiable air bubbling, the tube may be removed after 12 to 24 hours. The tube is withdrawn rapidly and aseptically. Pressure should be applied to the incision with gauze coated with an appropriate antibiotic ointment or petroleum jelly to prevent entrance of air through the chest tube incision. The gauze should then be taped in place. A chest radiograph should be obtained after withdrawal of the tube to check for recurrence of a pneumothorax.

III. **Diaphragmatic hernia.** Congenital diaphragmatic hernia occurs as a result of a defect in the developing diaphragm, known as the foramen of Bochdalek. The incidence is approximately 1 in 2000 to 1 in 5000 births. It occurs on the left side in 85% of cases, on the right in 13%, and bilaterally in 1% to 2%. Occurrence in female infants predominates by a 2:1 ratio. Diaphragmatic hernia within a fetus may be suspected in pregnant women with polyhydramnios and an intrathoracic mass on fetal ultrasonography. Herniation through the diaphragm may be identified on prenatal ultrasound as early as 12 weeks gestation but may not become evident until the third trimester.

A. **Diagnosis.** The infant with a diaphragmatic hernia who has not been diagnosed prenatally will present with respiratory distress most commonly at birth or occasionally up to several days afterward. The initial signs and symptoms include

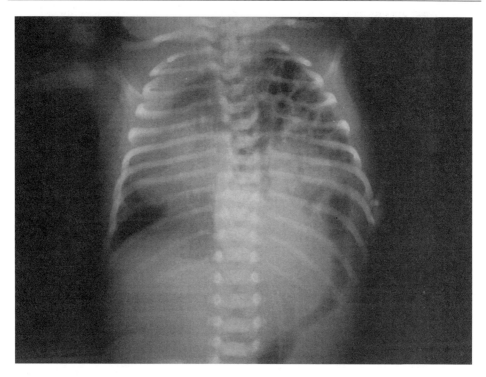

Figure 10-9. Congenital diaphragmatic hernia.

cyanosis, labored respirations, and retractions. Heart sounds may be displaced and breath sounds may be decreased on the involved side. A chest radiograph is usually diagnostic. On occasion this may show only an opacity until the intrathoracic loops of bowel become air filled (Fig. 10-9).

B. **Treatment.** Rapid initiation of therapy is imperative. Immediate endotracheal intubation should be accomplished, followed by transport to a facility capable of providing the acute care necessary for these infants to survive. Bag-and-mask ventilation should be avoided because of the large amount of air that can be swallowed and introduced into the gastrointestinal tract with that technique. In addition, an orogastric tube should be placed to decompress the stomach and bowel within the chest to minimize additional pulmonary compression.

Current protocols for acute management of infants with congenital diaphragmatic hernia focus on the stabilization of the associated pulmonary hypertension that these infants inevitably exhibit. These infants no longer undergo immediate surgical repair. They are stabilized by correcting their acid-base imbalance, avoiding hypothermia, and optimizing oxygenation to minimize exacerbations of pulmonary hypertension. Extracorporeal membrane oxygenation (ECMO) may be utilized to aid in the oxygenation of these infants during periods of severe pulmonary hypertension, which results in right-to-left shunting through a patent ductus arteriosus and foramen ovale. Once stable from the respiratory standpoint, these infants may then undergo operative repair of the diaphragmatic defect.

Postoperatively, the prognosis depends on the degree of lung hypoplasia of both lungs. Large hernias, which occur early in intrauterine life, can cause incomplete development of the lung, leading to severe hypoxia and inadequate ventilation. The overall mortality for infants who present with severe respiratory distress within 24 hours of birth remains 40% to 50%, whereas the survival for those infants presenting later is more favorable (80% to 90%).

IV. **Eventration of the diaphragm.** Eventration of the diaphragm refers to a weakness or attenuation of the central portion of the diaphragm. The lesion can be congenital in origin from unknown causes or acquired as a result of birth trauma with phrenic nerve

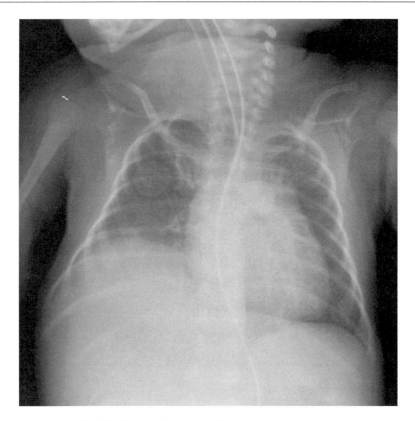

Figure 10-10. Right-sided diaphragmatic eventration.

injury. This latter form is commonly associated with Erb palsy (brachial plexus injury) and torticollis.

  A. **Diagnosis.** The affected diaphragm, usually on the left, is greatly elevated into the chest, causing loss of intrathoracic volume, paradoxical motion of the diaphragm, and respiratory embarrassment (Fig. 10-10). This paradoxical motion is diagnostic on airway fluoroscopy for diaphragmatic eventration.

  B. **Treatment.** In children who are initially asymptomatic in infancy, more than 50% will subsequently develop recurrent pulmonary infections. Therefore the more severe eventrations should undergo operative repair early in life despite being asymptomatic.

V. **Esophageal atresia and tracheoesophageal fistula.** These lesions represent one of the more common congenital anomalies encountered by pediatric surgeons, occurring in one in 3000 births. There are five anatomic variants recognized: esophageal atresia without fistula, esophageal atresia with a fistula from the proximal pouch to the trachea, esophageal atresia with distal fistula (the most common form, representing 86% of cases), esophageal atresia with fistulae from both proximal and distal pouches, and an "H"-type cervical fistula from an intact esophagus to the trachea (Fig. 10-11). Approximately one-third of infants with esophageal atresia and tracheoesophageal fistula will experience respiratory distress shortly after birth, both from aspiration of saliva that collects in the blind proximal pouch and from gastric reflux up the distal fistula into the lungs. Mild to severe pulmonary infiltrates can result, increasing the morbidity and overall mortality for these infants.

  A. **Diagnosis.** Diagnosis is suggested early after birth by excessive salivation and drooling. Oral feedings are met with gagging and coughing episodes or severe desaturation episodes from aspiration. Attempts to pass an orogastric tube will be met by obstruction (Fig. 10-12), making the injection of contrast materials such as barium usually

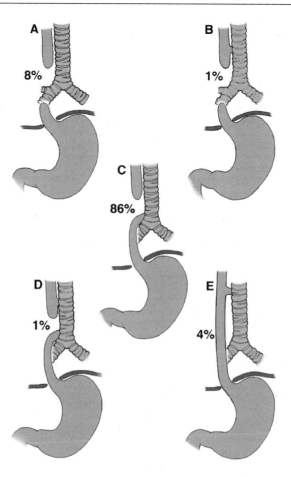

Figure 10-11. Type and frequency of esophageal atresia and/or tracheoesophageal fistulas. (Courtesy of Office of Visual Media, Indiana University School of Medicine, 2004.)

      unnecessary. Pulmonary infiltrates, atelectasis, or lobar collapse may already be present at the time of the first chest radiograph.

B. Treatment. Emergency care of these infants includes aspiration of the proximal esophageal pouch. A double-lumen suction tube (Replogle) on low continuous suction will clear saliva and other secretions. The infant should be positioned with an elevated head of bed, using gravity to prevent reflux of gastric contents into the trachea. An intravenous line and antibiotics are begun, and the infant is transported to a center equipped to handle these seriously ill neonates. Shortly after arrival, early primary repair is performed or a gastrostomy is placed under local anesthesia to keep the stomach empty.

      The overall management of these infants is challenging and exacting; thus, these procedures should be performed only at tertiary neonatal intensive care facilities with experienced pediatric surgeons and neonatologists. Associated cardiac, gastrointestinal, renal, and musculoskeletal anomalies are common in these patients and these associated anomalies often complicate care and must be screened for diligently.

VI. Chylothorax. Chylothorax refers to an abnormal accumulation of chyle or lymph within the pleural space. It is a relatively rare condition. Respiratory distress presents within the first week of life in the majority of cases but can be apparent immediately after

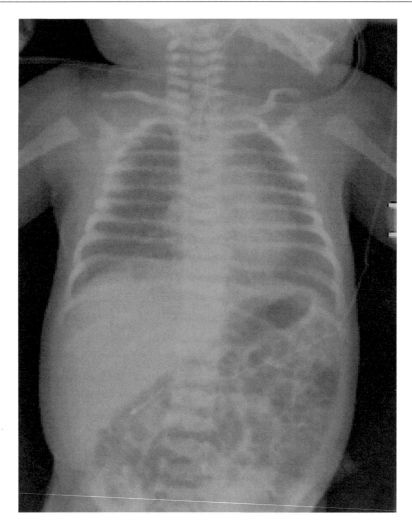

Figure 10-12. Failure of orogastric tube to pass in patient found to have type-C tracheoesophageal fistula.

birth. Absent breath sounds on the side of fluid accumulation is the obvious clinical finding; however, this is also present in several other conditions (pneumothorax, diaphragmatic hernia, etc.).

A. **Diagnosis.** Chest radiographs demonstrate an opacified hemithorax that will usually lead to thoracentesis, which may show clear fluid if the infant has not received fat-containing formula. Once long-chain fats are ingested, however, the fluid becomes milky in appearance. Respiratory distress is produced by atelectasis and compression by the space-occupying fluid. Mediastinal shift is unusual but possible.

B. **Treatment.** Immediate treatment consists of thoracentesis with needle and syringe, which is diagnostic as well as therapeutic. The infant is then placed on a diet free of long-chain triglycerides, with repeat thoracentesis performed as necessary. If a restricted diet is unsuccessful, a trial of strict parenteral nutrition should then be attempted. Tube thoracostomy is occasionally necessary until the flow of lymph slows to a level sufficient to allow a spontaneous seal of the lymphatic leak. Surgical repair is rarely necessary.

VII. **Cystic adenomatoid malformation.** Cystic adenomatoid malformations represent hamartomatous overgrowth of elements representing bronchioles and alveolar ducts (Fig. 10-13).

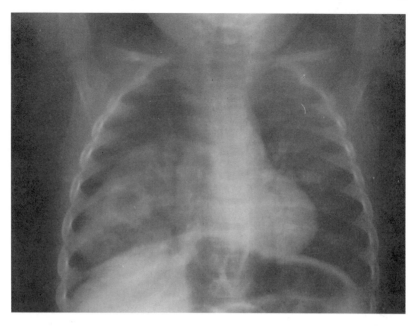

Figure 10-13. Congenital cystic adenomatoid malformation.

    A. Diagnosis. Cystic and adenomatous elements are present histologically, which gives rise to the typical radiographic appearance of a "Swiss cheese wedge" on chest radiograph. A single upper lobe is usually affected, and severe respiratory distress may be present, even at birth.

    B. Treatment. Because nonoperative therapy is generally morbid from recurrent pulmonary infections and possibly fatal, thoracotomy and lobectomy is the procedure of choice.

VIII. Congenital lobar emphysema. Lobar emphysema is marked by massive air trapping and stiff lung from over-distention of alveolar spaces, resulting in compression of the remaining lung and mediastinal shift (Fig. 10-14).

    A. Diagnosis. The majority of infants will present with respiratory distress. The left upper lobe is most frequently affected, followed by right middle and right upper lobes. Histologically, cartilaginous dysplasia is present in some specimens, whereas others show diffuse changes in small bronchi. In the majority of cases, however, the etiology is unknown.

    B. Treatment. Lobectomy is the treatment of choice and is curative in most instances. Occasionally, reoperation and pneumonectomy have been necessary, primarily for cystic degeneration and emphysema of the remaining lobe on the ipsilateral side.

IX. Choanal atresia. The nares form as a posterior deepening of the olfactory pits, eventually joining with the oral cavity. Failure of complete canalization results in a bony palate that obstructs one or both nares and can result in significant respiratory embarrassment, as the newborn is an obligate nose breather.

    A. Diagnosis. Diagnosis can be made rapidly by attempting to pass a nasogastric tube through both nares.

    B. Treatment. Should obstruction be found bilaterally, establishment of an oral airway is mandatory with surgical correction to follow.

X. Micrognathia. Micrognathia, as seen in the Pierre Robin sequence, is a common cause of respiratory distress.

    A. Diagnosis. The hypoplastic mandible, evident on physical examination, leads to a small oral cavity and allows the tongue to fall posteriorly, occluding the airway with resulting respiratory distress.

    B. Treatment. Various degrees of hypoplasia may be present, and, thus, therapy is dependent on the extent of respiratory distress present. Maintaining the infant in the prone position is useful. The more severe cases may require anterior traction on the

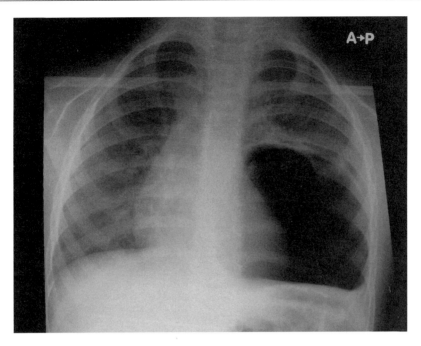

Figure 10-14. Left hemithoracic lucency from congenital lobar emphysema.

tongue with suture fixation, and tracheostomy may be required until more complicated mandibular reconstruction is undertaken.

XI.   **Laryngeal atresia/stenosis.** Laryngeal atresia is always fatal unless tracheostomy is performed shortly after birth. Fortunately, this anomaly is quite rare. Laryngeal stenosis or web is a more common anomaly and usually presents with stridor, sternal retraction, and labored breathing occurring shortly after birth.

    A. Diagnosis. Diagnosis is made by laryngotracheoscopy.

    B. Treatment. Depending on severity of symptoms, it may require tracheostomy. Repeated dilatations or resection with electrocautery, cryotherapy, or laser are the procedures available.

XII.   **Vascular ring.** The embryologic development of the great vessels (aorta, pulmonary arteries, subclavian, and carotid arteries) is rather complicated, and a variety of anomalies may result. The term vascular rings has been used when the vascular malformations surround the trachea and/or esophagus, thus producing partial obstruction. The common anatomical configurations include double aortic arch with ligamentum arteriosum, anomalous innominate artery, anomalous left carotid artery, aberrant right subclavian artery arising from the descending aorta, and aberrant left pulmonary artery (pulmonary sling).

    Symptoms range from mild to severe and may be episodic in nature. Stridorous or croup-like breathing, choking episodes while eating, and expiratory wheezing are commonly observed. Recurrent pneumonitis from aspiration is unusual but occasionally occurs. Chest radiographs frequently show bilateral hyperaeration as a result of air trapping.

    A. Diagnosis. Diagnosis is suggested by barium esophagram, which may show anterior or posterior indentation on the esophagus by the aberrant vessels. Tracheal compression or indentation by a pulsatile vessel is frequently seen at bronchoscopy. Definitive diagnosis is often made by echocardiography or occasionally by angiography.

    B. Treatment. Treatment is surgical.

XIII.   **Clinical pearls.**

    • A pneumothorax cannot be excluded by clinical examination; therefore, a chest radiograph is mandatory in any infant with respiratory distress.

- Acute management of infants with congenital diaphragmatic hernias focuses on the stabilization of the associated pulmonary hypertension prior to surgical repair.
- Cystic adenomatoid malformations represent hamartomatous overgrowth of elements representing bronchioles and alveolar ducts.
- Lobar emphysema is marked by massive air trapping and over-distention of alveolar spaces, resulting in compression of the remaining lung and mediastinal shift.

BIBLIOGRAPHY

Boloker J, Bateman DA, Wung JT, et al. Congenital diaphragmatic hernia in 120 infants treated consecutively with permissive hypercapnea/spontaneous respiration/elective repair. *J Pediatr Surg* 2002;37(3):357–366.

De Lorimier AA. Respiratory problems related to the airway and lung. In: O'Neill JA, Rowe MI, Grosfeld JL et al. eds. *Pediatric Surgery*, 5th ed. St. Louis, MO: Mosby–Year Book, 1995: 873–898.

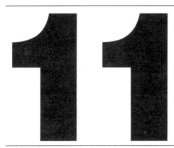

Oxygen: Use and Monitoring

Matthew E. Abrams and
Neal Simon

I. **Description of the issue.** Oxygen is an important and frequently used therapy in the care of ill newborns. This chapter addresses oxygen physiology, the risks and benefits of oxygen therapy, blood gas analysis, oxygen delivery systems, blood sampling techniques, and noninvasive blood gas monitoring.

II. **Oxygen physiology.** The amount of oxygen available to body tissues depends, in part, on the environmental oxygen concentration, the amount of oxygen in the airways, and, ultimately, the amount of oxygen in the blood. FIO_2 refers to the fraction of oxygen in inspired air and is expressed as a percentage, for example, 21%, or in decimal form, for example, 0.21. PAO_2, measured in mm Hg, is the partial pressure of oxygen in the gas mixture delivered to the alveoli, whereas PaO_2, also measured in mm Hg, is the partial pressure of oxygen in the arterial blood. Oxygen is transported in blood either freely dissolved or bound to hemoglobin (Hb) within the red blood cell. The oxyhemoglobin saturation (SaO_2) is the percentage of Hb that is carrying oxygen.

The amount of oxygen available to the tissues is determined not only by the amount of oxygen in the blood, that is, oxygen content, but also by how effectively the oxygen is supplied to the tissues, that is, oxygen delivery. Both oxygen content and oxygen delivery and the factors that influence them are defined in the following paragraphs.

The total oxygen content of the blood is the sum of the oxygen bound to Hb plus the dissolved oxygen. Because the amount of dissolved oxygen contributes little to the total oxygen content, the simplified equation for oxygen content of the blood is:

$$O_2 \text{ content} = 1.34 \times Hb \times SaO_2$$

By increasing the oxygen saturation, for example, from 80% to 100% at a constant Hb level, the oxygen content will increase by approximately 25%. In most instances, the oxygen saturation can be elevated by increasing the amount of supplemental oxygen the infant receives. Alternatively, increasing the amount of Hb, as occurs with a blood transfusion, may also significantly increase the oxygen content of the blood.

The relationship between PaO_2 and the amount of oxygen bound to Hb can be seen from the oxygen-Hb dissociation curve (Fig. 11-1). Increasing the PaO_2 above 50 to 80 mm Hg will result in a minimal increase in the oxygen saturation. However, small increases in the PaO_2 in the steep part of the curve will result in a significant increase in oxygen saturation and, therefore, a significant increase in the total oxygen content of the blood. In contrast, there are a number of factors that decrease the amount of oxygen that Hb will bind, with subsequent shift of the oxyhemoglobin curve to the right. These factors include acidosis, hypothermia, increased partial pressure of carbon dioxide ($PaCO_2$), an increase in 2,3-diphosphoglycerate (2,3-DPG), and adult Hb. Minimizing these factors will improve oxygen saturations.

Hypoxia, defined as inadequate tissue oxygenation, results from either a decrease in the delivery of oxygen to tissues or an increase in the tissue oxygen requirement beyond the ability of the infant to meet those demands. Oxygen delivery to the tissues is dependent on four factors: (1) adequate alveolar ventilation; (2) adequate gas diffusion between the alveoli and the blood; (3) sufficient concentration of Hb; and (4) adequate cardiac output to ensure homeostatic transport of oxygen to the tissues. The first three are important determinants of the oxygen content of the blood. For oxygen to reach the periphery so that it can be utilized, there needs to be adequate cardiac output. The cardiac output is dependent upon the stroke volume of the heart and the heart rate. Hence:

$$\text{cardiac output} = \text{stroke volume} \times \text{heart rate}$$

If something interferes with either stroke volume or heart rate (e.g., pneumothorax, congenital complete heart block, or obstruction to ventricular output as may occur in

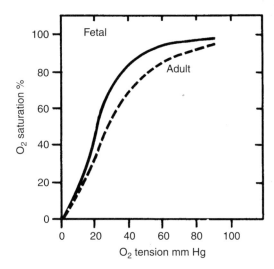

Figure 11-1. Oxyhemoglobin dissociation curves for fetal and adult hemoglobin (Hb).

congenital heart disease), cardiac output may be diminished. This will result in a decrease in delivery of oxygen, even though oxygen may be present in the blood in high concentration.

Oxygen delivery to the tissues is thus dependent on both the content of oxygen in the blood and the cardiac output. Hence:

$$\text{oxygen delivery} = \text{cardiac output} \times \text{oxygen content}$$

Some of the more common clinical conditions affecting oxygen delivery are listed in Table 11-1.

One of the most common causes of hypoxemia is the mismatch of ventilation (V) and perfusion (Q) within the lung. Oxygen must be effectively delivered to the alveolar unit and then be picked up by the circulating blood. V/Q mismatch may result from intrapulmonary shunting of blood caused when capillary blood perfuses collapsed alveoli and no gas exchange occurs. Alternatively, the lungs may ventilate well but there is a perfusion defect. This may occur with right-to-left shunting of blood through a septal defect in the heart or the presence of a ductus arteriosus. This shunted blood subsequently does not come into contact with alveoli, and therefore does not pick up oxygen.

III.   **Oxygen excess and deficiency.** Both hypoxia and hyperoxia can lead to short- and long-term complications. Oxygen should be given in quantities sufficient to eliminate central cyanosis. Whenever there is a question concerning the amount of oxygen required, one should err on the side of too much rather than too little oxygen until further objective assessments can be made.

The 2002 *Guidelines for Perinatal Care,** a joint publication of the American Academy of Pediatrics (AAP) and the American College of Obstetrics and Gynecology (ACOG), makes the following recommendations regarding the use of oxygen in newborns:

- Supplemental oxygen should not be used without a specific indication, such as cyanosis, low PaO_2, or low oxygen saturation.
- The use of supplemental oxygen other than for resuscitation should be monitored by regular assessment of PaO_2 and oxygen saturation.
- The duration of time that oxygen therapy should be administered in nurseries unequipped to monitor PaO_2 or oxygen saturation, before consideration of transfer to a higher level unit, is contingent on the gestational age of the neonate and the severity of oxygen deficit. In general, neonates delivered at less than 36 weeks gestation or those requiring more than 40% ambient oxygen should be stabilized and transferred promptly.
- For neonates who require oxygen for acute care, measurements of blood pressure, blood pH, and $PaCO_2$ should accompany measurements of PaO_2. In addition, a record of blood gas measurements, details of oxygen delivery system, and ambient oxygen concentrations should be maintained.

*Cited with permission from the AAP and ACOG.

Table 11-1. Conditions that affect oxygen delivery

Amount of oxygen in blood
 Hemoglobin concentration
 Partial pressure of oxygen (PaO_2)
 Oxygen–hemoglobin affinity
 Delivery of oxygen
Cardiac output
 Blood pressure
 Peripheral vascular resistance
 Venous return to the heart

- When supplemental oxygen is administered to a preterm neonate, attempts should be made to maintain the PaO_2 at 50 to 80 mm Hg. Oxygen tensions in this range should be adequate for tissue needs, given normal Hb concentrations and blood flow. Even with careful monitoring, however, PaO_2 may fluctuate outside of this range, particularly in neonates with cardiopulmonary disease.
- It is prudent when oxygen therapy is needed for a preterm neonate to discuss the reasons for using supplemental oxygen and the associated risks and benefits with the parents.
- Hourly measurement and recording of the concentration of oxygen delivered to the neonate is recommended.
- Except for an emergency situation, air–oxygen mixtures should be warmed and humidified before being administered to newborns.

Retinopathy of prematurity (ROP) and bronchopulmonary dysplasia (BPD) are serious complications of prolonged or excess oxygen therapy in premature infants. However, factors other than hyperoxia may contribute to the pathogenesis of both ROP and BPD. While attempts should be made to maintain the PaO_2, at 50 to 80 mm Hg, it may be acceptable to use higher concentrations of oxygen for brief periods of time during resuscitation and efforts to stabilize an infant after an acute clinical deterioration. Prolonged use of oxygen should not continue without objective assessment.

IV. **Blood gas analysis.** Blood gases are among the most frequently utilized tests in the evaluation and management of sick neonates. A thorough understanding of blood gas analysis and accurate interpretation of results is essential in providing optimal care to these infants. Blood gas measurements including pH, $PaCO_2$ and PaO_2 are helpful in assessing the adequacy of pulmonary ventilation and the efficiency of the lungs in exchanging gas. Blood gas measurements may be obtained by different methods, including percutaneous peripheral artery sampling, umbilical artery sampling, capillary heelstick sampling, or by noninvasive transcutaneous monitoring. Table 11-2 outlines an approach to blood gas interpretation. Normal or "target" neonatal blood gas values are listed in Table 11-3.

A. **Acid–base balance (pH).** The regulation of acid–base balance involves the lungs, kidneys, and blood buffers. Rapid changes in pH are most often under the control of the respiratory system. Renal compensation occurs more slowly. Acid–base derangements are outlined in Table 11-4.

Acidosis may have a respiratory or metabolic cause. Respiratory acidosis is diagnosed by an elevated $PaCO_2$ with a resultant decrease in pH. As the basic underlying pathophysiology is hypoventilation, treatment should be directed at establishing effective ventilation. Ventilatory assistance must be provided if primary lung disease exists. If hypoxemia is present as a result of V/Q mismatch, increased inspired oxygen concentration in addition to ventilatory support may be needed.

Metabolic acidosis is characterized by a decreased serum bicarbonate concentration and a low pH. This results from a loss of bicarbonate or the accumulation of acid. Respiratory compensation may occur by hyperventilation with a resultant decrease in $PaCO_2$. Correction of a metabolic acidosis is accomplished by treating the underlying cause. In the rare instance where the cause of acidosis cannot be determined, symptomatic treatment with sodium bicarbonate may be indicated. Because of the high osmolality of standard bicarbonate solution (approximately 1500 mOsm/liter), bicarbonate therapy should be done with caution to avoid dramatic fluctuations in serum osmolality. Bicarbonate should be diluted to a concentration of 0.5 mEq/mL and infused slowly over 5 minutes. If rapidly infused (less than 5 minutes), the fluid shifts caused by the osmolar load may increase intravascular volume and may contribute to intracranial hemorrhage.

Table 11-2. Interpretation of blood gases

Is the patient ALKALOTIC or ACIDOTIC?

If the pH >7.45 = alkalotic
If the pH <7.30 = acidotic

What direction did the Pco_2 change?

For acidosis:
Pco_2 >40 = respiratory acidosis
Pco_2 <40 = metabolic acidosis
For alkalosis:
Pco_2 >40 = metabolic alkalosis
Pco_2 <40 = repiratory alkalosis

Does the change in Pco_2 fully account for the change in pH?

For every 10 mm Hg increase in Pco_2, the pH will decrease by 0.08.
For every 10 mm Hg decrease in Pco_2, the pH will increase by 0.08.
For every increase in the HCO_3^- by 10, the pH will increase by 0.15.
For every decrease in the HCO_3^- by 10, the pH will decrease by 0.15.

Is the measured Pao_2 appropriate for the patient's Fio_2?

This can be determined by calculating the gradient between the calculated pressure
of oxygen in the alveolar sacs (Pao_2) and the measured pressure of oxygen in the
bloodstream (Pao_2). This is called the A-a gradient and is measured in mm Hg.
A normal value is <20 mm Hg.

$$\text{A-a gradient} = Pao_2 - Pao_2$$

Pao_2 is measured by arterial blood gas.

Pao_2 is calculated by the following equation (assuming a sea level barometric
pressure of 760 mm Hg and water vapor pressure of 47 mm Hg at 37°C). $Paco_2$ is
measured by arterial blood gas.

$$Pao_2 = [Fio_2 \times (760 \text{ mm Hg} - 47 \text{ mm Hg})] - (Paco_2/0.8)$$

or, more simply

$$Pao_2 = (Fio_2 \times 713 \text{ mm Hg}) - Paco_2/0.8)$$

Table 11-3. "Target" neonatal blood gas values

	Arterial	Capillary
pH	7.30–7.45	7.25–7.35
Pco_2 (mm Hg)	35–50[a]	40–55
Po_2 (mm Hg)	50–80	35–50
HCO_3^- (mmol/L)	20–24	18–24

[a]In certain infants, such as the extremely premature infant or the infant with chronic lung disease, even higher PCO_2
values may be tolerated if accompanied by an acceptable pH.

The following formula may be used as a guideline for calculating the amount of bicarbonate to be administered to correct a metabolic acidosis:

$$\text{base deficit} \times \text{weight (kg)} \times 0.3 = \text{mEq NaHCO}_3$$

The $Paco_2$ may increase if sodium bicarbonate is given to a patient with impaired
pulmonary function. As the $Paco_2$ level is inversely related to the pH, the elevation
in carbon dioxide tension reduces the drug's effectiveness in normalizing the acidosis. Therefore, close attention must be paid to the respiratory status of the patient
when treating a metabolic acidosis. Other complications that may result from the
administration of bicarbonate include hyperosmolality, hypernatremia, and tissue
necrosis associated with intravenous (IV) infiltration.

Respiratory alkalosis is diagnosed whenever the $Paco_2$ is decreased. It may be a
primary respiratory alkalosis or compensatory for a metabolic acidosis. Metabolic

Table 11-4. Acid-base derangements and common causes

Respiratory acidosis	Metabolic acidosis
Lung disease with alveolar hypoventilation	Tissue hypoxia (accumulation of lactic acid)
Cardiac disease with congestive heart failure	Sepsis
Central nervous system depression with resultant hypoventilation (narcotics, intracranial hemorrhage)	Necrotic tissue (e.g., necrotizing enterocolitis)
	Hyperalimentation with excess protein intake
	Diarrhea
Recurrent apnea	Inborn errors of metabolism

Respiratory alkalosis	Metabolic alkalosis
Spontaneous hyperventilation	Diuretic therapy
Iatrogenic mechanical hyperventilation	Iatrogenic secondary to administration of excess bicarbonate
Compensated severe metabolic acidosis	
Central nervous system injury (hypoxic or ischemic injury with neuronal edema)	Compensated respiratory acidosis (common in premature babies with chronic lung disease)
	Abnormal gastric losses
	Adrenal disorders (adrenal hyperplasia, cortisol-secreting tumor)

alkalosis is diagnosed by elevated serum bicarbonate. The primary abnormality in this condition is the loss of acid or the gain of base.

B. $Paco_2$. Accurate measurement of alveolar ventilation is best done by measuring $Paco_2$. Unlike Pao_2, which may be affected by diffusion defects and distribution of ventilation and blood flow to the lungs, carbon dioxide is a highly soluble gas and is therefore a good indicator of the status of alveolar ventilation. Infants with acute respiratory disease may hypoventilate, which is reflected in an elevation of their $Paco_2$. Assisted ventilation may be necessary to correct the hypoventilation.

If the $Paco_2$ is <35 mm Hg, the infant is either hyperventilating or is being iatrogenically over-ventilated. The $Paco_2$ may be low or remain normal early in the course of mild respiratory disease, when tachypnea occurs and CO_2 can still easily diffuse. Spontaneous hyperventilation may be caused by a central nervous system lesion or in response to a metabolic acidosis.

Cerebral blood flow is responsive to changes in $Paco_2$, pH, and Pao_2. Cerebral vasodilatation occurs in response to a high $Paco_2$, with vasoconstriction occurring in response to a low $Paco_2$. An infant who is artificially hyperventilated may not breathe spontaneously because of the low $Paco_2$ and diminished central respiratory drive.

C. Pao_2. The goal in monitoring Pao_2 is to maintain levels between 50 and 80 mm Hg. These ranges are somewhat arbitrary and have been selected in order to decrease the risk of hypoxic damage as well as to prevent complications that can result from hyperoxia. However, some infants may benefit from maintaining a Pao_2 higher than 50 to 80 mm Hg. Hyperoxia, or a Pao_2 >100 mm Hg, may be necessary in some infants with persistent pulmonary hypertension. These infants are often particularly sensitive to changes in oxygen tension, and lowering oxygen tension can result in pulmonary vasoconstriction with an increased right-to-left shunt. The high Pao_2 decreases the chance of further pulmonary vasospasm via a direct effect of dilating the pulmonary arterioles and decreasing pulmonary hypertension.

V. Oxygen delivery systems. Each hospital involved in the care of newborns should have appropriate equipment for the delivery of oxygen. Oxygen may be delivered via a number of different systems. It is important to know the benefits and limitations of each system, as they are not equal.

Regardless of the mechanism of delivery, oxygen should be warmed to 32°C to 34°C and humidified. Inadequate humidification causes fluid loss from the respiratory tract and impedes tracheal ciliary activity. Cold oxygen administered to a newborn may cause apnea and hypothermia, resulting in increased oxygen requirement, increased metabolic demands, and metabolic acidosis. Oxygen blenders are useful when delivering oxygen to infants in order to obtain the appropriate mixture of air and oxygen.

A. Nasal cannula. The nasal cannula is relatively noninvasive and easily applied. However, the fractional concentration of inspired oxygen F_{IO_2} varies with the baby's inherent inspiratory flow. In a newborn, a nasal cannula can only deliver a maximal F_{IO_2} of approximately 45% even when 100% oxygen is used at a flow rate of two liters per minute. Flow rates greater than two liters per minute are not recommended in a newborn. There are newer systems that provide improved humidification of oxygen by nasal cannula.

B. Nasopharyngeal catheters. Nasopharyngeal catheters may also be used, but are less common. The catheter should be inserted into the baby's nose to a depth slightly above the uvula. The delivered FIO_2 will also vary with the baby's inspiratory flow.

C. Simple oxygen masks. Simple oxygen masks are designed to fit over the baby's nose and mouth. The mask serves as a reservoir. There are holes on the sides of the mask to provide an escape for exhaled gases. The delivered FIO_2 will also depend on the baby's inspiratory flow. CO_2 accumulation due to rebreathing can occur with inadequate O_2 flow. Simple masks can deliver up to approximately 50% FIO_2.

D. Partial rebreathing masks. Partial rebreathing masks are similar to simple masks but contain a reservoir at the base of the mask. The reservoir receives fresh gas plus exhaled gas. Partial rebreathing masks can deliver up to 60% FIO_2.

E. Nonrebreathing masks. Nonrebreathing masks do not allow mixing of fresh gas with exhaled gases. There are one-way valves at the reservoir opening and on the side ports. These ensure a fresh oxygen supply. These masks can deliver up to 90% FIO_2.

F. Oxygen hoods. Oxygen hoods can deliver up to approximately 90% FIO_2 at flows of approximately 7 L per minute. The oxygen sensor should be placed near the baby's head because layering of oxygen may occur. Adequate heat and humidification are also important.

G. Venturi masks. Venturi masks offer a more precise control of oxygen concentration. They deliver oxygen at high flow rates and thus provide a fixed amount of oxygen. This type of mask can deliver only the maximum FIO_2 recorded on the mask. For example, a Venturi mask labeled 24% at 4 L delivers 24% oxygen at that oxygen flow rate and can achieve only a slightly higher FIO_2 at higher flow rates. Because Venturi masks deliver a fixed oxygen percentage, they are generally not very practical in the delivery room or in acute situations. There are some situations, however, when a Venturi mask may be useful, especially in the stable infant on lower oxygen concentrations or during procedures in which an infant must not be removed from oxygen.

H. Continuous positive airway pressure. Continuous positive airway pressure (CPAP) is another means of delivering oxygen. Because positive airway pressure is provided throughout the respiratory cycle, CPAP helps to prevent complete collapse of the alveoli at the end of expiration. CPAP can improve oxygenation by increasing the functional residual capacity, increasing compliance of the lung, recruiting alveoli for gas exchange, and improving the ventilation-perfusion relationship. The infant on CPAP must exhibit spontaneous respiratory effort. CPAP may be delivered through specialized devices or a ventilator. Babies on CPAP must be monitored for worsening respiratory distress, air leak syndromes, and apnea.

I. Endotracheal tube. A failure to respond to the above devices may be an indication for endotracheal intubation. An individual trained in neonatal intubation should be readily available at any institution that cares for newborns. Most importantly, there should be an individual skilled in bag-and-mask ventilation of infants.

J. Laryngeal mask airway. Laryngeal mask airways (LMAs) come in a range of sizes. Their use in neonates is still being evaluated. The LMA should be placed only by a properly trained healthcare provider and only if endotracheal intubation is not successful.

VI. Arterial blood sampling. Monitoring the arterial PaO_2, $PaCO_2$, and pH can provide valuable information about the clinical status of a baby. However, this can be technically difficult, especially in small, premature infants. Possible sites of arterial blood sampling include peripheral arteries, umbilical arteries, and capillaries.

Pulse oximetry and transcutaneous monitoring of PO_2 and PCO_2 may provide an alternative to arterial catheterization. However, these advances do not replace the need for intermittent arterial samples during infant stabilization and for verification of the accuracy of transcutaneous methods.

A. Peripheral artery puncture. Peripheral artery puncture may be performed in the radial, brachial, temporal, dorsal pedal, and posterior tibial arteries. Unlike the other arteries, there is no vein or nerve immediately adjacent to the radial artery, which decreases the risk of obtaining venous blood or damaging a nerve. Therefore, the radial artery is the preferred initial choice for intermittent arterial sampling.

Before radial artery puncture is attempted, one should be aware of the anatomy of the arteries and nerves of the wrist (Fig. 11-2). Only the radial artery is used for arterial puncture in order to preserve the collateral circulation to the hand via the ulnar artery.

When preparing for a radial artery puncture, one may use a specially prepared blood gas syringe or a heparinized tuberculin syringe. The amount of heparin coating

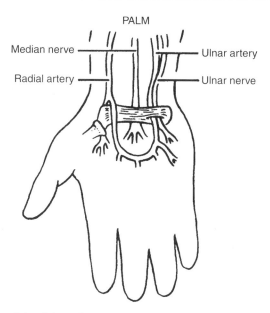

Figure 11-2. Anatomy of the right wrist (palm side).

the barrel of the syringe is adequate to anticoagulate the sample. Excess heparin may result in inaccurate $Paco_2$ or pH determinations. A 23- or 25-gauge butterfly needle is attached to the syringe.

- Grasp the infant's wrist and hand in your left hand (if right-handed) and palpate the radial artery just proximal to the transverse wrist creases (Fig. 11-3).
- Cleanse the area with alcohol.
- Penetrate the skin at a 30 degree to 45 degree angle (Fig. 11-4).
- While pulling on the plunger of the syringe, advance the needle slightly deeper until the radial artery is punctured or until resistance is met; at the same time provide continuous suction on the plunger of the syringe. Confirmation of radial artery puncture occurs when blood appears in the hub of the needle. If resistance

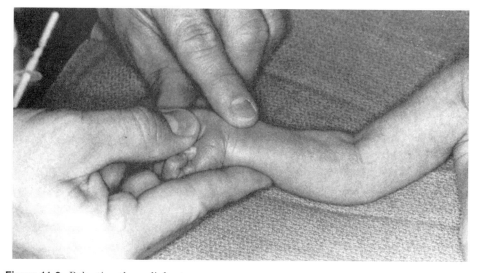

Figure 11-3. Palpating the radial artery.

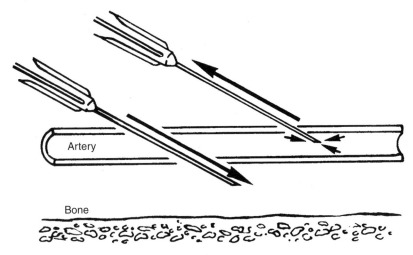

Figure 11-4. Insert needle under the skin at a 30 degree to 45 degree angle.

is met while the needle is pushed deeper, slowly withdraw the needle, staying beneath the skin, and repeat the procedure.

- After 0.3 mL blood is obtained (or the volume required by the clinical laboratory to perform analysis), withdraw the needle and apply pressure to stop the bleeding.

  Complications of radial artery puncture include hematoma formation, and rarely, infection and nerve damage. With the use of proper technique, the complication rate should be extremely low. It is important to remember that with any peripheral arterial puncture in the newborn, the baby may start to cry before blood is obtained, thus changing the PaO_2 and $PaCO_2$ from that present in the quiet state.

B. **"Capillary" sticks.** There is a limit to the number of times that extremely small arterial vessels can be successfully punctured by a needle. Because of the limitations of arterial blood sampling techniques, capillary specimens are an alternative. These samples are usually obtained from the heel. There is reasonably good correlation between the arterial and capillary sample for the pH and $PaCO_2$ when the patient is well perfused. However, the measurement of PaO_2 is not equally reliable by both procedures. The capillary (heelstick) PaO_2 correlates poorly with the actual arterial PaO_2, particularly when the latter is greater than 60 mm Hg. In any individual case, one does not know how close the capillary value is to the arterial value.

Many sources of error in capillary samples could contribute to the observed variations. Inadequate warming of the extremities, excessive squeezing of the heel resulting in venous contamination, and exposure of the blood to ambient oxygen concentrations have been implicated as causes for the repeated discrepancies. In infants receiving supplemental oxygen it is mandatory that the arterial PaO_2 be monitored accurately by a means other than capillary measurement.

To obtain a blood specimen by a heelstick properly, it is necessary to be familiar with the anatomy of the heel (Fig. 11-5) and to follow the steps as outlined.

- Wrap the infant's foot with a warming pack for 3 minutes and then cleanse the heel with alcohol.
- Puncture the skin on the lateral portion of the foot just anterior to the heel with a commercially available heelstick device (Fig. 11-6). The commercially available devices will minimize size of the laceration and local trauma.
- Discard the first drop of blood and then carefully "milk" blood into a heparinized capillary tube (Fig. 11-7). Place the tip of the tube as near the puncture site as possible to avoid exposure of the blood to environmental oxygen. Avoid collecting air in the tube. Avoid excessive squeezing of the foot, as tissue damage as well as red blood cell hemolysis may result.
- Collect a 0.3 mL sample (or the volume required by the clinical laboratory for analysis) and then apply a bandage to the puncture site once bleeding has stopped.

Heelsticks may cause infection and scarring. Lacerations are rare when trained persons perform the procedure. As with samples obtained by radial arterial puncture,

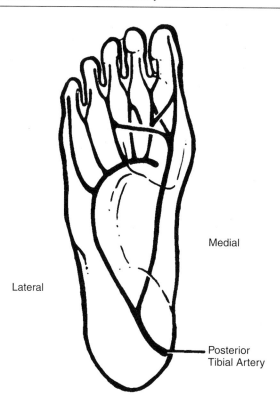

Figure 11-5. Anatomy of heel.

too much heparin may falsely lower the $PaCO_2$ or pH. Heelstick blood gases probably should not be used when the infant is hypotensive, when the heel is markedly bruised, or when there is evidence of peripheral vasoconstriction. While capillary samples provide a reliable means for obtaining pH and $PaCO_2$ determinations in most newborns, the inherent variability in PaO_2 measurements from heelstick samples precludes their use for effectively monitoring the need for supplemental oxygen.

C. **Umbilical vessel catheterization.** Catheterization of the umbilical vessels is sometimes necessary in the care of ill neonates. Umbilical artery catheterization (UAC) is indicated when frequent measurements of arterial blood gases are required and for continuous blood pressure monitoring. Additionally, certain medications and IV fluids may be infused by this route. It may also be used for exchange transfusions and for neonatal resuscitation, although the umbilical vein is preferred for these procedures. Umbilical venous catheterization (UVC) is useful for the administration of medications, IV fluids, and to obtain blood specimens. A discussion of venous catheter placement follows the discussion on arterial catheter placement.

1. **Equipment.** Prepackaged umbilical line kits and individually packaged umbilical lines are available. Clinicians should become familiar with contents of their hospital's kits. All equipment should be assembled prior to catheterization to validate its availability and working condition. Supplies and equipment are listed in Table 11-5.

2. **Procedure for umbilical artery catheterization.**
   - Place the infant supine and restrain the arms and legs to preserve the sterile field. Reposition any monitor leads and temperature probes out of the working field.
   - Open the umbilical line kit in a sterile fashion; ensure that all necessary contents are present.
   - Put on sterile hat and mask and then scrub hands and arms in a surgical fashion. Put on sterile gown and gloves.
   - Prepare the umbilical catheter by attaching the stopcock to the end of the catheter.
   - Flush the stopcock, catheter, and sideport of the stopcock with sterile saline solution. Pay close attention not to introduce any air bubbles. Close the stopcock to the patient.

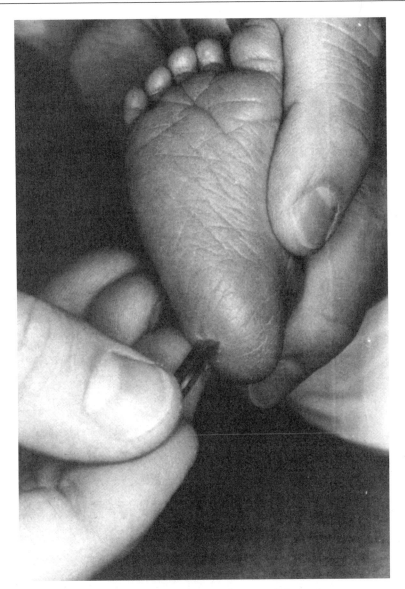

Figure 11-6. The heelstick is performed on the lateral aspect of the heel.

- Clean the umbilical cord area with antiseptic solution. An assistant will be needed to hold up the umbilical cord at its cut end so that sterile technique can be maintained while cleansing and subsequently cutting the cord. Place the umbilical tape around the cord to provide hemostasis (Fig. 11-8). Cut the cord about $\frac{1}{2}$ to 1 cm above the umbilicus making sure not to cut the skin. Then place sterile drapes around the umbilicus.
- Three vessels should be visualized. The vein has a thin floppy wall, is larger than the arteries, and enters the abdomen at the 12-o'clock position (if estimated as the face of a clock). The two arteries are smaller, thick-walled, and enter the abdomen at 4- and 8-o'clock positions, respectively.
- Using the curved hemostat, grasp the firm covering of the umbilicus for stability.
- Use the special, curved forceps to slowly penetrate, then open and dilate the artery (Fig. 11-9). This is a very slow and tedious process. One must be patient or the vessel may perforate and cause the catheter to track down a false passage.

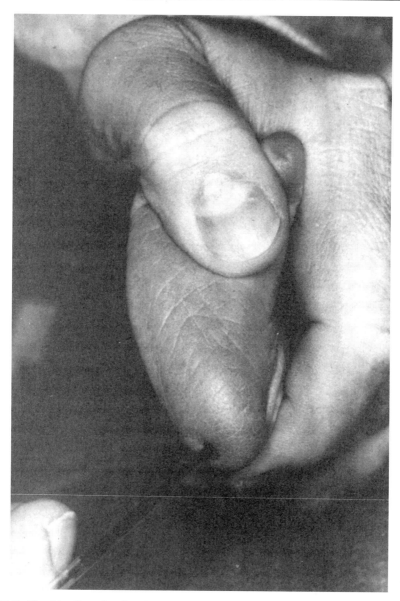

Figure 11-7. Blood is allowed to flow into the capillary tube, avoiding air bubbles.

- Once the artery is sufficiently dilated, insert the catheter (Fig. 11-10A) *very gently*. If you meet resistance, apply slow, steady, and continuous pressure until you feel a give. On insertion of the catheter, tension is placed on the cord in the cephalad direction, and the catheter is advanced with slow, constant pressure toward the feet. Resistance is occasionally felt at 1 to 2 cm, the junction of the artery and the fascial plane, and can be overcome by gentle sustained pressure. If the catheter passes 4 to 5 cm and meets resistance, this generally indicates that the catheter has perforated the vessel wall and created a false passage just outside the lumen of the vessel. Occasionally,

Table 11-5. Supplies needed for the placement of an umbilical vessel catheter

Umbilical catheter (No. 3.5 French for infants <1.0 kg; No. 5 French for infants >1.0 kg)
Sterile gloves
Sterile hat, mask, and gown
3-way stopcock
3–5cc syringe
Sterile saline 3–5cc (may add 1 unit heparin/mL fluid)
Umbilical tape
Sterile drapes
Suture scissors
Hemostat
Forceps
Scalpel
3.0 silk suture
Sterile gauze pads
Antiseptic cleansing solution
Arm and leg restraints
Line fluids: 0.25% or 0.45% normal saline with 1 unit heparin/mL fluid (avoid using a dextrose
    containing solution for umbilical artery lines as this will interfere with laboratory
    interpretations of serum glucose)

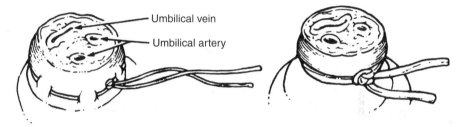

Figure 11-8. A purse-string suture or umbilical tape around the base of the cord provides hemostasis.

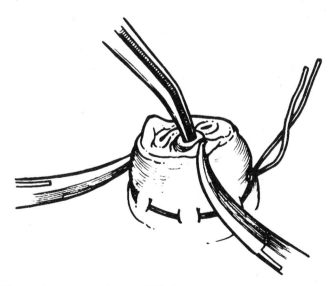

Figure 11-9. Dilating the artery with curved iris forceps.

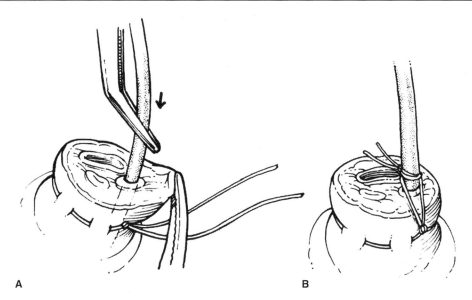

A   **B**

Figure 11-10. **(A)** Introduction of a catheter into a dilated artery; **(B)** Catheter is tied with suture.

one may bypass the perforation by attempting catheterization with the larger 5 French catheter or by carefully introducing a second catheter into the same vessel.

- **Catheter position:** The catheter may be positioned in two ways. A "high-lying catheter" should have the tip between thoracic vertebrae 6 and 9 (T6-T9). A "low-lying catheter" should have the tip positioned at the level of lumbar vertebrae 3 and 4 (L3-L4). The catheter tip should not be positioned between T9 and L3 because of the risk to the major arterial vessels that originate from the aorta in this area. To estimate the position of a high-lying catheter, multiply the neonate's weight (in kg) by 3 and add 9. For example, for a 2-kg baby, the distance of insertion should equal $(2 \times 3) + 9 = 15$ cm. For a low-lying catheter, measure two-thirds the distance from the umbilicus to the midportion of the clavicle. High-lying catheters are associated with less lower extremity vasospasm.
- Once the catheter is in position, aspirate to verify blood return.
- There are multiple ways to secure the catheter. It may be secured as in Fig. 11-10B, or rather than place a purse-string suture around the base, one may suture an anchor near the artery at the edge of the cord and then tie the suture around the line.
- Silk or surgical tape is used to fix the catheter to the abdominal wall (Fig. 11-11).
- Obtain chest and abdominal radiographs to verify the position of the line. Once sterile technique is broken, the line may not be advanced, so it is preferable to position the catheter too high and withdraw as necessary according to the x-ray. X-rays of an arterial catheter will show the catheter proceeding from the umbilicus down toward the pelvis, making an acute turn into the internal iliac artery, proceeding into the bifurcation of the aorta toward the head, and then moving up the aorta slightly to the left of the vertebral column (Fig. 11-12). In contrast, a catheter in the umbilical vein is directed cephalad and is anterior (when viewed via a cross-table lateral x-ray in the supine infant) until the catheter dips posteriorly via the ductus venosus into the inferior vena cava (Fig. 11-13).
- If catheterization with a 3.5 French catheter fails, a 5 French catheter might be tried for the other artery. The end of the tip of a 5 French catheter is blunter than the end of a 3.5 French umbilical artery catheter.
- When an umbilical artery catheter is to be removed, it should be withdrawn slowly to 3 cm and left there for 5 to 10 minutes without infusion to allow spasm of the artery to occur, which will prevent bleeding when the remainder of the catheter is removed. The stump should be observed for oozing for 10 minutes after catheter removal.

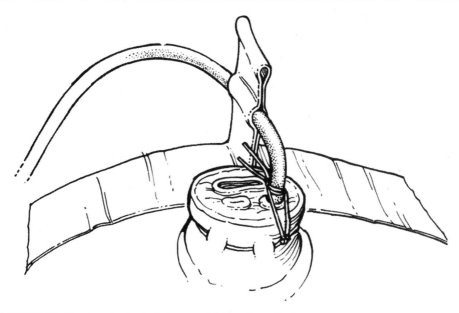

Figure 11-11. The tape is pleated above and below the catheter.

3. Complications of umbilical arterial catheters.
- Bleeding. Bleeding can be prevented by providing good hemostasis.
- Infection. A catheter that has already been positioned should never be advanced. It is recommended to remove umbilical catheters within 7 to 10 days after placement to reduce the risk of infection.

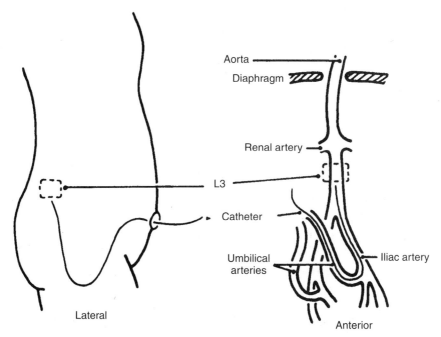

Figure 11-12. The umbilical artery catheter makes a loop downward before heading in the cephalad direction.

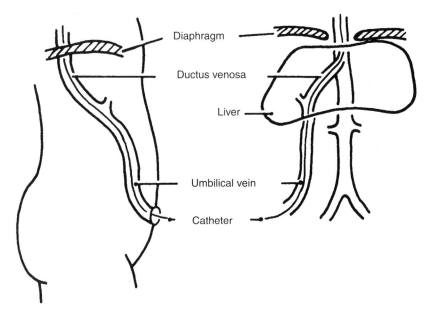

Diaphragm

Ductus venosa

Liver

Umbilical vein

Catheter

Figure 11-13. The umbilical vein catheter is directed in the cephalad direction and remains anterior until it passes through the ductus venosus into the inferior vena cava.

- Thrombolic or embolic phenomenon. Air should never be allowed to enter the catheter and one should never attempt to flush a clot from the end of a catheter.
- Vasospasm. Extremity loss can occur.
- Renal artery stenosis. Renal artery stenosis may occur with an improperly placed low-lying catheter.

4. **Withdrawing blood.** Blood is obtained from an umbilical catheter in the following manner. Using a sterile tuberculin syringe, slowly aspirate the infusing fluid from the tubing (Fig. 11-14). Withdraw an additional 0.5 mL after the first blood is obtained (Fig. 11-14A). If blood is being withdrawn for chemistry studies, more "dead space" blood (3 mL) should be withdrawn, which is set aside on a sterile surface for reinfusion later. Using a second 1-mL heparinized syringe, withdraw 0.3 mL blood for pH, $PaCO_2$, and PaO_2 analyses (Fig. 11-14B) and then slowly reinfuse the blood previously withdrawn (Fig. 11-14C). Flush the line with approximately 0.3 mL flush solution so that no blood remains in the line and leave this syringe attached to the stopcock until the next sample is drawn (Fig. 11-14D). Be sure that all connections are tight.

5. **Procedure for umbilical vein catheterization.** The technique for umbilical vein catheterization (UVC) is similar to UAC.
   - UVC is useful for the administration of intravenous fluids, especially hyperalimentation and medications. They are also useful for exchange transfusions, during delivery room resuscitation, and for central venous pressure monitoring. Double lumen catheters are available and may be preferred for very ill neonates.
   - The umbilical vein wall is larger and floppier than the arteries and is much easier to dilate and cannulate.
   - A 5 French catheter is suitable for all infants. An 8 French catheter should be used for term newborns that require an exchange transfusion. A 3.5 French catheter may be appropriate for the extremely premature infant (birth weight <500 g).
   - The UVC should be placed 0.5–1.0 cm above the diaphragm (assuming normal lung expansion) at the level of the inferior vena cava/right atrial junction (Fig. 11-13). This may be approximated by adding 6 cm to the patient's weight. (For example, for a 2-kg infant, insert the catheter 8 cm). An umbilical venous catheter will proceed directly toward the head without making the downward loop (Fig. 11-13).

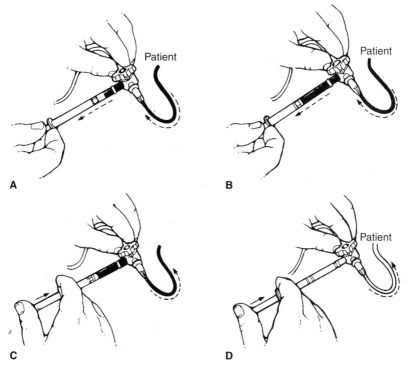

Figure 11-14. Technique of withdrawing blood from an umbilical artery catheter. See text for details.

- If you meet resistance during attempted insertion and detect a "bobbing" motion and cannot advance the catheter to the desired distance, the catheter has likely entered the portal vein. The catheter cannot be left in this position. To avoid this, try injecting flush as you advance the catheter, which sometimes makes it more likely to go through the ductus venosus or apply gentle external abdominal pressure in the right upper quadrant over the liver as you are advancing the catheter.

6. **Complications of umbilical venous catheters.**
   - Infection. A catheter that has already been positioned should never be advanced. It is recommended to remove umbilical lines within 7 to 10 days after placement to reduce the risk of infection.
   - Thrombolic or embolic phenomenon. Air should never be allowed to enter the catheter and one should never attempt to flush a clot from the end of a catheter.
   - Cardiac arrhythmias. Cardiac arrhythmias may occur when a line is inserted too far and rests near the sinus node.
   - Portal hypertension and hepatic necrosis. These may occur with lines that are malpositioned on insertion and left in the portal vein.

VII. **Noninvasive blood gas monitoring.** Noninvasive blood gas monitoring is a growing and developing field in intensive care. The modality that is most widely available is pulse oximetry. Oxygen saturation monitoring relies on the measurement of absorption of specific wavelengths of light by Hb and oxyhemoglobin as they pass through tissue and blood. In order to measure oxygen saturation, measurements are recorded with reference to the change in light transmittance that occurs with each arterial pulse of blood flowing through the tissues. The ratio of the light transmitted at each of the two wavelengths, 660 nm or red, and 940 nm or infrared, varies according to the percentage oxygen saturation of Hb. The instrument is then programmed to calculate and display percentage oxygen saturation during each pulse. Pulse oximeters offer some advantages over transcutaneous monitors (discussed below) in that they do not heat or burn the sensitive skin of the neonate and they can be left in place for extended periods of time. Their response time is more rapid. However, clinicians must remember that pulse oximeters do not allow precise measurements of PaO_2 at saturations $>90\%$. In this range, small oxygen saturation changes are associated with relatively large PaO_2 changes because, at this point, the patient is located on the flat part of the oxygen-Hb dissociation curve. This problem is particularly important in preterm infants with high Hb F concentrations. It is important, therefore, to make some correlation between the O_2 saturation from the pulse oximeter and the measured arterial PaO_2.

Transcutaneous oxygen monitoring is another noninvasive technique. Transcutaneous oxygen and carbon dioxide monitoring provides clinicians with an instantaneous evaluation of the infant for whom they are caring. The reported incidence of complications from transcutaneous monitoring is extremely low and consists almost exclusively of a transient erythema. The transcutaneous monitors employ electrodes that are similar to those used in most blood gas analyzers. The transcutaneous electrodes are heated to facilitate diffusion of oxygen and carbon dioxide through the tissue to the skin surface. The electrodes must be prepared properly as well as calibrated correctly and applied appropriately to the patient. After the electrode is placed, a 10- to 20-minute stabilization period follows. After the stabilization period, it is important to correlate the values that are being obtained with arterial blood gas samples. The method used to obtain the arterial sample needs to be taken into account when transcutaneous and arterial samples are compared. Poor correlation between the transcutaneous value and the arterial blood gas value may be due to failure to calibrate the electrode appropriately, due to the presence of an air bubble under the electrode, or it may be related to an inadequate degree of local hyperemia. If local circulation is compromised for any reason, transcutaneous monitoring will deviate from arterial values while continuing to accurately reflect local tissue oxygenation. Shock, severe anemia, hypothermia, and acidosis may all be accompanied by microcirculatory changes that can alter transcutaneous readings.

VIII.   Clinical pearls.
- Oxygen is a powerful therapeutic agent and the potential risks associated with its use must be appreciated as complications occur with both hypoxia and hyperoxia.
- The oxygen delivered to body tissues depends both on the oxygen content of the blood and on cardiac output.
- Continuous monitoring is warranted when supplemental oxygen is being administered.
- Capillary blood gases are useful in monitoring pH and $PaCO_2$ but are not a reliable estimate of PaO_2.
- Umbilical arterial catheters can cause vasospasm. If an infant with an umbilical arterial catheter in place develops duskiness in one lower extremity, a heat pack can be applied to the opposite lower extremity in an attempt to induce reflex vasodilation on the affected side. In contrast, if a lower extremity blanches white, the catheter must be removed *immediately*.

BIBLIOGRAPHY

American Academy of Pediatrics/American College of Obstetricians and Gynecologists. *Guidelines for perinatal care*, 5th ed. Elk Grove Village, IL: American Academy of Pediatrics, 2002:244–248.

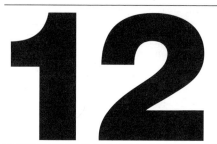

Apnea

Jo Ann E. Matory

I. **Description of the issue.** Apnea is defined as the cessation of breathing for greater than 20 seconds or the cessation of breathing accompanied by a decrease in heart rate and/or the presence of cyanosis. It is noted primarily during active sleep. In contrast to apnea, periodic breathing is defined as the cessation of breathing for less than 15 or 20 seconds without cyanosis or bradycardia. Periodic breathing is a normal phenomenon that occurs in as many as 95% of infants weighing less than 1500 g and one-third of babies weighing more than 2500 g. It typically presents as recurrent pauses in respiration for 5 to 10 seconds followed by rapid respiratory efforts for 10 to 15 seconds.

   During initial normal transition following delivery, respiratory effort may cease if the newborn is deprived of oxygen. This period of apnea may be either primary, in which respiratory effort will improve with stimulation, or it may be secondary and require positive pressure ventilation for resolution. These two forms of apnea require specific managements outlined in the *Textbook of Neonatal Resuscitation,* 4th edition. For purposes of this discussion, management for infants with apnea beyond the immediate post-delivery period will be presented.

   A. **Epidemiology.** Approximately 25% of all infants weighing less than 2500 g and 80% of all infants weighing less than 1000 g experience apnea some time during their neonatal course; more than half of surviving newborns with birth weights less than 1500 g will require management for apnea to ensure avoidance of hypoxia associated with persistence of these events.

   B. **Classification.** Three types of apnea have been described: central, which is characterized by cessation of airflow and respiratory efforts; obstructive, which is described as absence of airflow despite continued respiratory effort; and mixed, which consists of both central and obstructive components. Airway closure is frequently identified in cases of central apnea, suggesting that these categories may not be separate entities but actually be interrelated.

   C. **Etiology.** Several aspects of normal development of chemical and reflex controls for breathing in the newborn have been identified. An active respiratory pattern has been described in the fetus beginning at approximately 11 weeks gestation. Three mechanisms are subsequently important for control of breathing in the newborn: chemical receptors, pulmonary reflexes, and respiratory muscles.

   Although input from all three components is crucial for the development of normal respiratory patterns, their effectiveness is variable based on gestation, sleep state, and clinical status. In both full term and premature newborns, an increase in carbon dioxide concentration will result in an increase in minute ventilation. However, this increase, which reflects central medullary chemoreceptor response and carotid body chemoreceptor activity, is less developed in the premature infant. There also exists a hypoxemic response that is biphasic and characterized by an initial increase in ventilation followed by depressed respiratory effort. In the premature infant, if hypoxia continues, the hypercarbic response is further diminished. Changes in respiratory effort are also associated with sleep states, with apnea seen mostly during active (rapid eye movement) sleep when compared with quiet sleep. During active sleep, chest wall movements are paradoxical, particularly in premature infants, and diminished functional residual capacity along with hypoxia exists, both of which can result in apnea and eventual respiratory compromise and failure. With decreased respiratory effort and/or impaired pulmonary function due to immaturity or to failure of either of these normal respiratory responses, apnea along with subsequent desaturation and reflex bradycardia can develop.

II. **Making the diagnosis.**

   A. **Signs and symptoms.** Apnea in newborns may present alone or in combination with other generalized symptoms caused by multisystem involvement. Although apnea may be a consequence of the infant's immature cardiorespiratory or neurologic system, it is not a benign disorder. Any infant experiencing apnea for the first time or who has apnea during the first 24 hours of life should be considered to have a pathologic process. As always, a complete history and physical are imperative. The history should include a review of the maternal prenatal course and perinatal events including maternal drugs, evidence of bleeding or meconium staining, duration of rupture of membranes, and Apgar scores. The postnatal period should be reviewed for complications associated with the delivery, initial resuscitation and stabilization, and nursery course, such as difficulty with feedings. On physical examination, one should look for signs of respiratory distress, heart disease, or evidence of congenital malformations. Sucking movements, eye deviation, or abnormal posturing of the infant may be indicative of a seizure. The abdomen should be examined for hepatomegaly, as a result of infection or congestive heart failure, and distention or visible loops of bowel, suggesting necrotizing enterocolitis, sepsis, or ileus.

  B. Differential diagnosis. Apnea can be a symptom of several different disorders in the newborn owing to interference with normal development and function of chemical and reflex controls for breathing. Common causes of apnea are presented in Table 12-1 and can be divided into two categories: acute illness and nonacute conditions.

    1. Acute illness. Apnea can be a sign of serious illness, such as bacterial sepsis, in a newborn. If infection is considered, it must be managed appropriately with antibiotics and in a timely fashion as it is usually fatal if untreated. Associated findings of necrotizing enterocolitis, seen in up to 20% of very low birth weight infants, may also present with apnea and require not only antibiotic coverage but also cessation of feedings and adequate fluid resuscitation. Metabolic disturbances, in association with sepsis or isolated in the form of hypoglycemia, hypocalcemia, hyponatremia, or temperature instability, can present as apneic events. Along with lower respiratory tract symptoms, infants with hyaline membrane disease, pneumonia, or air leak syndromes may demonstrate apnea. Perinatal depression resulting from either asphyxia or secondary to maternal drugs, such as analgesics, anesthetics, or maternal tocolytics such as magnesium sulfate, may result in decreased respiratory effort and apnea shortly after birth. Central nervous system (CNS) disease (e.g., meningitis, intracranial hemorrhage, and seizure activity) may manifest as apnea in the newborn period, perhaps initially without any additional evidence of CNS involvement or instability. Apnea may be present in newborns with CNS pathology including tumors, hypoxic-ischemic encephalopathy, and structural anomalies in addition to changes in vital signs and abnormalities of neonatal reflexes.

    2. Nonacute conditions. A number of chronic conditions may cause apnea in infants who appear otherwise normal. Gastroesophageal reflux (GER) has been documented to occur simultaneously with episodes of apnea; however, the majority of infants who experience GER do not have apnea. In those infants who do develop this symptom, unusual sensitivity of the laryngeal and esophageal receptors to gastric contents seems to inhibit inspiration. Clinical symptoms can be significant and, in addition to apnea, may include cough, stridor, aspiration pneumonia, and failure to thrive. Neurologically mediated reflexes may also precipitate apnea in the newborn period, presumably because of immaturity of the CNS. For example, placement of an orogastric tube into the posterior pharynx may result in a vagal response with bradycardia and apnea along with pallor and hypotonia. Neck flexion due to poor head control and upper airway obstruction due to congenital facial anomalies such as macroglossia and micrognathia can result in apnea because of ineffective airflow.

Table 12-1. Common causes of apnea

Acute illness
Infection
Metabolic disturbances
Cardiorespiratory disorders
CNS pathology

Nonacute/chronic conditions
GER
Congenital anomalies
Immature CNS
Apnea of prematurity

In premature infants without an identifiable specific cause, apnea is most likely related to immaturity, usually described as apnea of prematurity. Because premature infants spend 90% of their total sleep time in active sleep, compared with 50% at term gestation, apnea of prematurity is one of the most common respiratory disorders seen during this period. It is defined as sudden lack of respiratory effort that lasts for at least 20 seconds or along with bradycardia or desaturation in infants who are less than 37 weeks gestation. Several mechanisms have been proposed to explain apnea of prematurity. One frequently described proposal suggests that disturbances of mechanisms required for control of breathing results in abnormal breathing patterns owing to immature and inadequate neuronal brainstem, synaptic connections, and peripheral chemoreceptor activity. Premature infants can also experience apnea following irritant stimulation near the carina, probably caused by an immature vagal response; this is in contrast to term infants, who will respond with an increase in respiratory efforts. Another potential cause for apnea in premature newborns results from chest wall instability with resultant collapse of airways and loss of sustained functional residual capacity following inspiration. As systems and controls for an adequate respiratory drive mature, this form of apnea disappears. It is inversely related to gestational age, with resolution noted between 34 and 52 weeks postconceptional age (PCA), generally by 43 weeks PCA.

C. **History.** Key questions to be raised in evaluating an infant with apnea include the following:
- Was consistent prenatal care obtained?
- Were there any hospitalizations, infectious illnesses, or preterm delivery?
- Were there any chronic illnesses, medications, or illicit drug use during pregnancy?
- Was any resuscitation required at delivery?
- Was any respiratory instability noted immediately following delivery?
- Are there any risk factors for sepsis?
- Are there any unstable vital signs or color changes (cyanosis or pallor)?
- Is there any relationship of event to feedings?
- What type of feedings is the newborn receiving? Bolus or continuous gavage, bottle, or breast?
- Is there any relationship to change in respiratory support or procedures (i.e., postextubation, suctioning)?
- Are there any abnormal neurologic findings suspicious for seizures, such as irritability, limpness, or unusual posturing?

D. **Laboratory evaluation and tests.** The initial laboratory evaluation should include the following: complete blood count, blood culture, urine culture, glucose, cerebrospinal fluid culture, calcium, magnesium, electrolytes, and arterial blood gas. Although this evaluation is not indicated for every instance of apnea in each patient, it should be considered in every infant less than 24 hours of age with apnea, in every infant with the first episode of apnea, and in any infant with evidence of acute illness. To evaluate potential intrauterine drug exposure, drug screens (urine or meconium) should be ordered. A chest radiograph may not be helpful in the absence of clinical symptoms referable to the chest; however, it may demonstrate cardiomegaly resulting from recurrent hypoxia or diffuse pulmonary infiltrates due to chronic aspiration. If apnea persists and a diagnosis is not established, additional laboratory testing may be required, such as evaluation of serum and urine for metabolic screening and serum ammonia levels. An electrocardiogram (EKG) may demonstrate ventricular hypertrophy or conductance disturbances indicative of congenital heart disease. If the history of the apneic episode suggests the possibility of seizures, an electroencephalogram (EEG) should be performed. A normal EEG, however, will not eliminate the possibility of a seizure disorder; additional studies including cranial ultrasound, computerized axial tomography (CAT), or magnetic resonance imaging (MRI) may be necessary to evaluate the CNS for intracranial hemorrhages or structural abnormalities. If the apneic episodes are associated with feedings, a barium swallow to evaluate pharyngeal function and the possibility of reflux might be indicated. A radionuclide scintiscan, oximetry swallow study, or an esophageal pH probe may also be helpful in the evaluation of GER.

Three continuous recording cardiorespiratory studies are available to evaluate infants with apnea, namely, the polysomnogram or PSG/sleep study, the pneumogram, and the oxypneumocardiogram or OPCG (also known as multichannel recording). Availability of these studies will vary among different institutions.

1. **Polysomnogram.** The PSG or sleep study evaluates airflow, chest, and abdominal wall motion, as well as EKG, EEG, oxygen saturation with pulse corroboration,

expired CO_2 (EtCO_2), eye muscle movement (EOG), and chin muscle movement (EMG). Video and audio are recorded also. This study stages sleep and evaluates respiratory parameters. A 3-hour study can be requested for newborns that sleep longer and spend 50% to 90% of this time as active sleep. It is the test of choice when looking for obstructive sleep apnea. With the addition of a pH probe, the infant can also be evaluated for possible GER associated with the apneic events.

2. **Pneumogram.** The pneumogram is a 12- to 24-hour evaluation that is simple to perform. Standard leads are placed on the infant's chest; documentation of respiratory effort, heart rate, and chest wall movement by impedance are recorded on a cassette tape that is connected to the monitor. When interpreting a pneumogram recording, one must realize that obstructive apnea cannot be identified because only chest wall motion and not airflow is detected.

3. **Oxypneumocardiogram.** The oxypneumocardiogram (OPCG) or multichannel recording is an unobserved test that evaluates heart rate, EKG, oxygen saturation, and chest wall movement over a 12- to 18-hour period. Nasal airflow and pH probe can also be added. Central apnea can be detected but is probably only significant if associated with neurologic disease; obstructive apnea will not be identified unless airflow is evaluated. This test can be used to evaluate the effect of oxygen therapy for infants requiring long-term supplemental oxygen.

The decision to order any of these tests rests on the experience of the clinician and availability of reliable interpretations. The results must then be used in conjunction with the clinical course and response to overall managements; therapeutic decisions should not be made solely based on the results of the recording tests.

Table 12-2 provides an overview of a systematic approach for the evaluation of an infant with apnea.

III. **Management.**

A. **Treatment goals.** Treatment of apnea is aimed at the prevention of hypoxia to avoid subsequent asphyxial changes and potential for adverse neurologic injury.

B. **Treatments/management.** One should investigate and provide appropriate treatment for specific disorders such as sepsis, hypoglycemia, anemia, neonatal birth depression, respiratory compromise, seizures, and temperature instability. Occasionally, management for apnea must target the clinical situation in which it occurs. For example, if the infant's apnea is associated with such maneuvers as placing an orogastric tube, suctioning, or flexion of the neck, these should be eliminated or minimized. If the infant

Table 12-2. Approach to patient with apnea

History and physical examination

Maternal drugs

Maternal bleeding

Risk factors for infection

Perinatal asphyxia

Evidence of cardiorespiratory or neurologic disease

Temperature instability

Association of apnea with feeding, stooling, suctioning

Laboratory workup (initial)

CBC

Glucose, electrolytes, calcium

Arterial blood gas

Blood and spinal fluid cultures (urine culture if indicated)

Chest x-ray

Urine or meconium drug screen

Laboratory workup (more extensive, if indicated by history or exam)

Serum/urine for metabolic screen (amino acids, organic acids)

Serum ammonia level

Magnesium

EEG

Head ultrasound, CAT scan, MRI

Barium swallow, scintiscan, esophageal pH

Sleep study

becomes apneic with nipple feeding, it may be helpful to use a different feeding technique (e.g., gavage feedings, gravity, or perhaps prolonged feeding via timed pump) until a mature suck-swallow pattern develops. Some premature infants seem to have more frequent apnea if their hematocrit is less than 40%, for which transfusion to a hematocrit greater than 40% may be therapeutic, particularly if the infant requires supplemental oxygen, has a low birth weight, or has a patent ductus arteriosus. In some infants, increasing the supplemental oxygen to allow a PaO_2 to be in the 70 to 80 mm Hg range will eliminate the apnea. Hyperoxia should be avoided particularly in the premature infant to prevent potential damage to retinal vessels with resultant signs of retinopathy of prematurity and in all newborns to minimize effects of potential oxygen toxicity, which may contribute to the development of chronic lung disease. Transcutaneous oximetry monitoring should be used for any patient requiring supplemental oxygen; typically, oxygen saturations for term infants should be greater than 95% and between 88% and 92% for premature infants.

Nasopharyngeal continuous positive airway pressure (NCPAP) has been shown to be effective in the treatment of apnea. This may be partly because of improved oxygenation but is also thought to work through distention of pulmonary stretch receptors, stimulation of the nasopharyngeal area, and decreased work of breathing. With persistence of significant apneic events and potential for hypoxic events in spite of these managements, intubation and initiation of mechanical ventilation may be necessary.

For the management of apnea of prematurity, two medications, namely, caffeine and theophylline have been found to be effective. Caffeine and theophylline are both methylxanthines for which several proposed mechanisms of action have been suggested, including enhancement of respiratory drive receptors, improved diaphragmatic contraction, and an antagonistic action toward adenosine, a neurotransmitter that can cause respiratory depression. Both caffeine and theophylline are metabolized in the liver and have similar toxic effects, including tachycardia, sleeplessness, vomiting, cardiac arrhythmias, and diuresis. They may also lower the threshold for seizures, which will therefore require close monitoring of infants at risk of apnea due to perinatal depression or hypoxic events.

Theophylline is metabolized in part to caffeine. Caffeine, available as caffeine citrate, has a longer half-life than theophylline; therefore, doses may be given less frequently. Metabolism of both drugs is much slower in newborns than in older children and infants. Because of the long half-life of both drugs, a therapeutic level will be attained only after 2 or more days on maintenance dosages; serum levels are typically checked following a loading dose and 7 days of maintenance dosing to ensure the establishment of a steady state (Table 12-3). Caffeine citrate is preferable to caffeine sodium benzoate, as sodium benzoate may displace bilirubin from albumin binding sites.

Caffeine appears to be relatively safe when used under well-monitored conditions. The major complications are dose related and reversible on discontinuation of the drug. The therapeutic range for caffeine is 5 to 20 $\mu g/mL$ with serious toxicity seldom encountered at blood levels below 20 to 30 $\mu g/mL$. Of note, methylxanthines can also decrease lower esophageal tone, so GER may be exacerbated by their use. Methylxanthines also increase the basal metabolic rate, thereby increasing caloric demand.

It is often necessary to increase the dosage because of the increasing clearance of the drug as the infant matures. It is anticipated that caffeine can usually be discontinued by a corrected gestational age of 35 to 37 weeks, with monitoring for any further events off medication for 5 to 7 days.

Doxapram, another respiratory stimulant, is no longer recommended for the treatment of apnea of prematurity because of potential toxicity related to its preservative, benzyl alcohol.

C. **Follow-up strategies/home monitoring.** The development of apnea and bradycardia monitors for home use has created many concerns regarding the treatment of an infant who has experienced an apneic episode. Home monitoring has certainly allowed some children who previously would have required prolonged hospitalization to be safely cared for at home. However, the use of home cardiorespiratory monitors in term healthy infants to reduce anxiety about sudden infant death syndrome

Table 12-3. Dosage schedule for caffeine citrate for apnea

	Loading dose	Maintenance dose
Caffeine citrate (IV or p.o.)	20 mg/kg	5 mg/kg/dose given every 24 h

(SIDS) seems inappropriate. Although several potential risk factors for SIDS, such as maternal smoking during pregnancy, prematurity, prone sleeping position, and late or no prenatal care have been identified, at this time there is no definitive test capable of predicting susceptibility of an infant to SIDS. The most effective means of reducing the incidence of SIDS, to date, has been the institution of programs in accordance with the American Academy of Pediatrics recommendations published in 1992, which promote placement of infants to sleep on their backs.

In accordance with recommendations from the American Academy of Pediatrics, infants for whom home monitoring may be warranted include those who have experienced an apparent life threatening event (ALTE), infants with tracheostomies or anatomic abnormalities with potential for airway compromise, infants with neurologic or metabolic disease and potential for respiratory compromise, and infants with chronic lung disease, particularly if home supplemental oxygen or mechanical ventilation is required.

It must be recognized and emphasized to families that home monitoring equipment will not prevent a fatal event; however, it may allow the earlier institution of resuscitation measures. Before home monitoring is instituted, it is important to consider all the ramifications. Home monitoring is expensive, currently costing $200 to $300 per month. Caretakers must be capable of hearing the alarms at all times, which may disrupt routine schedules. Child-care arrangements become more difficult, as all involved with the child must be proficient in maintenance of the monitor as well as in infant cardio-pulmonary resuscitation skills. Home monitoring is not without risk to the patient as well as to other children. The monitor represents potential hazards, such as cord entanglement, electrocution, or electrical burns if the lead wires or electrical cords are handled inappropriately or if young children are left with equipment without proper adult supervision. If home monitoring is warranted and provided for infants, adequate instruction and support must be provided for the family. Support staff (medical, nursing, and respiratory therapy) and systems should be available on a 24-hour-a-day basis. The duration of home monitoring must be individualized to the needs of each infant and requires close outpatient follow-up and medical supervision by the primary care physician and additional subspecialty support staff, including pulmonary services, allied health support personnel, and home health care.

IV. **Clinical pearls.**
- Apnea is defined as the cessation of breathing for greater than 20 seconds or the cessation of breathing accompanied by a decrease in heart rate and/or the presence of cyanosis.
- Three types of apnea have been described: (a) central, defined as the cessation of airflow and respiratory efforts; (b) obstructive, defined as the absence of airflow despite continued respiratory efforts; (c) mixed, which contains both central and obstructive components.
- Possible pathophysiologic mechanisms of action responsible for apnea in the newborn include abnormal control of breathing due to immaturity of the brainstem and of the dendritic connections from peripheral chemoreceptors.
- Medications used for treatment of apnea of prematurity include the following:
  - theophylline, which is metabolized to caffeine.
  - caffeine, which has a longer half-life than theophylline, therefore allowing less frequent dosing.
- Apnea of prematurity usually resolves between 34 and 52 weeks PCA.
- The test of choice to identify obstructive apnea is PSG.
- Costs of home apnea monitoring are $200 to 300 per month.

BIBLIOGRAPHY

American Academy of Pediatrics, Committee on Fetus and Newborn. Apnea, sudden infant death syndrome and home monitoring. *Pediatrics* 2003;111:914–917.

American Academy of Pediatrics, Task Force on Infant Sleep Position and Sudden Infant Death Syndrome. Changing concepts of sudden infant death syndrome: implications for infant sleeping environment and sleep position. *Pediatrics* 2000;105:650–656.

Fanaroff AA, Martin RJ. *Neonatal-perinatal medicine: Diseases of the fetus and infant*, 7th ed. Vol 2. St. Louis: Mosby, 2002:1038–1043.

Infectious Diseases

David E. Hertz

I. **Description of the issue.** Infectious diseases of the newborn remain a significant cause of neonatal morbidity and mortality; therefore, it is imperative that the clinician maintain a high degree of vigilance in assessing not only symptomatic infants but also asymptomatic infants who may be at risk.

A. **Epidemiology.** Neonatal sepsis occurs at every level of neonatal care and is estimated to affect 1 to 5 per 1,000 newborns; it is four times more common in low-birth-weight infants. Although the incidence of sepsis caused by group B streptococcus, the most common cause of neonatal sepsis, has decreased in recent years due to intrapartum antibiotic strategies, the incidence of sepsis from other pathogens has increased at least in part due to the increasing survival of the very premature infant.

B. **Pathogenesis.** There are several factors that predispose newborns to sepsis:
- prematurity
- immune system immaturity
- rupture of amniotic membranes greater than 18 hours prior to delivery
- maternal infection
- the presence of congenital anomalies that include the disruption of normal barriers to infection such as skin and/or mucous membranes
- the presence of foreign bodies, such as intravascular catheters, endotracheal tubes, chest tubes, etc.

The neonate may acquire infection before delivery (*in utero*), during delivery, or in the postpartum period. *In utero*, infections may be acquired transplacentally, or from organisms that ascend from the vaginal canal either across intact amniotic membranes or following their rupture. Infections caused by cytomegalovirus (CMV), rubella, toxoplasmosis, syphilis, and varicella zoster are examples of those that can be acquired by transplacental passage. Infants with these infections may or may not be symptomatic at the time of birth. Infections acquired during labor and delivery are caused by organisms found in the maternal genital tract, such as group B streptococcus, *E. coli*, herpes simplex virus (HSV), and enteroviruses. Infants infected with these organisms may present with symptomatology shortly after birth or any time for several weeks following delivery. Postnatal infections may be acquired from breast milk, family members, nursery staff, or medical equipment. In addition, infections such as hepatitis, CMV, and human immunodeficiency virus (HIV) can be transmitted by blood transfusion. Early-onset sepsis has been described as that occurring in the first week of life, whereas late-onset sepsis presents any time between 1 week and 3 months of life.

II. **Diagnosis.**

A. **Clinical signs of infection.** The signs of infection in a newborn are subtle and nonspecific and are often the same signs seen in other neonatal diseases. It is not uncommon for the first sign noted by a caretaker to be that the infant is "not doing well" or "not acting right." Early signs also include temperature instability, apnea, tachypnea, glucose instability, poor feeding, lethargy, irritability, and poor perfusion. A list of signs is outlined in Table 13-1. It should be noted that neurologic signs can be seen in infants without central nervous system (CNS) involvement and, therefore, sepsis must be considered in any infant presenting with neurologic symptomatology. Similarly, early on it is difficult to differentiate respiratory distress caused by pneumonia versus that caused by noninfectious processes such as surfactant deficiency or retained amniotic fluid. A chest radiograph can appear the same with any of these entities, and so, it is important to consider an infectious etiology and treat infants presenting with respiratory distress with antibiotics until infection has been ruled out. The evolution of the pneumonic process on subsequent chest radiographs can be helpful in determining which disease process is occurring, as changes secondary to

Table 13-1. Clinical signs and symptoms of neonatal sepsis

General	"Not doing well"
	"Not acting right"
	Temperature instability
	Jaundice
	Hypoglycemia
	Hyperglycemia
Neurologic	Lethargy
	Irritability
	Seizures
Respiratory	Apnea
	Tachypnea
	Increased work of breathing
Cardiovascular	Tachycardia
	Bradycardia
	Cyanosis
	Poor perfusion
	Hypotension
	Congestive heart failure
Gastrointestinal	Poor feeding
	Gastric residuals
	Abdominal distention

surfactant deficiency and retained amniotic fluid occur rapidly over several days while infiltrates caused by an infectious pneumonia persist.

B. Laboratory evaluation.

1. **Blood culture.** Isolation of a pathogen from a normally sterile body fluid such as blood or cerebral spinal fluid (CSF) is the definitive test in the diagnosis of infection, and techniques for obtaining these specimens are described throughout this chapter. In the absence of maternal antibiotic therapy, greater than 96% of neonatal blood cultures that contain true pathogens will be positive for bacterial growth within 48 hours of culture incubation. The use of culture media with antibiotic-binding resins increases the yield of those cultures obtained from infants whose mothers have received intrapartum antibiotics.

   At least 1 mL of blood should be obtained by a percutaneous venous or arterial puncture for a blood culture. Strict adherence to sterile technique while obtaining the specimen will decrease if not eliminate the growth of skin contaminants. To prepare the skin, the area can first be wiped with alcohol. An antiseptic such as a provodine-iodine solution should then be generously applied to the site and allowed to air dry. The antiseptic solution need not be rubbed in and it should not be wiped off prior to obtaining the specimen as the drying process itself achieves maximal bactericidal effect of the antiseptic. Once the specimen has been obtained, the provodine-iodine solution should be cleansed from the skin. A 23-gauge or 25-gauge butterfly needle are most commonly used to obtain neonatal blood specimens. A new sterile needle should be used to inoculate the culture bottle. Obtaining a blood culture from an umbilical venous or arterial catheter under sterile technique at the time of catheter insertion may be an acceptable alternative in cases where obtaining a peripheral specimen is not feasible; however, these catheters are not acceptable sources of blood for culture after the sterile technique of initial insertion has been broken.

2. **Lumbar puncture.** The lumbar puncture (LP) is part of the evaluation of any symptomatic infant with suspected sepsis. If the infant is critically ill, and there is concern that the procedure may compromise the infant's clinical status, then the procedure can be deferred until the infant is more stable. There is debate whether or not to perform an LP on the asymptomatic infant who is being evaluated in the first 24 hours of life for sepsis based on risk factors. It is imperative, however, that any neonate whose blood culture becomes positive undergoes an LP if one was not performed as part of the initial evaluation.

   When specimens of CSF are obtained, aliquots are sent for culture and sensitivity studies, glucose and protein concentrations, and cell count. Generally a normal value for CSF glucose concentration is three-fourths of the serum glucose concentration. A decrease is usually found with infection. Protein concentrations are more variable and, in the preterm infant during the first week of life, the protein concentration may be as high as 200 mg per dL compared with 150 mg per dL in the term infant. Elevations in CSF protein may be associated with infection.

The normal white blood cell (WBC) count in the cerebrospinal fluid is usually less than 30 cells per mL in neonates during the first 4 weeks of life. The red blood cell count should be zero and the presence of red cells implies a CNS hemorrhage or a traumatic tap (i.e., contaminating blood from a surrounding vessel). Definitive diagnosis of a CNS hemorrhage requires other diagnostic tests such as ultrasound or CT scan. Clearing of red blood cells in the spinal fluid during the procedure or clotting of the blood in the specimen suggests a traumatic tap. Interpretation of CSF results is complicated with a traumatic tap. However, a quick rule of thumb is to attribute one WBC as a contaminant for every 500 contaminating red blood cells. For example, if the red blood cell count in the CSF following a traumatic tap is 20,000, then one could attribute up to 40 WBCs as "contaminants" from the peripheral blood. If the WBC count in the CSF in this example was found to be 240, then 200 WBCs would not be accounted for as contaminants and would support the diagnosis of meningitis.

Performing an LP requires a skilled assistant who should immobilize the infant in either the lateral decubitus or sitting position (Figs. 13-1 and 13-2). Care must be taken to ensure that neonate's respirations are not compromised. The assistant must play close attention to the infant's clinical status during the entire procedure. Unrecognized cyanosis is a potential complication. Continuous monitoring of the vital signs and transcutaneous oxygen saturation monitoring may prevent serious complications.

The clinician should localize the L3-L4 intervertebral space. This is usually the interspace along the line connecting the posterior-superior portion of the iliac crests (Fig. 13-3). In a difficult or traumatic tap, it may be beneficial to move cephalad one interspace.

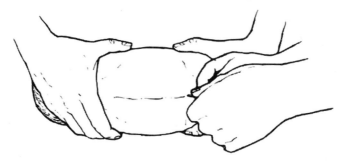

Figure 13-1. The lateral decubitus position for performing a lumbar puncture.

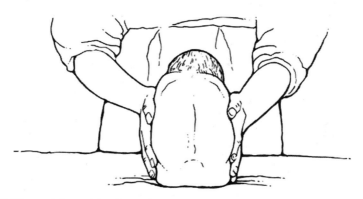

Figure 13-2. The upright position for performing a lumbar puncture.

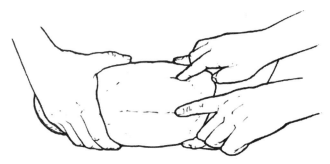

Figure 13-3. Localization of the L3-L4 interspace between the iliac crests.

The clinician should scrub his or her hands and put on sterile gloves. The infant's back should be prepped with a provodine-iodine solution applied in a concentric circular motion. As with a blood culture, maximal bactericidal effect will be achieved by allowing the antiseptic solution to air dry. The infant's back should then be draped with sterile towels.

A 22- or 24-gauge spinal needle with stylet is then introduced into the interspace directed cephalad, pointing toward the umbilicus, but perpendicular to the lateral axis of the spine. The needle is advanced until a decrease in resistance is noted, usually 1 to 1.5 cm, and this is sometimes associated with a "pop" as the needle enters the subarachnoid space. The stylet is removed so that the clinician can visualize the cerebrospinal fluid. If no fluid is obtained, the stylet can be reinserted and the needle is once again cautiously advanced. If the spinal canal is traversed and bone is encountered, bleeding from the anterior venous plexus almost always occurs, which will result in bloody CSF (traumatic tap).

Once CSF is visualized, 0.5 to 1 mL is allowed to drip into each of three sterile test tubes. One tube should be sent for culture, sensitivity, and gram stain, one for glucose and protein concentrations, and one for cell count, including red blood cells, WBCs, and differential. Collecting the CSF to be sent for cell count last allows the CSF to clear to some degree if the tap has been traumatic. The stylet is then reinserted into the needle, and the needle is then removed.

A number of minor alterations in technique may be responsible for the success or failure of an LP. It is essential to have the infant well immobilized. An infant LP needle with a short bevel and clear hub is helpful. The needle should be inserted into the interspace slowly and without lateral deviation. The most common cause of a traumatic LP is over advancement of the needle with penetration of the venous plexus on the anterior side of the spinal canal. When this occurs, a repeat attempt one interspace higher or lower may yield clear fluid.

The LP is usually well tolerated by the neonate and complications are rare. Although brainstem herniation has been reported in older children with papilledema at the time of LP, this complication is uncommon in the neonate because the open fontanelles disperse pressure. Spinal epidermoid tumors have been reported years after LPs performed with an open spinal needle (one without a stylet), theoretically resulting from displacement of a core of epidermis into the spinal canal by the open end of the needle.

3. **Urine culture.** It is rare for a neonate to develop a urinary tract infection in the first few days of life; however, a urine culture should be part of the evaluation for sepsis in any neonate who is over 48 to 72 hours old. The culture must be obtained using sterile technique by either a suprapubic bladder aspiration or a sterile "in and out" bladder catheterization. The diagnosis of urinary tract infection is supported when there is any bacterial growth from a urine specimen obtained by suprapubic bladder aspiration or when there is growth of greater than 1000 organisms per mL from a specimen obtained from sterile "in and out" catheterization. It is not appropriate to obtain urine for culture from a bagged specimen because of the high rate of contamination.

Suprapubic bladder aspiration is considered the gold standard for obtaining uncontaminated urine specimens. The complication rate with this procedure is low when carefully performed. Complications include microscopic hematuria, gross hematuria, suprapubic hematoma, and bowel perforation. Most complications are thought to result from performing the procedure in the presence of contraindications. Probably the most common mistake is using the technique in an infant with an empty bladder. To avoid this error, the bladder should be palpated or percussed prior to needle aspiration. The presence of urine in the bladder is also suggested by a history of no voids in the preceding hour and can be confirmed by ultrasound if there is doubt. Dehydration is a contraindication to suprapubic bladder aspiration. Other major contraindications include abdominal distention, abdominal anomalies, genitourinary anomalies, and hemorrhagic disorders.

Performing a suprapubic aspiration requires an assistant to immobilize the infant. The bladder is then palpated, although it is not always possible to feel the bladder in a neonate. The suprapubic area is prepped with an antiseptic solution such as provodine-iodine solution. Aspiration is performed with a suitable needle and syringe (e.g., 1.5 to 3 cm, 23 gauge needle on a 3 to 5 mL syringe). Puncture is performed 1 to 1.5 cm above the symphysis pubis in the midline (Figs. 13-4 and 13-5). The needle is inserted perpendicular to the examining table or angled slightly (10 degrees) toward the head and to a distance of 1 to 2 cm, until a slight decrease in resistance is felt when the bladder is penetrated. Urine is aspirated with minimal suction, and the needle is withdrawn. Gentle pressure is applied over the puncture site until any bleeding stops. If no urine is obtained, the needle should be withdrawn. Aimless probing or repeated attempts should be avoided.

The most common mistakes in performing a suprapubic tap are (1) attempting to aspirate an empty bladder, (2) insertion of the needle too close to the pubis, and (3) insertion of the needle angled toward the feet rather than perpendicular to the table or angled slightly toward the head.

4. **Viral culture.** When viral infection is suspected, specimens can be sent for viral culture. Nasopharyngeal, conjunctival, and rectal swabs are transported to the laboratory in viral transport media. Stool, urine, cerebrospinal fluid, and other body fluid specimens are sent to the laboratory in sterile, leakproof containers and should not be diluted with viral transport media. Polymerase chain reaction (PCR) assays are available for the detection of certain viral pathogens such as HIV, herpes simplex, and enteroviruses.

5. **Complete blood cell count.** A complete blood cell count (CBC) can be helpful in the evaluation of an infant with suspected sepsis. However, no single parameter of the CBC is diagnostic of sepsis. Parameters that can be useful in the evaluation of suspected sepsis include total neutrophil count (TNC) and ratio of immature to total neutrophils (I:T ratio) (Table 13-2). An elevated total WBC count in the newborn is not uncommon and may be reflective of stress rather than sepsis.

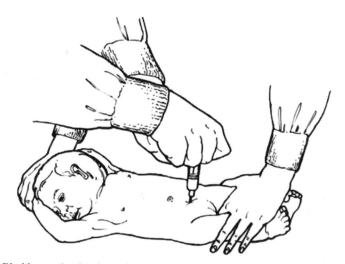

Figure 13-4. Bladder aspiration is performed 1 to 1.5 cm above the symphysis pubis. The needle is directed perpendicular to the table and inserted 1 to 2 cm until urine is aspirated.

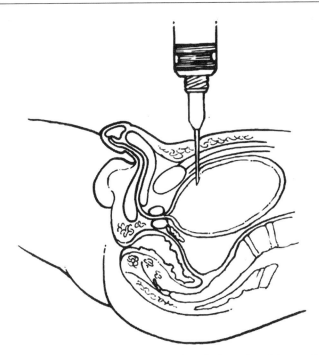

Figure 13-5. Cross-sectional view of the abdomen showing the insertion of the needle into the bladder.

Table 13-2. Calculations of neutrophil counts

TNC (total neutrophil count) = WBC × (% PMN + % bands + % metamyelocytes)

INC (immature neutrophil count) = WBC × (% bands + % metamyelocytes)

I:T ratio (immature: total neutrophil) = INC divided by TNC

TNC, total neutrophil count; INC, immature neutrophil count.

A low WBC count, especially less than 5000 per mm^3, is more ominous in the symptomatic infant. However, low WBC counts can be seen in infants who are not septic but who have suffered hypoxia or who have been born to hypertensive mothers. The TNC, comprised of the polymorphonucleocyte and its immature forms, is of concern when it is less than 1750 per mm^3. The I:T ratio is suggestive of sepsis when it is greater than 0.2. In any case, it must be remembered that the septic infant may have a normal CBC, at least initially, and it is helpful to obtain a second blood count 12 to 24 hours later.

6. **Chest radiograph.** A chest radiograph revealing diffuse infiltrates or a reticulogranular pattern may represent pneumonitis, retained amniotic fluid, or surfactant deficiency. The chest radiograph alone is never diagnostic of any of these entities. More useful clinically is the evolution of the chest radiograph over time as changes due to retained amniotic fluid and surfactant deficiency will clear over several days, whereas the infiltrates due to infectious pneumonias will persist, even lagging behind clinical improvement. The presence of pleural effusions is suggestive of bacterial pneumonias, especially those due to group B streptococcus.

III. **Pathogens causing neonatal infection.** A wide array of microorganisms can cause infection in the neonate. Bacterial agents are outlined in Table 13-3. Viral agents such as herpes simplex, HIV, and CMV can cause neonatal infection, as can spirochetes such as *Treponema pallidum*. The more common organisms encountered are described in the following sections.

A. **Bacterial pathogens.**

1. **Group B streptococcus.** Group B streptococcus (GBS) remains a predominant cause of neonatal sepsis, although the incidence of disease caused by this organism

Table 13-3. Bacteria causing neonatal sepsis

Common organisms
    Group B *streptococcus*
    E. Coli
    Coagulase-negative staphylococcus
Less common organisms (usually seen in high-risk neonatal populations)
    Enterococcus
    Staphylococcus aureus
    Haemophilis influenzae
    Klebsiella pneumonia
    Enterobacter species
    Streptococcus pneumoniae
    Pseudomonas
    Proteus
    Bacteroides
    Listeria monocytogenes

has decreased by 70% with the institution of intrapartum antibiotic strategies. GBS are gram-positive diplococci that are divided into nine serotypes based on capsular polysaccharides. Serotypes Ia, Ib, II, III, and V account for the vast majority of neonatal disease.

GBS commonly inhabit the gastrointestinal and genitourinary tracts and the colonization rate in pregnant women ranges from 15% to 40%. Intrapartum antibiotic administration can decrease the incidence of neonatal disease in the infant born to a colonized mother. Both a culture screening method and a risk-based method have been utilized to identify women who should receive chemoprophylaxis. The culture screening method has been shown to be more efficacious and the current recommendation is that all pregnant women be screened for vaginal and rectal colonization at 35 to 37 weeks gestation. Women identified as colonized during screening should receive chemoprophylaxis with the onset of labor or with rupture of membranes. The only exceptions to this universal screening are those women who have had GBS bacteriuria during the current pregnancy or those women who have had a prior infant with invasive GBS disease, as these women should automatically receive intrapartum chemoprophylaxis. Following the institution of intrapartum chemoprophylaxis strategies, the incidence of GBS disease has dropped from approximately 1 infant per 100 to 200 colonized women to 0.5 infants per 1000 colonized women.

GBS may cause early-onset disease, which occurs during the first week of life and usually within the first 24 hours, or late-onset disease, which may occur any time from 1 week to 3 months of age. Early onset disease most often presents with respiratory symptoms or cardiovascular instability and shock. Therefore, sepsis should be considered in any infant who presents with respiratory distress, apnea, or hypotension. Risk factors for early onset disease are listed in Table 13-4. Management of the neonate whose mother received intrapartum chemoprophylaxis or who had chorioamnionitis is outlined in Fig. 13-6. Late-onset disease is more likely to present as meningitis. Early-onset meningitis and most late-onset disease are

Table 13-4. Risk factors for early onset sepsis

Prematurity (<37 wk gestation)
Rupture of membranes >18 h
Intrapartum fever (>100.4° F)
Chorioamnionitis
GBS bacteriuria during pregnancy
Low or absent maternal concentration of serotype-specific serum antibody
High maternal genital GBS inoculum
Maternal age <20 years
Black or hispanic ethnicity

Figure 13-6. An approach to the neonate born to a mother who has received intrapartum antibiotic prophylaxis (IAP) for GBBS prophylaxis[1] or chorioamnionitis.

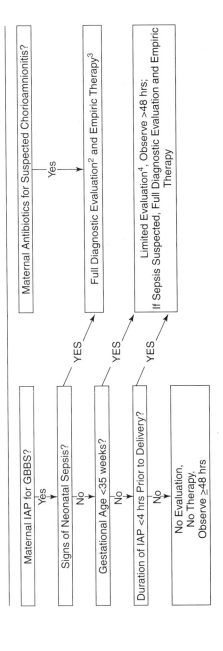

1 If indications for GBS prophylaxis were present but no therapy administered, approach must be individualized.

2 Full diagnostic evaluation includes a blood culture, complete blood cell count with differential, a chest radiograph if respiratory symptoms present. A lumbar puncture should be included in symptomatic infants.

3 Empiric therapy usually includes ampicillin and gentamicin. In the asymptomatic infant, antibiotics are continued until blood cultures have remained negative for a least 48 to 72 hours.

4 Limited evaluation includes a blood culture and a complete blood cell count with differential.

(From American Academy of Pediatrics. Group B Streptococcal Infections. In: Pickering LK, ed. Red Book: 2003 Report of the Committee on Infectious Diseases. 26th ed. Elk Grove Village, IL: *American Academy of Pediatrics*, 2003;590, with permission.)

caused by serotype III. GBS can also cause infection at other sites resulting in otitis media, osteomyelitis, septic arthritis, cellulitis, or conjunctivitis.

Initial treatment of the infant with suspected GBS disease should include ampicillin and an aminoglycoside. Once the organism has been identified and clinical and microbiologic responses have been documented, penicillin G can be used alone. For infants with bacteremia without a defined focus, treatment should continue for 10 days. For uncomplicated meningitis, 14 days of treatment is recommended. Four weeks of treatment are required in cases of osteomyelitis or ventriculitis.

2. **Escherichia coli.** *E. coli*, a gram-negative bacillus, is the second most common bacterial cause of neonatal sepsis. In addition to previously noted risk factors for infection, metabolic abnormalities such as hypoxia and galactosemia have been implicated as predisposing factors for gram-negative infection. The K1 capsular antigen strain of *E. coli* is responsible for the majority of cases of *E. coli* meningitis. Treatment of non-meningeal *E.coli* infections includes ampicillin and an aminoglycoside or an expanded-spectrum cephalosporin for 10 to 14 days. Meningitis requires a minimum of 21 days of treatment. With the widespread use of intrapartum ampicillin for women colonized with GBS, the emergence of ampicillin resistant *E. coli* is of increasing concern.

3. **Coagulase-negative staphylococcus.** Historically considered a contaminant because of its presence as normal skin flora, the coagulase-negative staphylococcus has now become the most common cause of late-onset sepsis in the low-birth-weight infant (<1,500 g). *S. epidermidis, S. haemolyticus,* and *S. hominis* are examples of coagulase-negative staphylococci; however, most microbiology laboratories do not routinely identify the species. These organisms have an affinity for the synthetic plastics in catheters, cannulas, and shunts, making them a common cause of nosocomial infection. Some of these organisms secrete a polysaccharide "slime" layer that makes them less susceptible to host defenses and antibiotics. Many of these organisms are resistant to ampicillin and, therefore, vancomycin should be considered when initiating treatment of an infant at risk for coagulase-negative staphylococcal infection, for example, a 10-day-old, low-birth-weight infant with an indwelling catheter. Treatment duration for catheter-related infections ranges from 3 to 7 days if the catheter can be removed. Longer courses may be considered if the catheter is left in place.

4. **Neisseria gonorrhoeae.** Neonatal infection caused by *Neisseria gonorrhoeae*, a gram-negative diplococcus, most commonly involves the eyes (ophthalmia neonatorum). Topical ocular antimicrobial prophylaxis should be administered to all neonates immediately after delivery. Commonly utilized agents include 1% silver nitrate, 0.5% erythromycin ointment, and 1% tetracycline ointment. Less common sites of infection include scalp abscess, vaginitis, arthritis, meningitis, or bacteremia with disseminated disease. The newborn with gonococcal disease should be evaluated with cultures of blood, cerebrospinal fluid, and discharge from any other sites of involvement. The infant should also be tested for *Chlamydia trachomatis*, syphilis, and HIV.

Infants born to mothers with active gonorrhea but who are themselves without any evidence of clinical disease are treated with a single dose of ceftriaxone, 125 mg, intramuscularly (IM) or intravenously (IV); or cefotaxime, 100 mg per kg, IM or IV. Low-birth-weight infants should receive cetriaxone, 25 to 50 mg/kg, IM or IV. A single dose of systemic therapy is considered adequate treatment of ophthalmia neonatorum and as prophylaxis for systemic disease.

Infants with clinical gonococcal disease should be hospitalized. Treatment consists of ceftriaxone, 25 to 50 mg/kg/day, IM or IV, as a single daily dose (not to exceed 125 mg per day as a single daily dose) or cefotaxime, 50 to 100 mg/kg/day, divided into two doses every 12 hours. Cefotaxime is suggested for infants with hyperbilirubinemia. Infants with disseminated disease should receive at least 7 days of antimicrobial therapy, and those with meningitis should receive a minimum of 10 to 14 days.

5. **Chlamydia trachomatis.** *Chlamydia trachomatis* is a common sexually transmitted disease. Maternal infections are often asymptomatic and 50% of infants born to infected mothers become colonized. Conjunctivitis develops in 25% to 50% of infected infants, with a purulent ocular discharge developing several days to weeks following delivery. Chlamydial pneumonia can occur in 5% to 20% of infected infants and classically presents at several weeks of age with a "staccato

cough." Diagnosis is by cell culture, direct fluorescent antibody staining, DNA probe, or PCR (the most sensitive). The recommended treatment is a 14-day course of oral erythromycin (50 mg/kg/day divided in four doses). The effectiveness of erythromycin therapy is approximately 80% and a second course may be necessary. An association between oral erythromycin and hypertrophic pyloric stenosis has been observed in infants less than 6 weeks old. Infants born to infected mothers who have not been treated or who have been inadequately treated are at risk for infection and should be monitored closely; however, prophylactic antibiotic treatment is not indicated.

6. **Listeria monocytogenes.** *Listeria monocytogenes* is an aerobic gram-positive bacillus that is a rare cause of neonatal sepsis. The organism can be transmitted transplacentally, by ascending route from the vaginal canal, or during passage through the vaginal canal. Maternal infection, which can be associated with a "flu-like illness," is usually the result of contamination of food, especially dairy products and undercooked meats. Transplacental infection has been associated with spontaneous abortion, preterm delivery, and even fetal death. Infection acquired perinatally can result in an "early-" or "late"-onset sepsis presentation indistinguishable from GBS. Definitive diagnosis is by culture. Treatment is with ampicillin and an aminoglycoside. A 10- to 14-day course is recommended for invasive disease without meningitis and a 14- to 21-day course is recommended for meningitis.

7. **Mycobacterium tuberculosis.** The incidence of tuberculosis in pregnant women is rising and in some areas may be as high as 1 per 1,000. In most cases, neonatal infection occurs after birth by inhalation of droplets produced by a person with a primary infection. In rare instances, congenital infection can result from transplacental spread or by aspiration of the tubercle bacilli from infected amniotic fluid.

   If a mother is suspected of having tuberculosis but is asymptomatic and has a negative chest x-ray, no separation of the infant and mother is necessary and the newborn needs no evaluation or therapy. If a mother is suspected of having tuberculosis and has an abnormal chest x-ray, she and the infant should be separated until she undergoes evaluation and is begun on antituberculosis therapy if needed. If a mother has an abnormal chest x-ray but has no evidence of disease, she should undergo further testing to see if the abnormality represents a quiescent focus of tuberculosis. If testing is positive and she has not had therapy, she should be treated (in this scenario, the risk to the infant would be low and separation is not necessary). If a mother has evidence of active disease, clinical or radiographic or both, and is possibly contagious, the health department should be notified so that an investigation of all contacts may be initiated. The infant should be evaluated for congenital infection and the mother and infant should be separated until both are receiving appropriate treatment. Treatment of a newborn for tuberculosis should be done in consultation with an expert in pediatric infectious disease.

B. **Viral pathogens.**
   1. **Herpes simplex virus.** Herpes simplex virus (HSV) is a significant viral cause of sepsis in the neonate. In the United States, approximately 75% of neonatal infections are caused by HSV-2, and 25% of cases are caused by HSV-1. *In utero* infection with intact membranes is extremely rare. Most commonly the infant contracts the infection from an ascending infection following rupture of membranes or during passage through the birth canal. Infection by postpartum contact can occur. The majority of infants who acquire infection are born to mothers with no prior history of herpes infection. In fact, the risk of acquiring infection during vaginal delivery to a mother with a primary infection is 30% to 50%, whereas the risk to the infant born to a mother experiencing a recurrence is <5%.

      Neonatal infections are classified into three groups:
      • disease localized to the skin, eyes, and/or mouth.
      • encephalitis with or without involvement of the skin, eyes, and/or mouth.
      • disseminated infection involving multiple organs, such as the CNS, liver, lung, adrenals, skin, eyes, and mouth.

      Initial presentation and prognosis with or without treatment depend on the group. Disease localized to the skin, mouth, and eyes accounts for approximately one-third of neonatal herpes infections and is characterized by discrete vesicles that are 1 to 2 mm in diameter and have an erythematous base. Coalescence of clusters of these lesions is characteristic. Infants with localized disease usually present toward the end of the second week of life. Early institution of therapy can minimize progression of localized disease. Recurrences of the skin lesions for months or years are common in these children.

One-third of neonates with herpes infection present with encephalitis alone. The mechanism of CNS involvement is thought to result from axonal transport of the virus into the CNS. Onset of illness in these infants is not until the second or third week of life and sometimes as late as the sixth week. Seizures, lethargy, tremors, poor feeding, and temperature instability are common clinical manifestations. Many of these infants exhibit no skin lesions at the time of initial presentation. Without treatment, approximately 60% of infants with encephalitis will develop lesions later in their course.

Disseminated disease also accounts for approximately one-third of cases of neonatal herpes infections and has the worst prognosis. These infants usually present in the first week of life with symptoms that may include irritability, seizures, respiratory distress, jaundice, disseminated intravascular coagulation, and shock. The short incubation period and multi-organ involvement suggests an acute viremia that results in widespread seeding of multiple organ beds. The characteristic vesicular rash is usually not present at the onset of symptoms and 20% of infants with disseminated disease never develop the exanthema.

Evaluation of the symptomatic infant should include the following: a swab of skin vesicles, if present, to be sent for both culture and direct immunofluorescence testing; stool, urine, and cerebrospinal fluid specimens for viral culture; swab of conjunctivae, nasopharynx, and rectum for viral culture; and CSF for PCR. The infant should be placed in isolation and managed with contact precautions. Management of infants born at risk but who are asymptomatic is outlined in Table 13-5.

The goal of treatment of neonatal HSV infection is to prevent progression of the disease. Localized disease initially limited to the skin, eye, and/or mouth will progress to involve the CNS or become disseminated in 70% of cases if untreated; however, with treatment, progression decreases to less than 20%. Treatment of infants with CNS disease reduces their mortality from 50% to 10%, but the majority of survivors suffer neurologic sequelae. Of those with disseminated disease, treatment decreases mortality from more than 80% to less than 60%, but nearly all survivors are neurologically impaired. Treatment consists of acyclovir 60 mg/kg/day divided in three doses for 2 weeks for localized disease and for 21 days for CNS and disseminated disease. When there is ocular involvement, topical ophthalmic treatment with an antiviral agent such as 1% to 2% trifluridine should be initiated in addition to systemic treatment.

2. **Human immunodeficiency virus.** Perinatal acquisition of HIV can occur in infants born to HIV-infected mothers. The rate of transmission can be greatly decreased with treatment of the mother with zidovudine (ZDV) during pregnancy and delivery and subsequent treatment of the newborn with ZDV for 6 weeks following delivery. For the infected mother who has received no treatment during pregnancy, the rate of transmission can be reduced by cesarean section prior to the onset of labor and prior to rupture of membranes.

Infants born to mothers infected with HIV should be evaluated for possible infection. HIV antibody testing is not diagnostic in the newborn as it may represent maternal antibody that has crossed the placenta and this maternal antibody may be detected for as long as 18 months. Diagnosis is accomplished by viral culture for HIV or HIV DNA PCR. Testing should be performed at birth and again at 1 to 2 months of age. If these tests do not indicate infection, testing should be repeated at 4 months of age. If at any time testing is positive, whether it is culture or PCR, the test should be immediately repeated and confirmed before a diagnosis of HIV infection is made. The infant who is 4 months old and has had no positive HIV test has a greater than 95% chance of being noninfected. These infants should have serologic testing after 6 months of age to document the disappearance of antibody. The HIV-exposed infant is considered noninfected if all early testing is negative and if two or more HIV antibody tests performed at least 1 month apart after 6 months of age are negative.

A CBC count and differential should be monitored at birth and monthly in the HIV-exposed infant for 4 months. This should continue beyond 4 months in those infants who are infected or whose status is unclear. A T cell profile should be obtained at 1 and 3 months in all exposed infants and again at 6 months in those infants found to be infected or whose status remains unclear.

Table 13-5. Management of asymptomatic[a] infants born at risk for herpes simples infection

Maternal status	Mode of delivery	Evaluation	Treatment	Isolation
Primary maternal infection—active lesions or positive genital cultures at delivery	Vaginal delivery or delivery by cesarean section after rupture of membranes	Obtain herpes simplex virus (HSV) cultures 24 to 48 h following birth—include urine and stool and swabs from rectum, mouth, and nasopharynx. Some experts recommend that cultures be repeated weekly for 4 to 6 wk.	Empiric treatment (acyclovir 60 mg/kg div q 8 h) is controversial. If the decision is made to institute empiric therapy, cultures should be obtained prior to initiation of therapy.	Isolation is recommended for the duration of the hospitalization. It is acceptable for the infant to room in with the mother. Contact precautions should be observed. (Some experts believe isolation is not necessary if the infant is born by cesarean section less than 4 h following rupture of membranes.)
Primary maternal infection—active lesions or positive genital cultures at delivery	Cesarean section prior to rupture of membranes	Obtain HSV cultures 24 to 48 h following birth—include urine and stool and swabs from rectum, mouth, and nasopharynx.	None unless cultures become positive or symptoms develop[b]	No
Recurrent maternal infection—active lesions	Vaginal delivery or delivery by cesarean section after rupture of membranes	Obtain HSV cultures 24 to 48 h following birth—include urine and stool and swabs from rectum, mouth, and nasopharynx. Some experts recommend that cultures be repeated weekly for 4 to 6 wk.	None unless cultures become positive or symptoms develop[b]	Isolation is recommended for the duration of the hospitalization. It is acceptable for the infant to room in with the mother. Contact precautions should be observed. (Some experts believe isolation not necessary if the infant is born by cesarean section less than 4 h following rupture of membranes.)
Recurrent maternal infection—active lesions	Cesarean section prior to rupture of membranes	Obtain HSV cultures 24 to 48 h following birth—include urine and stool and swabs from rectum, mouth, and nasopharynx.	None unless cultures become positive or symptoms develop[b]	No
History of recurrent maternal infection—no active lesions	Vaginal delivery or cesarean section with or without prior rupture of membranes	None	None unless symptoms develop[b]	No

[a]Symptomatic infants born to mothers with herpes infection should undergo complete evaluation (see text) and therapy should be initiated (see text).
[b]Because symptomatology can develop as late as 6 weeks of age, it is imperative that parents and caretakers be educated in the signs and symptoms of the disease and remain vigilant.

Management of HIV-exposed infants should be done in conjunction with the consultation of a pediatric infectious disease specialist. Treatment of the HIV-exposed neonate consists of oral administration of ZDV in a dose of 2 mg per kg of body weight per dose every 6 hours for the first 6 weeks of life, with the first dose optimally to be administered within 6 to 12 hours following delivery. The treatment interval for premature infants is longer and should be decided in consultation with a pediatric infectious disease expert. If exposure is recognized at any time during the first week of life, ZDV therapy should be initiated even if the mother did not receive ZDV. A transient anemia has been reported with ZDV therapy and the hematocrit of the infant receiving ZDV should be monitored. Prophylaxis for *Pneumocystis carinii* pneumonia should be initiated at 6 weeks of age and continued until an infant is considered noninfected. Infants born to HIV-infected mothers should not breastfeed.

3. **Enteroviruses.** The nonpolio enteroviruses include groups A and B coxsackie virus, the echoviruses, and the enteroviruses. These viruses are common and spread via the respiratory and fecal-oral route. If maternal antibody is lacking, infection in the neonate can be severe and can include pneumonia, meningitis, encephalitis, and myopericarditis. Diagnosis can be made by isolation of the virus from swabs from the throat or anus and from samples of the stool, spinal fluid, or blood. PCR can be performed on the spinal fluid and is more sensitive than culture. Treatment is supportive care and contact precautions should be observed.

4. **Cytomegalovirus (CMV) infection.** CMV is a herpes virus and is the most important cause of congenital viral infection in the United States. Transmission of the virus occurs person to person via contact with saliva, urine, or other bodily fluids. The virus can be transmitted in breastmilk and, rarely, by blood transfusion. Infection in infants and children is most often asymptomatic, whereas infection in adolescents and adults may result in a mononucleosis-like illness with prolonged fever and evidence of hepatitis. Primary maternal infection during pregnancy can have devastating effects on the developing fetus. The incidence of primary CMV infection in pregnant women in the United States is between 1% and 3%. When primary maternal infection occurs during pregnancy, 40% of infants will become infected. Of those, approximately 10% will exhibit manifestations at birth, which may include intrauterine growth retardation, jaundice, hepatosplenomegaly, purpura, retinitis, microcephaly, and intracranial calcifications. Of the 90% of infected infants who are asymptomatic at birth, 10% to 15% will later develop long-term sequelae that may include the following:
   * sensorineural hearing loss
   * motor defects
   * mental retardation
   * chorioretinitis
   * dental defects

   In both symptomatic and asymptomatic infants, virus can be shed for years in urine and saliva.

   Diagnosis of congenital CMV is made by isolation of the virus in tissue culture from specimens of either saliva or urine. Urine specimens have the highest sensitivity because of the high titers of virus concentrated in those specimens. Treatment is supportive. There is insufficient efficacy data to recommend the routine use of ganciclovir to treat congenital CMV infection and its use should be considered only in consultation with an expert in pediatric infectious disease.

5. **Hepatitis A virus.** Hepatitis A virus has little impact on pregnancy. Transplacental infection is extremely rare as is perinatal acquisition. Vaccines are available and effective. Although the safety of these vaccines in pregnancy has not been established, the theoretical risk is low and vaccination of high-risk mothers might be considered. These would include the following: mothers with intravenous drug addiction, those with chronic liver disease, recipients of liver transplants, those traveling to endemic areas, and those with clotting disorders who receive factor concentrate.

6. **Hepatitis B virus.** Hepatitis B virus (HBV) is a common cause of viral hepatitis and transmission of HBV from mother to infant can occur during delivery. Neonates born to women who are HBV antigen positive are at risk for infection and, therefore, routine maternal prenatal testing includes serology for hepatitis B surface antigen. Universal immunization of all neonates is recommended. The first dose of HBV vaccine is administered prior to release from the hospital following delivery or by 2 months of age. The second is administered 1 to 2 months

later with the third dose being administered between 6 and 18 months of age. In low-risk preterm infants, the initial dose of vaccine should be held until the infant weighs 2 kg or is 2 months of age.

For infants, both term and preterm, born to hepatitis B surface antigen positive mothers, the initial dose of vaccine and a dose of Hepatitis B immunoglobulin (HBIG) should be given within the first 12 hours of life. These injections should be administered at different sites. The initial dose given to the preterm infant does not count in the three-dose immunization schedule. After their initial postnatal injection, those preterm infants should subsequently follow the schedule that begins when they reach 2 kg body weight or 2 months of age. For term infants, the usual dosing schedule is followed. Testing to ensure response should be conducted in all infants born to hepatitis B surface antigen positive mothers 1 to 3 months following completion of the immunization schedule.

If the hepatitis B status of the mother is unknown, the neonate should receive the hepatitis B vaccine within 12 hours of birth and the mother's blood should be tested for HBV serology. If the mother is found to be positive, the neonate should receive HBIG within 7 days of birth and should then continue with routine immunization schedule at 1 to 2 months and at 6 months. Mothers who are hepatitis B surface antigen positive can breastfeed with no additional risk to their infants.

7. **Hepatitis C virus.** Hepatitis C virus (HCV) is transmitted by exposure to blood and blood products of HCV-infected persons. Diagnosis is made serologically by detection of HCV RNA or the presence of HCV antibodies. Routine testing in pregnant women is not recommended and is reserved for those at high risk. The rate of transmission from mother to fetus is less than 10% but appears to be increased for HIV-positive mothers. Antiviral agents and immunoglobulin are likely not effective and are not recommended for postexposure prophylaxis for infants born to HCV-positive mothers. Children born to HCV-positive mothers should be tested for infection but testing should be deferred until at least 12 months of age when levels of passively acquired antibody have decreased to levels below detection. Transmission of HCV via breast milk is theoretically possible and the decision to breastfeed should be made following an informed discussion between the mother and her healthcare provider.

8. **Human papillomavirus (HPV).** HPV is the cause of genital warts and is sexually transmitted. Infection with HPV appears to predispose to the subsequent development of genital neoplasms. Although the development of laryngeal papillomatosis has been reported in infants born to mothers infected with HPV, the risk is low and delivery by cesarean section for the prevention of transmission is not indicated. Infants born to mothers with HPV require no special isolation precautions.

9. **Rubella.** Although rubella infection during pregnancy is usually a mild, self-limiting disease for the mother, the effects on the fetus can be devastating, especially if the infection occurs during the first half of gestation. Because of widespread vaccination, congenital rubella infection is rare but when it does occur it can result in severe multiorgan anomalies including retinitis, cataracts, sensorineural hearing loss, meningoencephalitis, mental retardation, and congenital heart disease. Clinical manifestations that may be noted at birth include intrauterine growth restriction, hepatosplenomegaly, and purpuric skin lesions referred to as "blueberry muffin spots." Neonates with suspected congenital rubella, either from clinical manifestations or by a maternal history of infection during pregnancy, should be placed in contact isolation and cared for by personnel known to be immune. Diagnosis of infection is made by viral culture or by detection of rubella-specific IgM in cord or neonatal blood. Neonates with documented infection should be presumed to be contagious for 1 year.

10. **Varicella-zoster (chickenpox).** Varicella-zoster infection during pregnancy can have significant effects on the developing fetus. First trimester maternal infection can result in spontaneous abortion, and second trimester infections may result in a syndrome that includes cutaneous scarring, limb hypoplasia, cataracts, chorioretinitis, cortical atrophy, and microcephaly.

When clinical maternal infection develops between 5 days before and 2 days after delivery, the infant should be given varicella-zoster immune globulin (VZIG). Following administration of VZIG, the mother and infant should be isolated together under airborne and contact precautions. If still hospitalized, these infants should remain in isolation until 28 days of age (or 21 days of age if no VZIG was given).

If signs of maternal infection do not develop until after 48 hours of delivery, VZIG is not indicated for the healthy, term neonate. In contrast, the preterm infant born earlier than 28 weeks gestation who is exposed to varicella-zoster postnatally should receive VZIG regardless of maternal history because of the poor transfer of antibody across the placenta early in gestation.

C. Spirochetal and parasitic infections.

    1. Treponema pallidum. Syphilis is caused by *Treponema pallidum*, a spirochete. Congenital infection of the neonate is usually the result of hematogenous transplacental infection of the fetus but can also result from direct contact with infectious maternal lesions during or after delivery. Intrauterine infection can result in still birth, hydrops fetalis, or premature delivery. The newborn with congenital syphilis may be symptomatic or asymptomatic. Manifestations of congenital infection that may be present at birth or that may occur in the first months of life are outlined in Table 13-6.

    All mothers should have serologic screening for syphilis early in pregnancy. Retesting later in pregnancy is indicated if a woman has been at risk for or treated for syphilis during pregnancy. Screening tests for syphilis are often referred to as "nontreponemal antibody tests" because they do not detect antibody to *T. pallidum*, but rather, they detect antibodies to mammalian membrane lipid cardiolipin found in the serum of patients with active syphilis. The antibodies detected by the nontreponemal antibody tests include both IgG and IgM antibody classes. The two most commonly used assays are the VDRL (Venereal Disease Research Laboratory) and the RPR (rapid plasma reagin). Nontreponemal test results usually become nonreactive 1 to 2 years following successful therapy.

    Because positive screening tests can be seen in patients with other disorders such as HIV, mycoplasma pneumonia, malignancy, Lyme disease, and autoimmune disorders, to name a few, the diagnosis must be confirmed by a "treponemal antibody test." Treponemal antibody tests detect antibody to *T. pallidum* and include the FTA-ABS (fluorescent treponemal antibody) and the TP-PA (*T. pallidum* particle agglutination test). The antibodies detected by the treponemal antibody tests include both IgG and IgM antibody classes. Patients with positive treponemal antibody tests usually remain reactive for life, even after successful therapy.

    No newborn should be released from the hospital without knowledge of the mother's syphilis serology status. Criteria for evaluation of a newborn for congenital syphilis are listed in Table 13-7. Evaluation of the infant with suspected infection is outlined in Table 13-8. A guide for interpretation of maternal and infant syphilis serologies is presented in Table 13-9.

    Treatment regimens are outlined in Table 13-10. For the asymptomatic infant born to a mother who received adequate therapy more than 1 month prior to delivery, in which there was a four-fold decrease in maternal nontreponemal antibody titers and no evidence of maternal reinfection or relapse, close clinical and serologic follow-up is necessary. Some experts would recommend that these infants receive penicillin G benzathine, 50,000 U per kg, IM, in a single dose.

Table 13-6. Manifestations of congenital syphilis

Hepatosplenomegaly
Jaundice
Lymphadenopathy
Edema
Mucocutaneous lesions (diffuse maculopapular rash; vesiculobullous rash of palms and soles)
Bony abnormalities (osteochondritis, periostitis, osteomyelitis)
Pneumonitis
Hemorrhagic rhinitis ("syphilitic snuffles")
Hemolytic anemia
Thrombocytopenia
Leukopenia/leukocytosis
Nephrosis
Pseudoparalysis (atypical Erb palsy)
Chorioretinitis

Table 13-7. Indications for the evaluation of congenital syphilis

Infants should undergo an evaluation for syphilis if they are born to mothers with a positive treponemal test result and have one or more of the following:
Syphilis or human immunodeficiency virus (HIV) infection.
Untreated or inadequately treated syphilis.
Syphilis during pregnancy treated with a nonpenicillin regimen.
Syphilis treated with an appropriate penicillin regimen that failed to produce the anticipated decreased in nontreponemal antibody titer following therapy.
Syphilis treated less than 1 month prior to delivery—treatment failures occur and efficacy of treatment cannot be documented.
Syphilis treatment not documented.
Syphilis before pregnancy that was treated but with insufficient follow-up during pregnancy to assess response to treatment and current status of infection.

From American Academy of Pediatrics. Syphilis. In: Pickering LK, ed. Red book: *2003 Report of the committee on infectious Diseases.* 26th ed. Elk Grove Village, IL: American Academy of Pediatrics, 2003;598, with permission.

Table 13-8. Neonatal evaluation for congenital syphilis

Physical examination
Quantitative nontreponemal and a treponemal serologic test for syphilis on infant serum[a]
CSF Venereal Disease Research Laboratory (VDRL), cell count and differential, and protein concentration
Long bone radiographs
CBC count
Other tests as clinically indicated (chest radiograph, liver function tests, etc.)
Pathologic examination of the placenta

CSF Cerebrospinal fluid; CBC, complete blood count.
[a] Because nontreponemal and treponemal tests detect both IgG and IgM, a positive test may reflect transplacental passage of maternal IgG without true infection of the infant; therefore, if available, include a determination of antitreponemal IgM antibody by a testing method recognized by the Centers for Disease Control and Prevention.
From American Academy of Pediatrics. Syphilis. In: Pickering LK, ed. Red book: *2003 Report of the Committee on Infectious Diseases.* 26th ed. Elk Grove Village, IL: American Academy of Pediatrics, 2003;598–599, with permission.

2. **Toxoplasmosis.** Congenital toxoplasmosis results from the transplacental passage of *Toxoplasma gondii* from an infected mother to her fetus. Maternal infection is the result of ingestion of tissue cysts in raw or poorly cooked meat or from exposure to oocysts in the feces of infected cats. Maternal infection is often asymptomatic and the majority of infants with congenital infection are asymptomatic. Congenital infection is most commonly seen following a primary maternal infection in the third

Table 13-9. Interpretation of syphilis serologies of mothers and infants

Nontreponemal test result (e.g., VDRL, RPR)		Treponemal test result (e.g., FTA-Abs, TP-PA)		
Mother	Infant	Mother	Infant	Interpretation
−	−	−	−	No syphilis or incubating syphilis in the mother or infant.
+	+	−	−	No syphilis in mother with passive transplacental transfer of IgG to infant.
+	+ or −	+	+	Maternal infection with possible infant infection; or mother treated during pregnancy; or mother with latent disease and possibly infected infant.
+	+	+	+	Recent or prior disease in mother and possible infant infection.
−	−	+	+	Mother successfully treated before or early in pregnancy; or false-positive serology.

From American Academy of Pediatrics. Syphilis. In: Pickering LK, ed. Red book: *2003 Report of the Committee on Infectious Diseases.* 26th ed. Elk Grove Village, IL: American Academy of Pediatrics, 2003;600, with permission.

Table 13-10. Recommended treatment of neonates with proven or possible syphilis

Proven or highly probable disease	Aqueous crystalline penicillin G, 100,000–150,000 U/kg/d, administered as 50,000 U/kg/dose, IV, every 12 h during the first 7 d of life and every 8 h thereafter for a total of 10 d.
	OR
	Penicillin G procaine, [a]50,000 U/kg per d, IM, in a single daily dose for 10 d.
	(With either regimen, if more than 1 d of therapy is missed, the entire course should be restarted).
Asymptomatic infant with normal cerebral spinal fluid (CSF) results, CBC and platelets, and radiographs and follow-up is certain with the following maternal treatment history:	Aqueous crystalline penicillin G, IV, for 10 to 14 d.
	OR
–no penicillin treatment, inadequate treatment, or no documentation of penicillin treatment[b];	Penicillin G procaine,[a]50,000 U/kg per d, IM, single daily dose for 10 d.
–mother was treated with erythromycin or other nonpenicillin regimen;	
–mother received treatment ≤4 wk prior to delivery;	OR
–fourfold or greater decrease in maternal nontreponemal antibody titers NOT demonstrated on sequential serologic tests	Clinical, serologic follow-up, and penicillin G benzathine, [a]50,000 U/kg, IM, single dose.

[a]Penicillin G benzathine and penicillin G procaine are approved for IM administration only.
[b]If any part of infant's evaluation is abnormal or not performed or if CSF is uninterpretable, the 10-d course of penicillin is required.
From American Academy of Pediatrics. Syphilis. In: Pickering LK, ed. Red book: *2003 Report of the Committee on Infectious Diseases*. 26th ed. Elk Grove Village, IL: American Academy of Pediatrics, 2003;602, with permission.

trimester but infections that occur in the first trimester result in the most severe sequelae, which may include microcephaly, hydrocephaly, chorioretinitis, and intracranial calcifications. Definitive diagnosis is made by serologic detection of specific antitoxoplamsa IgM and IgA antibodies. *Toxoplasma gondii* may also be isolated from the placenta, umbilical cord, or neonatal peripheral blood by mouse inoculation or PCR. Prolonged treatment with pyrimethamine and sulfadiazine in consultation with an infectious disease expert is recommended for treatment of symptomatic and asymptomatic infants with congenital infection.

IV. **Clinical pearls.**
- Neonatal sepsis remains a major cause of neonatal morbidity and mortality and, because the signs and symptoms are often subtle, the clinician must maintain a high degree of vigilance when assessing the newborn for possible infection.
- Septic neonates can exhibit both hypothermia and hyperthermia; however, a normal temperature does not exclude the possibility of sepsis.
- Neutropenia is as concerning, if not more so, as neutrophilia in the newborn with suspected sepsis.
- The neonate who presents *in extremis* in the first days or weeks of life should be presumed to have sepsis or cyanotic congenital heart disease until proven otherwise. Treatment for both entities should be initiated *immediately*.

BIBLIOGRAPHY

Pickering LK, ed. *Red book: 2003 report of the committee on infectious diseases*, 26th ed. Elk Grove Village, IL: American Academy of Pediatrics, 2003.
Wiswell TE. Neonatal septicemia. In: Polin RA, Yoder MC, Burg FD, eds. *Workbook in practical neonatology*. Philadelphia, PA: WB Saunders, 2001.

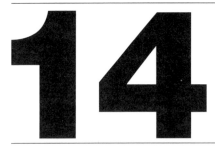

Congenital Heart Disease in the Neonate

Anne G. Farrell and
Randall L. Caldwell

I. **Description of the issue.** The incidence of congenital heart disease (CHD) is approximately 8 per 1000 (0.8%). This figure excludes children who have been shown by more sophisticated diagnostic methods to have a bicuspid aortic valve, which may be found in approximately 1% of the normal population. Table 14-1 lists the congenital defects that more commonly present in the first few days of life with congestive heart failure (CHF) or cyanosis, as opposed to those lesions that present later in the neonatal/infant period. Ventricular septal defect has the highest incidence of all congenital heart defects but accounts for a very small percentage of those infants who present with signs of CHF during the first week of life. Conversely, the hypoplastic left heart complex accounts for a very small percentage of all CHD but accounts for a high percentage of those infants who die from a congenital heart defect in the first month of life.

II. **Congestive heart failure.** CHF is initially evident only with exercise, but as it progresses, signs of CHF are present at rest. The major form of exercise for the newborn is feeding. During the first several months of life, the clinical signs are usually not identified until they are persistent at rest. Infection or metabolic stress may also be a precipitating factor. Infants with CHF may demonstrate dyspnea only with feeding. When the infant tries to feed, breathing is interrupted, and the process of sucking and swallowing may lead to exhaustion and respiratory distress. These signs should make clinicians suspicious of incipient CHF, particularly when these signs are associated with a history of poor weight gain. As CHF becomes more severe, the infant manifests tachypnea and dyspnea at rest and may have increased energy expenditure that may contribute to poor growth.

The venous pressure in the systemic and pulmonary circuits is elevated with CHF. It is difficult to assess jugular venous distention in the newborn; therefore, the most reliable sign of CHF is the size of the liver. The infant's liver is easily palpated, and the edge may be accurately measured from the costal margin. A liver that extends 2 cm or more below the costal margin usually indicates pathologic enlargement. With increased venous distention, the liver edge may appear more rounded than usual.

As left ventricular failure progresses, there may be fine pulmonary rales heard over the lung bases. Although this is a common finding in older children and adults, it is

Table 14-1. Common congenital heart defects

Early neonatal presentation with congestive heart failure and/or cyanosis
Transposition of the great vessels
Hypoplastic left heart syndrome
Tricuspid atresia
Pulmonary atresia
Pseudotruncus (pulmonary atresia with ventricular septal defect)
Aortic stenosis
Coarctation of the aorta
Total anomalous pulmonary venous return
Later neonatal or infant presentation
Ventricular septal defect
Atrial septal defect
Patent ductus arteriosus
Tetrology of Fallot
Atrioventricular canal
Total anomalous pulmonary venous return

much more difficult to appreciate in a small infant. With intrathoracic congestion and edema, the vital capacity and lung volume are further reduced, leading to tachypnea and dyspnea. The normal circulation time of young infants is 6 to 12 seconds, but as CHF becomes more severe, the circulation time may be prolonged by as much as 30 to 50 seconds. With this prolongation, there is increased oxygen extraction from the periphery, thereby yielding cyanosis.

Tachycardia (heart rate greater than 150 beats per minute) is partially mediated by catecholamine release caused by CHF. Cardiomegaly develops as a compensatory mechanism to increase cardiac output.

The signs associated with right heart failure are increased venous pressure, dyspnea, enlarged liver, and peripheral edema, whereas those associated with left ventricular failure are dyspnea, rales, a gallop rhythm, and radiologic evidence of cardiomegaly and congested lung fields. In the newborn, left ventricular failure may lead to elevated pressures in the pulmonary veins, pulmonary artery, and right ventricle, thus presenting a picture of right heart failure. It is therefore much more difficult to differentiate right heart failure from left heart failure in the neonate.

A. Causes of CHF other than CHD. Table 14-2 lists some of the more common causes of CHF in an infant who has a structurally normal heart. Infants born following a difficult labor or delivery may develop neonatal asphyxia, hypoxia, acidosis, or hypoglycemia. All of these may result in a transient myocardial ischemia with secondary tricuspid or mitral insufficiency. Sepsis, particularly group B streptococcal sepsis, may present with signs of CHF in the neonate. Viral infections (those acquired *in utero* and postnatally) may also present with myoendocarditis and secondary CHF. Such infections include rubella, toxoplasmosis, cytomegalovirus, and Coxsackie virus.

Hematologic abnormalities may present with CHF. These include polycythemia and severe anemia.

The pulmonary system itself does not typically lead to CHF, with the exception of persistent fetal circulation, in which there is a markedly elevated pulmonary arterial pressure and secondary right heart failure.

Numerous metabolic problems may also lead to CHF. A typical presentation is that of the infant of a diabetic mother who presents with hypoglycemia, although these infants also have a higher incidence of idiopathic hypertrophic subaortic stenosis. Hypo- or hyperthyroidism may present with signs of either bradycardia and secondary low-output heart failure or tachycardia and a high-output failure. There are also several types of storage diseases, the most common of which is Pompe's form of glycogen storage disease, in which abnormal metabolic products are stored within the myocardial tissue leading to significant biventricular hypertrophy and congestive heart failure. Patient's with cerebral or hepatic arteriovenous malformation (vein of Galen) may also present with high-output failure and have evidence of diastolic flow reversal in arch vessels as well as a bruit over the anterior fontanelle.

B. Congenital heart lesions presenting with CHF. Some of the more common heart lesions that present during the newborn period or in early infancy with signs of CHF are listed in Table 14-3. These may be divided into three major categories: The first

Table 14-2. Common causes of congestive heart failure other than congenital heart disease

Transient myocardial ischemia associated with hypoxia
Infections
Sepsis (bacterial or viral)
Congenital infection with myocarditis
Hematologic disorders
Polycythemia
Severe anemia
Pulmonary disorders
Persistent fetal circulation
Metabolic disorders
Infant of a diabetic mother
Hypoglycemia
Hypo- or hyperthyroidism
Glycogen storage disease
Hypocalcemia
Vascular malformation (head, liver)

Table 14-3. Common lesions that present with congestive heart failure

Left-to-right shunts	Obstructive lesions	Other disorders
Ventricular septal defect (Fig. 14-1)	Aortic stenosis (Fig. 14-5)	Arrhythmias, particularly supraventricular tachycardia (Fig. 14-9)
Patent ductus arteriosus (Fig.14-2)	Coarctation of the aorta (Fig.14-6)	Anomalous left coronary artery (Fig. 14-10)
Atrial septal defect (Fig. 14-3)	Hypoplastic left heart syndrome (Fig.14-7)	
Atrioventricular canal (Fig. 14-4)	Mitral stenosis	
Arteriovenous malformation	Cor triatriatum (Fig. 14-8)	

comprises the intracardiac left-to-right shunt with increased pulmonary vascular markings. These include a ventricular septal defect (Fig. 14-1), patent ductus arteriosus (Fig. 14-2), atrial septal defect (Fig. 14-3), atrioventricular canal (Fig. 14-4), single ventricle, single atrium, and arteriovenous fistula.

The second category includes severe left heart obstructive lesions, which may also be present with CHF. These lesions include aortic stenosis that may be subvalvar, valvar, or supravalvar (Fig. 14-5), coarctation of the aorta (Fig. 14-6), and interrupted aortic arch. The hypoplastic left heart syndrome (Fig. 14-7), mitral stenosis, and cor triatriatum (Fig. 14-8) all present with signs of both left and right heart failure. The impedance of pulmonary venous drainage in these lesions results in an elevated pressure in the pulmonary veins, pulmonary artery, and right heart, leading to right heart failure.

The third category includes other causes of CHF, including arrhythmias and other rare congenital cardiac anomalies. The most common arrhythmia leading to CHF is

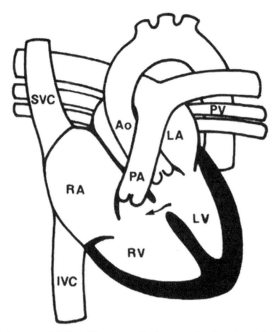

Figure 14-1. Ventricular septal defect. The *arrow* designates the flow from the left ventricle through the ventricular septal defect into the right ventricle. Superior vena cava (SVC), inferior vena cava (IVC), right atrium (RA), right ventricle (RV), pulmonary artery (PA), pulmonary vein (PV), left atrium (LA), left ventricle (LV), aorta (Ao).

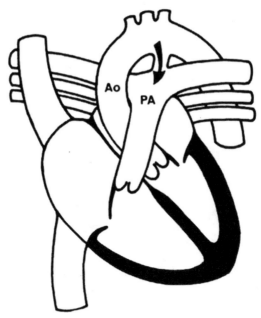

Figure 14-2. Patent ductus arteriosus. The *arrow* designates the flow from the aorta through the patent ductus into the pulmonary artery. Because of the higher pressure in the aorta compared with the pulmonary artery, the flow is from the aortic root into the pulmonary artery. Only if the pulmonary artery pressure is higher than the aortic pressure (persistent fetal circulation) is the flow reversed. Aorta (Ao), pulmonary artery (PA).

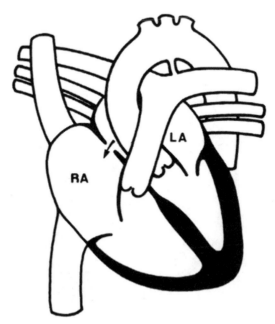

Figure 14-3. Atrial septal defect. The *arrow* depicts the flow from the left atrium through the atrial septal defect into the right atrium. The flow through an atrial septal defect is from the left atrium into the right atrium as a result of the increased compliance of the right ventricle. Right atrium (RA), left atrium (LA).

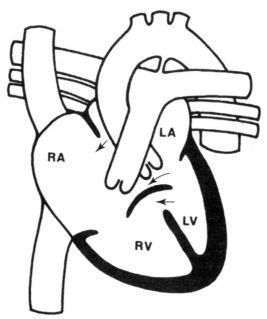

Figure 14-4. Atrioventricular canal. This complex congenital heart lesion consists of an atrial septal defect in the primum portion of the atrial septum (depicted by the *arrow* leading from the left atrium into the right atrium) and a ventricular septal defect (depicted by the *arrow* leading from the left ventricle into the right ventricle). There are also abnormalities of the atrioventricular valves in that a common anterior leaflet of the mitral and tricuspid valve spans through the septal defect. There is typically bidirectional intracardiac shunting. Right atrium (RA), right ventricle (RV), left atrium (LA), left ventricle (LV).

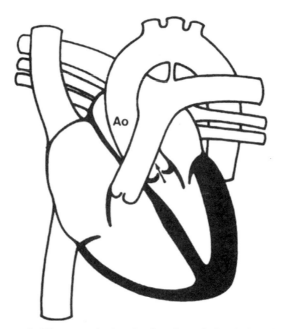

Figure 14-5. Aortic stenosis. The *arrow* depicts the flow through the thickened stenotic aortic valve. With moderate-to-severe aortic stenosis, there is left ventricular hypertrophy depicted by the thickened shading of the left ventricular wall. Aorta (Ao).

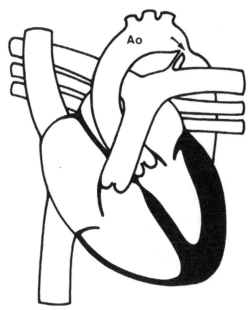

Figure 14-6. Coarctation of the aorta. The *arrow* depicts the flow through the narrowed segment of the thoracic aorta. Note the narrowing just distal to the ductus ligamentum arteriosum. The usual site of obstruction is just distal to the takeoff of the left subclavian artery. Aorta (Ao).

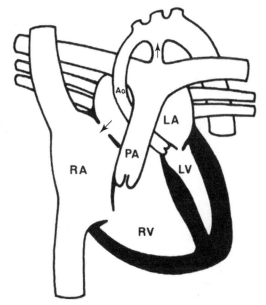

Figure 14-7. Hypoplastic left heart syndrome. In this complex congenital lesion, there is hypoplasia or atresia of the mitral and aortic valves with a markedly hypoplastic left ventricle. Note the small slit-like left ventricle and the very small ascending aorta. The majority of flow into the aorta is from the pulmonary artery through the ductus arteriosus, as emphasized by the *arrow* through the ductus arteriosus. Because of the obstruction at the level of the mitral valve, there is also a left-to-right shunt through the foramen ovale or an atrial septal defect from the left atrium into the right atrium (depicted by an *arrow* passing through an atrial septal defect). These infants also have a dilated right ventricle and a very prominent pulmonary artery segment. Right atrium (RA), right ventricle (RV), pulmonary artery (PA), left atrium (LA), left ventricle (LV), aorta (Ao).

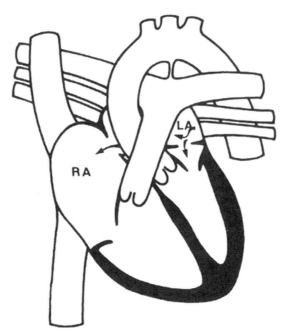

Figure 14-8. Cor triatriatum. This complex congenital lesion consists of a membrane or web within the left atrium that obstructs the blood flow normally returning from the pulmonary veins into the left atrium. The *arrows* within the left atrium depict the blood attempting to pass through this membrane. It finds significant resistance and therefore passes through an atrial septal defect into the right atrium. This membrane is located above the mitral valve. It is essential, but sometimes difficult, to differentiate this lesion from congenital mitral valve stenosis. Right atrium (RA), left atrium (LA).

paroxysmal supraventricular tachycardia (PSVT) (Fig. 14-9). Neonates, however, tend to have longer periods of stability and fewer symptoms than do older infants or children. The symptoms of CHF can sometimes take hours to days to develop. Patients having an anomalous left coronary artery arising from the pulmonary artery (Fig. 14-10) present with symptoms of myocardial ischemia or infarction and often a cardiomyopathy-like picture at 2 to 3 months of age. This time frame reflects the drop in pulmonary vascular resistance that normally occurs during this period but with this anomaly results in decreased perfusion at lower pressure through the left coronary artery.

III. **Cyanosis.** As noted earlier, infants with CHD typically present with CHF and/or cyanosis. Cyanosis in the infant generally originates from four major organ systems: cardiac, respiratory, hematologic, or neurologic, with the respiratory system leading the list as the most common source of cyanosis during the newborn period.

A. **Congenital heart lesions presenting with cyanosis.** Common cyanotic heart defects are listed in Table 14-4. There are four lesions presenting with severe cyanosis during the first 1 to 2 days of life. These include transposition of the great vessels (Fig. 14-11), tricuspid atresia (Fig. 14-12), pulmonary atresia with an intact ventricular septum, and pulmonary atresia with an associated ventricular septal defect (Fig. 14-13) (also called pseudotruncus arteriosus). Tricuspid atresia and pulmonary atresia present with signs and symptoms of decreased pulmonary vascularity. These infants may be neither tachypneic nor dyspneic but are quite cyanotic. Infants with transposition of the great vessels may have normal to increased pulmonary vascularity and, depending on associated lesions, may present with tachypnea in addition to severe cyanosis. Infants with this defect may need emergency balloon septostomy if the foramen ovale is small, as well as a prostaglandin infusion to keep the ductus arteriosus open to potentiate better mixing of oxygenated blood. If necessary, a septostomy can be performed at the bedside emergently with guidance by echocardiography. Some of these infants may have pulmonary hypertension as a complicating factor. Infants with

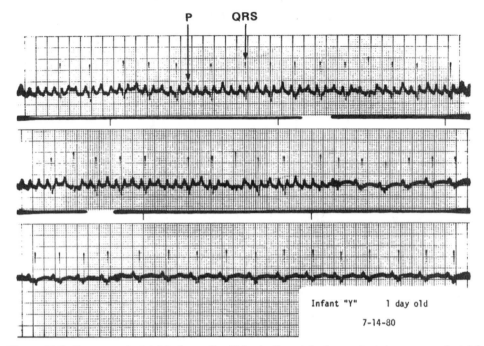

P   QRS

Infant "Y"   1 day old
7-14-80

Figure 14-9. Paroxysmal atrial tachycardia. This rhythm strip demonstrates paroxysmal atrial tachycardia with a variable atrioventricular (A-V) block. This is a continuous rhythm strip. On the middle portion, the infant converts spontaneously from paroxysmal atrial tachycardia with a variable block to a sinus rhythm. Note that the ventricular rate is approximately the same after the conversion as it was with the paroxysmal atrial tachycardia and the A-V block. The majority of infants presenting with paroxysmal atrial tachycardia do not have the A-V block as an infant. This strip was chosen to identify more clearly the P waves in this condition.

moderate-to-severe cyanosis and CHF may be found to have other lesions, including truncus arteriosus (Fig. 14-14), total anomalous pulmonary venous return (Fig. 14-15), or Ebstein's anomaly of the tricuspid valve (Fig. 14-16). Tetralogy of Fallot (Fig. 14-17) may present with moderate cyanosis during the newborn period, although typically it presents later in infancy.

Children with CHD may, unfortunately, have multiple defects involving the cardiovascular system. This is particularly common in cyanotic cardiac lesions such as transposition of the great vessels, where associated cardiac lesions such as situs inversus, dextrocardia, or systemic or pulmonary vein anomalies may be present.

Table 14-4. Common lesions presenting with cyanosis

Severe cyanosis in newborn	Moderate-to-severe cyanosis with congestive heart failure	Moderate-to-severe cyanosis during later infancy
Transposition of great vessels (Fig. 14-11)	Truncus arteriosus (Fig. 14-14)	Tetralogy of Fallot (Fig. 14-17)
Tricuspid atresia (Fig. 14-12)	Total anomalous pulmonary venous return (Fig. 14-15)	
Pulmonary atresia with intact ventricular septum	Ebstein's anomaly of tricuspid valve (Fig. 14-16)	
Pulmonary atresia with ventricular septal defect (Fig. 14-13)		

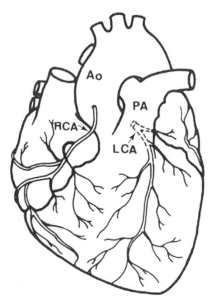

Figure 14-10. Anomalous origin of the left coronary artery from the pulmonary artery. Normally the left and right coronary arteries arise from the ascending aorta. In this condition, the right coronary artery arises normally from the aortic root; however, the left coronary artery arises anomalously from the pulmonary artery. Because the aortic pressure is higher than the pulmonary artery pressure, the flow is from the aortic root into the right coronary artery through collaterals into the left coronary artery and retrograde into the pulmonary artery. Right coronary artery (RCA), aorta (Ao), left coronary artery (LCA), pulmonary artery (PA).

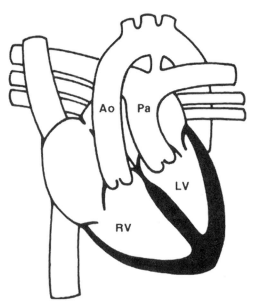

Figure 14-11. Transposition of the great vessels. This is the most common cyanotic congenital heart lesion presenting in the newborn period. The origins of the aorta and the pulmonary artery are reversed such that the aorta arises from the right ventricle. These infants are dependent on a patent ductus arteriosus or a patent foramen ovale to allow mixing between the two circuits. Right ventricle (RV), aorta (Ao), left ventricle (LV), pulmonary artery (Pa).

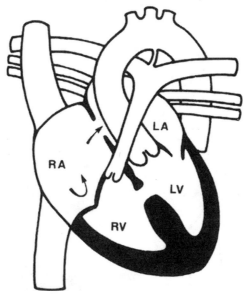

Figure 14-12. Tricuspid atresia. With this defect the blood returns from the systemic circuit into the right atrium and is unable to enter the right ventricle because of the atretic tricuspid valve. The flow is directed through a patent foramen ovale, as shown by the *arrows*. This allows the entire systemic flow to enter the left heart. Some infants with tricuspid atresia also have a ventricular septal defect. If no ventricular septal defect is present, the only route for the blood to enter the pulmonary artery is through a ductus arteriosus. Right atrium (RA), right ventricle (RV), left atrium (LA), left ventricle (LV).

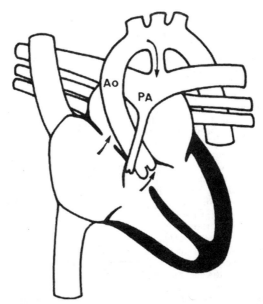

Figure 14-13. Pulmonary atresia. The entire systemic circulation enters the left heart through either an atrial septal defect or a ventricular septal defect. The only blood supply to enter the pulmonary artery is through a patent ductus arteriosus. The *arrows* depict the septal defects. There is also an *arrow* depicting flow from the aorta through a patent ductus arteriosus into the pulmonary artery. Note the small hypoplastic main pulmonary artery. Aorta (Ao), pulmonary artery (PA).

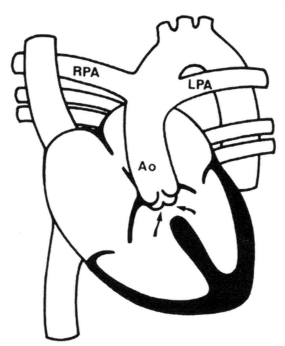

Figure 14-14. Truncus arteriosus. A common great vessel originates from the heart. The right and left pulmonary arteries arise from the ascending aorta. There is always an associated ventricular septal defect, with the aorta overriding the ventricular septum. The *arrows* depict the right and left ventricular flows entering the ascending aorta. Aorta (Ao), right pulmonary artery (RPA), left pulmonary artery (LPA).

Cyanosis in infancy and childhood is usually related to one of three factors. The first is that seen in CHD resulting from an intracardiac right-to-left shunt with desaturated blood reaching the systemic circulation and bypassing the pulmonary circulation. In the presence of CHF this shunt may be accentuated, bringing to the surface signs of desaturation in milder cases and a deepening of the cyanosis in severe defects. The second mechanism causing cyanosis is pulmonary congestion or disease in which there is inadequate oxygen exchange in the lungs. This may be seen in infants who have large left-to-right shunts or left heart obstructive lesions. These infants have decreased arterial and systemic venous oxygen saturation related to the degree of congestive heart failure and pulmonary edema. The third mechanism of cyanosis in the newborn period is vasomotor instability involving the small vessels and capillaries. Vasoconstriction yields a further desaturation of the hemoglobin, as it spends more time in the periphery. The venous return to the right heart has lower oxygen saturation, whereas the arterial oxygen saturation is normal. From reviewing these three common causes of cyanosis, it is apparent that a child may have one or more of these parameters functioning as the etiology of the cyanosis.

B. **Cyanosis: heart versus lung.** The differentiation of heart disease from pulmonary disease in the cyanotic newborn is sometimes very difficult. Several parameters may help in this evaluation, including the history, physical examination, chest x-ray, arterial blood gases, electrocardiogram (EKG), and echocardiogram. The history of the infant with lung disease may include prematurity, a difficult delivery with stress at the time of delivery, meconium staining, or low Apgar scores. On the other hand, infants with cyanotic CHD typically are born at term with relatively normal Apgar scores and are less likely to have undergone a difficult delivery. Unfortunately, some infants with cyanotic CHD also have lung disease such as meconium aspiration.

The physical examination may be divided into three major sections: the chest, heart, and abdomen. Infants with lung disease are frequently tachypneic and dyspneic with intercostal and suprasternal retractions. They may also have nasal flaring.

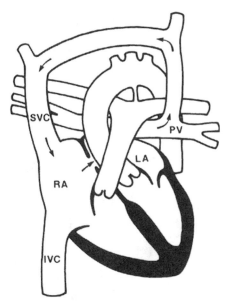

Figure 14-15. Total anomalous pulmonary venous return. In this condition the pulmonary veins do not enter the left atrium but, rather, enter the systemic veins. This may be a supracardiac connection, such as shown here, in which the pulmonary venous flow is directed through an azygous vein into the superior vena cava and down into the right atrium. Total anomalous pulmonary venous return may also be intracardiac, where the pulmonary veins enter directly into the right atrium through a coronary sinus, or it may be directed infracardiac, in which the pulmonary veins drain below the diaphragm into the inferior vena cava or portal system. Note that the only blood flow into the left heart is received from the right atrium through an atrial septal defect into a somewhat small left atrium. Pulmonary vein (PV), superior vena cava (SVC), right atrium (RA), inferior vena cava (IVC), left atrium (LA).

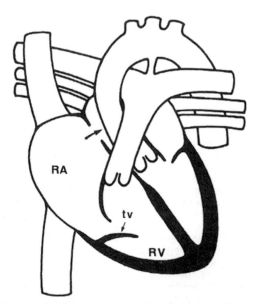

Figure 14-16. Ebstein's anomaly of the tricuspid valve. The tricuspid valve leaflets are displaced inferiorly into the right ventricle, creating a markedly dilated right atrium. Severe tricuspid insufficiency with decreased pulmonary arterial flow is usually associated. There is a large intracardiac right-to-left shunt from the right atrium into the left atrium, causing cyanosis. Right atrium (RA), right ventricle (RV), displaced tricuspid valve leaflet (tv).

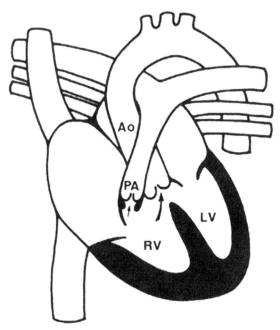

Figure 14-17. Tetrology of Fallot. This condition has four characteristic features: (1) a large ventricular septal defect, (2) pulmonary stenosis, primarily infundibular pulmonary stenosis, (3) aortic overriding, and (4) right ventricular hypertrophy. Note the *small arrow* demonstrating the diminished flow through the hypertrophied, obstructed subpulmonic area at the infundibulum. The flow from the right ventricle is therefore directed through a ventricular septal defect into the aorta. Note that the aortic root overrides the ventricular septum. Pulmonary artery (PA), right ventricle (RV), left ventricle (LV), aorta (Ao).

In contrast, infants with cyanotic CHD typically are not in severe respiratory distress. This is particularly true in infants with decreased pulmonary vascularity such as that seen in tricuspid or pulmonary atresia. Infants with severe cyanosis and increased pulmonary vascularity (e.g., those with transposition of the great vessels) may be tachypneic and dyspneic with retractions and nasal flaring, depending on the magnitude of pulmonary blood flow. Infants with left heart obstructive lesions such as hypoplastic left heart syndrome, critical aortic stenosis, coarctation, or total anomalous pulmonary venous return may also present with severe cyanosis and respiratory distress.

The cardiac examination of the infant with lung disease is typically normal. Usually no heart murmur is appreciated. The second heart sound is physiologically split, and the pulses are normal. Cardiac examination of the child with CHD may reveal heart murmurs, gallop rhythm, and abnormal peripheral pulses. The second heart sound may be single with no pulmonary component heard (e.g., transposition of the great vessels, pulmonary atresia, tricuspid atresia, or hypoplastic left heart syndrome).

The abdominal examination of infants with lung disease is usually normal. The abdominal examination of the child with congenital cyanotic heart disease, in contrast, may demonstrate an enlarged liver if congestive heart failure is present.

The chest x-ray may be helpful in differentiating lung from heart disease. Hyaline membrane disease has a typical ground-glass appearance of the lung fields, and pulmonary infiltrates may be seen. A diaphragmatic hernia is easily seen on the chest film. The heart size and pulmonary vascularity are usually normal with primary lung disease. Infants with cyanotic CHD have decreased pulmonary vascularity with lesions such as tricuspid atresia and pulmonary atresia. Infants with tricuspid atresia may demonstrate an increased right atrial size with a scaphoid pulmonary artery segment. In pulmonary atresia generally there is an upturned apex with a scaphoid pulmonary artery segment and decreased pulmonary vascularity. Transposition of the great vessels frequently presents with normal to slightly increased pulmonary vascularity and an "egg-shaped heart" with a narrow cardiac base (egg on a string). Total anomalous pulmonary venous return can have a "snowman" appearance if it is of the supracardiac type. Ebstein's anomaly can have a huge "wall-to-wall" heart, resulting from significant right atrial dilatation.

Arterial blood gases may be helpful in distinguishing lung disease from heart disease. Infants with lung disease frequently have decreased PaO_2 levels (which may increase with supplemental FIO_2), elevated $PaCO_2$ levels, and a variable pH. Infants with cyanotic CHD usually have a normal $PaCO_2$ with a decreased PaO_2 and a variable pH. One of the easiest ways to differentiate heart disease from lung disease is to obtain a blood gas on room air or on a lower supplemental FIO_2 and then place the infant in 100% oxygen to determine if there is any increase in the PaO_2. If little change occurs in the PaO_2 despite the higher FIO_2, cyanotic CHD with an intracardiac right-to-left shunt should be suspected. If there is a significant improvement of the PaO_2, this would suggest a primary lung process.

The electrocardiogram may be of use occasionally in differentiating lung from heart disease. Children who present with lung disease usually have a normal EKG. The EKG in tricuspid atresia typically has left axis deviation, left ventricular hypertrophy, and right atrial enlargement. Children with pulmonary atresia with an intact ventricular septum have right axis deviation and left ventricular hypertrophy. Those having pulmonary atresia and a ventricular septal defect (pseudotruncus arteriosus) have right axis deviation with right ventricular hypertrophy. Infants with transposition of the great vessels may have a normal EKG for a newborn or may have right axis deviation and right ventricular hypertrophy. Infants with hypoplastic left heart syndrome have right axis deviation, right atrial enlargement, and right ventricular enlargement secondary to the lack of leftward forces.

Echocardiography is very helpful in differentiating lung from heart disease. In infants with primary lung disease, a structurally normal heart is recorded. A persistent patent foramen ovale or a small patent ductus arteriosus may be demonstrated by Doppler echocardiography. This is important in lesions such as persistent fetal circulation, in which a right-to-left shunt at the foramen ovale or ductus arteriosus level may be shown. The majority of cyanotic congenital heart lesions are quite easily diagnosed by two-dimensional Doppler echocardiography. The echocardiogram evaluation allows accurate qualitative and quantitative assessment of all four cardiac valves and chambers; the spatial orientation of the great vessels arising from the heart can be determined to rule out transposition of the great vessels. The Doppler echocardiography evaluation is currently the most definitive noninvasive test available for evaluation of heart versus lung disease in the cyanotic newborn.

Cardiac catheterization is the definitive test to differentiate heart from lung disease. Children with suspected CHD undergo cardiac catheterization to confirm the anatomy and better establish which surgical procedures are indicated. Infants with persistent fetal circulation tend to tolerate cardiac catheterization poorly; thus, the previously mentioned noninvasive tests, particularly Doppler echocardiography, are preferable for differentiating heart from lung disease. In many tertiary newborn centers, infants, especially those with cyanotic lesions, are being sent to the operating suite for cardiovascular surgery based on a diagnosis established by noninvasive tests like echocardiography without undergoing a cardiac catheterization prior to surgery. When coronary artery anatomy needs to be defined or the question of venous drainage or collateral formation needs to be further defined, a cardiac catheterization may be needed.

IV. **Treatment of CHF.** The treatment of CHF is multifaceted. The arterial oxygen level may be increased by the administration of oxygen in most infants with CHF. If there is no systemic oxygen desaturation and the CHF is mild, it is unlikely that oxygen will be of benefit. Oxygen at high concentrations irritates the respiratory mucosa and occasionally favors the development of atelectasis by washing out nitrogen in the alveoli. It is therefore preferable to maintain the supplemental FIO_2 at the lowest therapeutic level that maintains adequate arterial saturations. Oxygen can also be detrimental in left heart lesions where pulmonary blood flow increases at the expense of systemic blood flow and can cause a cycle that can be difficult to break.

There is extensive evidence that digoxin improves myocardial function in patients with cardiomegaly and congestive heart failure. There is no evidence, however, that its administration improves the clinical condition if overt congestive heart failure is not present. During infancy, when rapid progression of untreated congestive heart failure is more common, early digitalization of patients with cardiomegaly is deemed advisable.

The major effects of digoxin on the failing myocardium are to increase the force of systolic contraction (inotropism) and increase the diastolic filling time by decreasing the heart rate (chronotropism). A beneficial but minor side effect of digoxin is its direct diuretic action, independent of its effects on the heart. Digoxin dosing is outlined in the appendix.

If CHF cannot be controlled with digoxin alone, diuretic therapy with an agent such as furosemide (Lasix) is added. A typical starting dose of furosemide is 1 mg/kg/day. This can be given either orally (p.o.), intramuscularly (IM), or intravenously (IV). The drug effect usually persists for 12 to 24 hours, and a once-daily dose is usually sufficient in mild CHF. With increasing CHF, the dose and frequency must be increased. Diuresis usually begins within 30 to 60 minutes, producing a significant loss of water, potassium chloride, and sodium. It is important to maintain adequate electrolyte balance when treating CHF. Following the introduction of diuretics, the urine contains a high concentration of chloride and sodium, more chloride than sodium (potassium or ammonium is excreted in place of sodium). The loss of chloride may produce alkalosis with a rise in the serum bicarbonate and a fall in the serum chloride level. Such hypochloremic alkalosis rarely itself produces symptoms, but it may cause a lack of responsiveness to further diuretics. Hypochloremic alkalosis may be corrected by administration of potassium chloride or occasionally by the administration of ammonium chloride. This generally restores responsiveness to diuretic therapy.

Hyponatremia may also be seen in patients with CHF. Dilutional hyponatremia may be associated with significant edema, thereby decreasing the concentration of sodium in the blood secondary to retention of greater quantities of free water in the body. This is corrected by restricting fluid intake. Acute sodium depletion may occur in the early stages of treatment if excessive or multiple methods of diuresis are used in association with salt restriction. Chronic sodium depletion may occur if a low-sodium diet and diuretics are employed. For this reason, low-sodium formulas are usually not used except in infants with refractory CHF. The symptoms of chronic sodium depletion include muscle weakness, lethargy, sleepiness, cramps, and poor tissue turgor. If these signs occur, a gradual or moderate increase in the dietary sodium generally alleviates this condition.

Potassium depletion may also occur with prolonged use of diuretics. The importance of hypokalemia is its propensity to increase the likelihood of digitalis intoxication. Therefore, infants with hypokalemia should be given supplemental potassium to prevent this complication. Spirtonolactone (Aldactone), a potassium-sparing diuretic, can also be useful. A typical dose of spironolactone is 1–3 mg/kg/day p.o. given once or twice daily.

It is essential to maintain adequate acid-base balance. Children with CHF, particularly those who are cyanotic or who have a left heart obstructive lesion (e.g., hypoplastic left heart syndrome, aortic stenosis, coarctation of the aorta), are prone to develop acidosis, which requires prompt correction.

Despite the need for fluid restriction and multiple medications for the control of CHF, it is imperative that adequate nutrition be maintained. Total energy expenditure has been shown to be significantly higher in infants with left-to-right shunts and CHF, as well as in patients with cyanosis; therefore, these infants benefit from higher caloric intake. It may be necessary to utilize formulas with caloric concentrations >20 calories per ounce. Smaller infants typically receive a 24-calories-per-ounce formula, although some may require as much as 27 to 30 calories per ounce to maintain adequate caloric intake without excessive fluid intake. It is important to guard against high renal solute load. This can be achieved by concentrating the formula to 24 calories per ounce and then adding supplemental calories in the form of a glucose polymer and/or medium-chain triglycerides. This can raise the concentration to as much as 30 calories per ounce.

V. **Cardiovascular surgery.** Corrective surgery is the ultimate goal for all congenital heart defects. Surgical procedures for the treatment of CHD may be divided into two groups: palliative and corrective.

    A. **Palliative procedures.** Palliative procedures are aimed primarily at either reducing or increasing pulmonary blood flow depending on the lesion. Infants with large left-to-right shunts and severe CHF may benefit from decreasing pulmonary blood flow, which aids in the control of CHF and protects against the development of pulmonary hypertension. However, the trend has been toward complete surgical repair earlier if possible. Pulmonary artery banding is performed in complex heart disease to prevent pulmonary hypertension when early repair is not an option. Single ventricle physiology surgical repairs are also considered palliative procedures, as complete correction is a 2- to 3-stage reconstruction (Fontan operation). Infants with cyanotic congenital heart lesions with decreased pulmonary artery blood flow may benefit from a systemic-pulmonary artery shunt. The most common systemic-to-pulmonary artery shunt is the Blalock-Taussig shunt, which consists of the anastomosis of a subclavian artery to the pulmonary artery. This can also be done by interposing a graft between the subclavian artery and the pulmonary artery. A central shunt is another option—it runs from the base of the brachiocephalic vessel to the pulmonary artery and provides better distribution of flow to both right and left pulmonary arteries.

Another palliative surgical procedure performed in some infants with cyanotic CHD is the balloon atrial septostomy. This procedure is performed on infants with complete transposition of the great vessels who require a large atrial septal defect to promote intracardiac mixing of desaturated and saturated blood in the atria. It is also performed on infants with tricuspid atresia, because the entire systemic venous return enters into the right atrium and then must pass through an atrial septal defect into the left atrium. The balloon atrial septostomy can be done emergently at the bedside under echocardiographic guidance or at initial cardiac catheterization if further diagnostic information (i.e., coronary artery anatomy) is needed prior to surgical repair. This procedure consists of passing a special catheter from the right atrium through the foramen ovale into the left atrium. A balloon at the tip of the catheter is then inflated with contrast solution. The catheter is pulled back through the foramen ovale resulting in a tear of the atrial septum.

B. Total corrective repair. Total repair is the only option for some congenital heart defects. These include transposition of the great vessels, truncus arteriosus, coarctation of the aorta, and total anomalous pulmonary venous return. These lesions require corrective surgery. There are several congenital heart lesions (e.g., ventricular septal defect, atrial septal defect, atrioventricular canal, tetralogy of Fallot) that may be repaired during early infancy but may have a higher operative mortality in the immediate newborn period than at a later date. Some would, therefore, attempt an early palliative procedure with the hopes of performing the corrective surgery some months later if necessary. On the other hand, with the improvement of cardiovascular surgical techniques, younger infants are undergoing successful early complete repair and thereby avoiding palliative procedures and the need for a second surgical procedure.

Many congenital lesions are also now being addressed in the cardiac catheterization lab and do not require surgical intervention at all. These include closure of a patent ductus arteriosus that is of the appropriate size by device closure or by coil embolization, device closure of secundum atrial septal defects, and balloon valvuloplasty of pulmonary and aortic stenosis.

VI. Arrythmias. The most common cause of a pathologic tachycardia in the newborn is paroxysmal supraventricular tachycardia (PSVT). This may occur *in utero* and lead to fetal hydrops. Neonates with paroxysmal atrial tachycardia may present with signs of CHF and cyanosis. Some infants have the electrocardiographic pattern of Wolff-Parkinson-White syndrome as the etiology of their PSVT. This is common in infants with Ebstein's anomaly. The long-term outlook for PSVT in the uncomplicated case is quite good. Digoxin is the drug of choice, but in infants with Wolff-Parkinson-White syndrome, it is usually safer to avoid digoxin as there may be a small risk for a rapid ventricular response. Usually a beta-blocker such as propranolol or atenolol or even amiodarone is a better choice. Electrocardioversion should be considered in the neonate who presents with PSVT and signs of severe congestive heart failure or cardiovascular collapse.

Although congenital heart block is a rare conduction abnormality in children, it presents frequently in the neonatal period. Most infants with a congenital complete heart block have no other anatomic cardiovascular defects. Detection may occur prenatally and, if it does, the mother should be tested for lupus. If hydrops, congenital heart block, and a heart lesion are detected prenatally, the prognosis for survival is very poor. Asymptomatic neonates may be discovered at routine examination to have a slower resting heart rate. Even without a structural heart defect, most infants with complete heart block have aortic systolic ejection murmur related to the increased stroke volume. Most infants with a resting heart rate of at least 70 beats per minute tolerate this quite well and usually do not require pacing. Those infants with resting heart rates below 50 beats per minute generally require long-term pacing. Other factors such as the presence or absence of CHF or associated congenital heart lesions determine whether pacing is required in infants with resting heart rates between 50 and 70 beats per minute.

VII. Clinical pearls and pitfalls.
- CHF usually presents in infants after 4 to 6 weeks of life as pulmonary vascular resistance drops. It can present simply as dyspnea or more severely with poor weight gain and failure to thrive.

- Common noncardiac causes of CHF include neonatal asphyxia, hypoxia, acidosis, hypoglycemia, sepsis, anemia, and polycythemia.
- Prolonged SVT in a newborn can present as CHF. However, many newborns are asymptomatic even after hours or days of persistent tachycardia.
- In newborns with cyanosis of suspected cardiac etiology, oxygen should be used only with significant hypoxia or desaturations (e.g., oxygen saturations lesser than 70%), as oxygen can be detrimental especially in infants with obstructed left heart lesions such as hypoplastic left heart syndrome and critical aortic stenosis. Oxygen in these situations can vasodilate the pulmonary vascular arteries and cause increased pulmonary blood flow at the expense of systemic perfusion.

BIBLIOGRAPHY

Allen HD, Gutgesell HP, Clark EB et al., eds. *Moss and Adams' heart disease in infants, children and adolescents*, 6th ed. Philadelphia, PA: Lippincott Williams & Wilkins, 2001.

Garson A, Bricker JT, Fisher DJ et al., eds. *The science and practice of pediatric cardiology*, 2nd ed. Philadelphia, PA: Lippincott Williams & Wilkins, 1997.

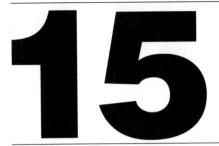

Fluid and Electrolyte Management

Vicki Powell-Tippit

I. **Description of the issue.** Management of fluid and electrolyte balance in the neonate is challenging. Although the same parameters are targeted as are in the older child and adult, several differences arise when addressing the newborn infant. Many of these differences are due to differences in gestational age, renal maturation, body composition, and endocrine influences governing fluid and electrolyte equilibrium. Developing an understanding of the mechanisms involved in maintaining body fluid homeostasis enables the practitioner to anticipate potential problems and prevent adverse circumstances from occurring.

II. **Physiology of body water and assessment of fluid balance in the neonate.** Total body water, the most abundant compound in the body, is contained in the intracellular and the extracellular compartments. In the adult, approximately two-thirds of total body water is contained in the intracellular compartment and accounts for nearly 70% of total body weight. This ratio differs significantly in the neonate, and fluctuation in body water distribution is dependent upon gestational age. Total body water composition in the developing fetus accounts for as much as 95% of total body weight, with the majority in the extracellular compartment. Total body water diminishes slowly as the fetus approaches term, when it comprises approximately 75% of total body weight. An alteration in fluid distribution occurs as well, with a shift into the intracellular compartment. However, even at term, intracellular water comprises only one-third of total body water, in contrast to two-thirds in the adult.

Following delivery, the term infant undergoes a period of diuresis resulting in a 5% to 10% loss of body weight during the first week of life. The premature infant also undergoes this physiologic diuresis; however, these infants often exhibit a greater body weight loss of 10% to 15%. Several factors, such as an increased extracellular fluid compartment, renal immaturity, and insensible water loss (IWL) influence this greater loss of body weight often observed in premature infants.

Renal function matures as gestational age increases, with complete nephrogenesis occurring at approximately 34 to 36 weeks gestation. Blood flow to the kidneys in the fetus is approximately 2% to 3% of cardiac output versus 15% to 18% in the adult. Following delivery, renal blood flow steadily increases as renal vascular resistance falls. The glomerular filtration rate, although enhanced by the increase in renal blood flow, remains reduced at birth in the term infant and even more so in the premature infant. By 2 weeks of age, the glomerular filtration has nearly doubled in the term infant; however, it remains decreased in those born prior to 34 to 36 weeks gestation, until nephrogenesis is complete.

Renal hormones, such as antidiuretic hormone and arginine vasopressin, in addition to the renin-angiotensin-aldosterone system, serve to alter the ability of neonates to maintain body fluid homeostasis. Immaturity of hormonal mechanisms also places neonates at risk for alterations in urine production and concentration, electrolyte disturbances, and under- or overhydration.

Fluid requirements in the neonatal population are influenced by a variety of factors and often fluctuate widely over the first few days following delivery. Close monitoring of laboratory values and clinical findings are important in the maintenance of fluid homeostasis. Inadequacy of proper hydration places the neonate at risk for dehydration, diminished vascular perfusion, and metabolic acidosis. On the other hand, excessive hydration may contribute to the development of congestive heart failure (CHF), a patent ductus arteriosus, and/or the development of chronic lung disease. The following parameters are useful in assessing fluid balance in the neonate.

A. **Body weight.** Total body weight is not always useful in determining fluid balance in the neonatal population, as internal shifts of body fluid may remain undetected. Nevertheless, the neonate should be weighed on a daily basis, and even more frequently if clinically indicated. Utilizing an electronic bed scale for the unstable or

165

premature infant will lessen the stress and decrease the cold exposure that can occur during the weighing process. Close attention should be paid to proper weighing techniques since variation may occur with the addition of supportive equipment such as ventilator circuits, intravenous (IV) tubing, and transducers.

B. Urine output. The amount of urine output varies with gestational age, fluid intake, perinatal events, and renal concentrating ability. The neonate usually voids within 24 hours following delivery, and the amount generally increases over the first 2 days of life. Neonates at risk for delayed spontaneous voiding include those exposed to maternal magnesium sulfate therapy and those requiring sedation. Attention should be directed to monitoring for bladder atony and distension that can result from these drug therapies. Normal urine output ranges from 1 to 3 mL/kg/hour. Oliguria is defined as urine output <0.5 to 1.0 mL/kg/hour.

Accurate collection and quantification of urine output in the neonatal population can be difficult. The most accurate means of urine collection is with an indwelling urinary catheter and collection chamber. However, routine use of indwelling urinary catheters may increase the risk of infection and trauma. The amount of urine can be reasonably quantified by the weighing of diapers. It is important to weigh diapers as soon as possible following the void as evaporation of urine decreases accuracy of measurement, especially in those infants under radiant warmers.

C. Clinical assessment. Performing a thorough physical examination that includes assessment of tissue turgor, anterior fontanelle fullness, moisture of mucous membranes, and presence of edema is helpful in determining fluid homeostasis. Edema alone may not be reflective of intravascular fluid excess. Extracellular edema may coexist with normal intravascular volume, and the restriction of fluid administration or the use of diuretic therapy in that case may compromise vascular perfusion. Additionally, frequent assessment of heart rate, blood pressure, and capillary refill time may also alert the clinician to changes in fluid status. Tachycardia and hypertension may be indicative of fluid excess, whereas, hypotension and delayed capillary refill time may indicate fluid depletion.

D. Blood chemistries. Blood chemistries should be analyzed, as these may be most reflective of changes in fluid status. In the determination of fluid status, blood chemistry analysis includes those entities listed in Table 15-1. In the ill or premature infant, the onset of blood sampling should begin at approximately 12 hours of age and continue regularly thereafter as clinically indicated. Initial measurements may reflect maternal electrolyte balance, and samples obtained after 12 to 24 hours are more reflective of the infant's fluid status. Blood samples may be obtained via heel stick; however, the risk of hemolysis is often greater with this type of sampling and may result in artificially elevated potassium levels. To ensure accuracy, a sample obtained via venipuncture or centrally placed intravascular catheter is optimal.

E. Fluid requirements. Fluid requirements vary depending upon the gestational age and size of the neonate in addition to the underlying disease process. For those neonates not receiving enteral feedings, the usual recommended intravenous fluid contains 10% dextrose. The endogenous glucose requirement of most neonates is 4 to 8 mg/kg/minute of glucose. The administration of 10% dextrose at 80 mL/kg/day will provide approximately 5 mg/kg/minute of glucose. In the term and near-term newborn, administration at this rate will usually provide an adequate amount of glucose to maintain normal serum glucose levels and conserve glycogen stores. The very premature infant may not tolerate this amount of glucose delivery secondary to a blunted response to insulin (see Chapter 7) and solutions containing 7.5% or 5.0% dextrose may be better tolerated. Table 15-2 outlines the recommended initial fluid recommendations for neonates during the first days of life.

F. Insensible water loss (IWL). IWL must be taken into consideration upon calculating the total fluid requirements in the neonate. The total fluid requirement is a summation of maintenance fluid requirements, replacement of fluid losses, and additional allowances to promote growth. IWL is reflective of water loss through the skin and from the respiratory tract, and may account for as much as a third of the total fluid requirement. IWL increases with decreasing size and gestational age of the neonate. Further, the proportional surface area from which evaporative water loss can occur is greater in the premature infant. The premature infant also experiences higher evaporative losses secondary to the increased permeability of the epidermis during the first weeks of life. Complications resulting from high IWL include hypernatremic dehydration, hypotension, diminished perfusion, metabolic acidosis, and renal failure. The factors that influence IWL are summarized in Table 15-3.

Table 15-1. Laboratory analysis of body fluid/hydration status

Common chemistries	Body fluid status	Influencing factors
Hematocrit	—	The hematocrit remains too variable in the neonatal period to provide an accurate reflection of body fluid status.
Urine specific gravity	—	Urine specific gravity may reflect urine osmolality; however, often it is unreliable if contaminated with blood, protein, or glucose.
Blood gas analysis	A metabolic acidosis may exist with underhydration	Acid–base balance can be affected by a variety of disease processes.
Serum sodium	Hypernatremia may be reflective of underhydration secondary to insensible fluid loss or inadequate fluid intake	Serum sodium levels are influenced by intracellular and extracellular fluid volume(s), hormonal regulation, and sodium delivery.
Serum creatinine	—	Early values are reflective of placental clearance and often remain elevated during the first few days of life, especially in those born prematurely.
Serum osmolality	Often increased with underhydration and decreased with overhydration	The value may be estimated by doubling the serum sodium level. In the syndrome of inappropriate antidiuretic hormone (SIADH), the serum osmolality is decreased in conjunction with hyponatremia. Additionally, the urine osmolality and sodium levels rise.
Blood urea nitrogen	May be increased with underhydration	Tissue catabolism, high protein intake, and renal hypoperfusion may increase levels as well.

Table 15-2. Initial fluid recommendations

Birth weight (g)	<24 h[a] (mL/kg/d)	24–48 h[a] (mL/kg/d)	>48 h[3] (mL/kg/d)
<1000	100–120	120–140	140–160
1000–1500	90–100	100–120	120–160
1500–2000	80–90	90–120	120–160
>2000	60–80	80–100	100–150

[a]During the first week of life, calculations are usually based on birth weight.

Table 15-3. Factors influencing insensible water loss

Increases insensible water loss
Radiant warmers
Phototherapy
High ambient temperature
Congenital defects (e.g., abdominal wall and neural tube defects)
Respiratory distress

Decreases insensible water loss
Plastic blanket with radiant warmer use
Incubators
High humidity (60%–70%)
Semipermeable dressings
Warmed and humidified inspired gases

III. **Electrolyte requirements and disorders of electrolyte balance.** Electrolyte requirements are somewhat variable in neonates, especially those born prematurely. Electrolytes are generally not added to IV fluids during the initial 24 to 48 hours following
birth. Diminished urinary excretion of sodium and potassium, in conjunction with IWL,
makes accurate assessment of electrolyte status difficult during the first few days of life.
Frequent serum electrolyte analysis in addition to frequent clinical assessment can be
helpful in the management of electrolyte balance.

A. **Sodium.** Sodium is the major extracellular cation and serves to play a role in the regulation of water balance. Sodium assists in controlling the osmotic equilibrium between the intracellular and extracellular compartments. A surplus of extracellular
sodium results in hypertonicity of intravascular fluid, causing the shift of fluid from
the intracellular to the extracellular compartment, which can result in cellular dehydration. Conversely, a deficit of extracellular sodium triggers the shift of fluid into
the intracellular compartment, resulting in cellular edema.

Neonates frequently experience a negative sodium balance during the first week
of life secondary to the shift of fluid from the extracellular compartment. This negative balance is often tolerated as long as the serum sodium levels remain within a
normal range. Following the first week of life, a positive sodium balance is important
to support the growth of new tissue. Because renal and hormonal maturation influence sodium balance, the sodium requirement varies inversely with gestational age.
The sodium requirement for the normal term infant is 2 to 3 mEq/kg/day. The premature infant, especially those weighing <1,500 g, experiences dramatic changes in
sodium requirements over the first few days of life and may require 4 to 6
mEq/kg/day due to renal immaturity and urinary loses.

1. **Hyponatremia.** Clinical manifestations of acute hyponatremia may include irritability, lethargy, apnea, tremors, or seizure activity. Many neonates remain asymptomatic; therefore, frequent blood serum analysis is important. Those suffering
from chronic hyponatremia, such as the "growing preemie," may remain clinically
asymptomatic, however, this may result in poor growth and poor weight gain.

Treatment of hyponatremia should focus on correcting the underlying cause. Mild
hyponatremia can often be corrected over a period of several days. However, when
severe or symptomatic hyponatremia is encountered, immediate action should be
taken toward correcting the disorder. One should attempt to raise the serum sodium
to 125 mEq/L using 3% normal saline (0.5 mEq Na$^+$/L) and the following equation:

Equation for sodium replacement therapy

$$[\text{desired serum Na}^+ \ (125 \ \text{mEq/L}) - \text{actual serum Na}^+] \times 0.6 \times \text{wt (kg)}$$

$$= \text{dose needed for correction in mEq of Na}^+ \ *$$

*Replace over 1 to 2 hours; check **Na$^+$** level at halfway point of correction (as full
dose may not be necessary).

Example: Five-day-old infant weighing 1.4 kg born at 30 weeks gestation with a
serum sodium of 119 mEq per L.
$(125 - 119) \times 0.6 \times 1.4 = 5 \ \text{mEq Na}^+$ required. Using 3% normal saline (0.5
mEq/mL), 10 mL of 3% normal saline will be required.

Once enteral feedings are established, the provision of an infant formula adequate
in meeting the electrolyte requirements for the targeted gestational age is necessary. In premature infants receiving breast milk, which is low in sodium, fortification should be initiated once full enteral feedings have been established and
subsequently continued until nephrogenesis is complete.

2. **Syndrome of inappropriate antidiuretic hormone.** The syndrome of inappropriate
antidiuretic hormone (SIADH) is the condition of excessive secretion of antidiuretic
hormone, that is, arginine vasopressin, in the absence of appropriate stimuli such
as high plasma osmolality or low blood volume. Conditions such as sepsis, asphyxia,
respiratory distress, and central nervous system pathology may trigger this excessive, inappropriate antidiuretic hormone secretion. Excess of the hormone results in
decreased urine output, increased urine sodium excretion, increased urine osmolality, and a dilutional hyponatremia with serum hypoosmolality.

Diagnosis of SIADH includes measuring serum and urine electrolyte levels,
and the analysis of serum and urine osmolality. The restriction of fluid intake
is the mainstay of treatment of SIADH when serum sodium levels remain stable at >120 mEq per L. When serum sodium levels are below 120 mEq per L,

the administration of furosemide and an infusion of hypertonic sodium chloride (3%) may become necessary.

3. **Hypernatremia.** Hypernatremia (serum Na >145 mEq per L) is often reflective of a deficit in total body water in relation to total body sodium content. Common etiologies may include an inadequacy in free water intake, increased IWL, and breastfeeding failure sometimes encountered in the term infant. Hypernatremia may also occur as a result of excessive sodium intake, for example, that which may follow the administration of sodium bicarbonate in the treatment of metabolic acidosis. Rarely, hypernatremia may result from a reduction in antidiuretic hormone production (diabetes insipidus), either of central or nephrogenic in origin.

Initial clinical manifestations of hypernatremia often coincide with those of dehydration, including weight loss, decreased urine output, tachycardia, hypotension, and metabolic acidosis. However, neonates suffering from diabetes insipidus may excrete urine in normal dilution and amount. Neurologic symptoms can occur with severe hypernatremia and may include irritability or lethargy, apnea, and seizure activity. Of great importance is the fact that alterations in sodium balance, or plasma osmolality, may increase the risk of intraventricular hemorrhage in the premature infant.

As with hyponatremia, treatment of hypernatremia should target the underlying cause of the disorder. Close attention to fluid and sodium intake is vital. When a deficit in fluid balance is encountered, an increase in free water administration should be considered. If sodium supplementation has occurred, then sodium intake should be gradually restricted in order to avoid rapid changes in plasma osmolality.

B. **Potassium.** Potassium functions with sodium in regulating cell membrane potential and it is the major cation residing within the intracellular space. The distribution of extracellular and intracellular potassium is governed by a sodium-potassium pump mechanism, the function of which is dependent on gestational age, renal maturity, and acid-base balance. Serum potassium levels often fail to accurately reflect total body potassium because the measurement reflects only the potassium in the extracellular compartment. Falsely elevated levels of serum potassium may be measured in specimens that contain hemolyzed red blood cells that have released their intracellular potassium during the hemolytic process. This is a common occurrence in specimens obtained by heel stick.

The premature infant of less then 32 weeks gestation is especially prone to alterations in potassium homeostasis secondary to catabolism and a decreased glomerular filtration rate. Within this population, the serum potassium level generally rises within the initial 24 to 72 hours, even in the absence of supplemental potassium administration and/or renal failure. This increase in serum levels is thought to result from the shifting of potassium from the intracellular compartment to the extracellular compartment. A fall in the serum level often occurs following 72 hours of age as the diuretic phase takes place. This decrease is thought to result from an increase in water and sodium delivery to the distal nephron, resulting in urinary potassium excretion. Premature and extremely-low-birth-weight infants, especially those under 28 weeks gestation and/or weighing <1,000 g, are particularly prone to significant alterations in potassium balance.

Potassium supplementation is not recommended until the second or third day of life and only when urinary output is well established. The usual daily requirement for potassium supplementation in the neonatal population is from 2 to 3 mEq/kg/day.

1. **Hypokalemia.** Hypokalemia, defined as a serum potassium (K^+) <3.5 mEq per L, signifies intracellular depletion as 90% of total body potassium resides in the intracellular compartment. If left untreated, a subnormal potassium level will adversely affect cell function, especially those found in the cardiac and gastrointestinal systems. Factors associated with hypokalemia include inadequate potassium intake, increased nasogastric and ileostomy drainage resulting in metabolic alkalosis, and the administration of certain medications such as insulin, bicarbonate, and certain diuretics.

Clinical manifestations may include hypotonia, abdominal distention and ileus, and cardiac arrhythmias. An electrocardiogram may be reflective of conduction defects such as a prolonged QT interval, the presence of prominent U waves, flattened T waves, or ST interval suppression.

Treatment of hypokalemia should focus on the underlying cause. Careful clinical assessment and frequent blood chemistry analysis should be performed. Potassium supplementation should be initiated following the second to third day of life once serum levels have stabilized (4 to 4.5 mEq/L) and adequate urine output has been established. Additional supplementation may become necessary for those infants at increased risk for hypokalemia, particularly those suffering from gastrointestinal losses or from the adverse effects of certain medications. Correction of hypokalemia is best accomplished by intravenous potassium supplementation that provides 2 to 3 mEq/kg/day via a constant infusion. Rapid administration, or a bolus dosing of potassium, is generally not recommended as potentially fatal cardiac arrhythmias may occur. Once potassium levels have normalized, supplementation may be continued by intravenous infusion or orally after enteral feedings have been established.

2. **Hyperkalemia.** Hyperkalemia, defined as a serum potassium >6.0 mEq per L, is one of most common life-threatening disturbances in electrolyte balance in the neonatal population, especially in premature infants. This imbalance is often secondary to a shift of potassium from the intracellular to the extracellular compartment. Because hyperkalemia can occur rather suddenly, close attention should be paid to those infants with the risk factors listed in Table 15-4.

Clinical manifestations of hyperkalemia are similar to those of hypokalemia and include hypotonia, abdominal distention, and cardiac arrhythmias. Electrocardiogram findings seem to correlate with the serum potassium level and include the peaking of T waves, flattening of P waves, widening of the QRS, and, ultimately, the development of ventricular tachycardia or sinus bradycardia, and fibrillation. When elevated serum potassium levels are encountered, the hyperkalemia should never be simply attributed to hemolysis of the specimen. A second blood sample should be obtained, preferably centrally rather than by heel stick, to verify the results in addition to performing other diagnostic studies that may prove helpful in identifying the underlying cause. Additional studies to consider include measurement of blood pH, serum ionized calcium, blood urea nitrogen, and serum creatinine.

Once the diagnosis of hyperkalemia has been made, all sources of exogenous potassium to the neonate should be discontinued. Treatment should then focus on rehydration, facilitating the intracellular uptake of potassium, and the prevention of cardiac arrhythmias. Initial interventions may include intravenous fluid resuscitation, correction of acid-base imbalance, the administration of diuretics, and/or certain aerosolized bronchodilators. A low-dose dopamine infusion might be considered to enhance renal perfusion. Additional interventions should be aimed toward reducing the effects of hyperkalemia on conducting tissues and enhancing cellular uptake of potassium. Calcium gluconate 10%, administered intravenously, will often serve to stabilize the cardiac cell membrane, and the initiation of a glucose and insulin infusion may enhance cellular uptake of potassium. The administration of a cation exchange agent (e.g., Kayexalate) may be considered, especially when severe hyperkalemia is encountered. Additional modalities to consider with severe hyperkalemia, particularly when changes involving cardiac conduction are encountered, may include a double-volume exchange transfusion or peritoneal dialysis.

Table 15-4. Risk factors significant for hyperkalemia

Condition	Causative mechanism
Extremely low birth weight, metabolic acidosis	Shift of potassium from intracellular to extracellular compartment in response to acidosis.
Trauma, tissue destruction, ecchymosis, disseminated intravascular coagulation, hemorrhage, intraventricular hemorrhage, hypoperfusion	Increased potassium release from traumatized or hemolyzed cells.
Renal failure	Decreased potassium clearance.
Excessive potassium supplementation, blood transfusion	Increased potassium delivery.

IV. **Renal failure.** Acute renal failure (ARF) in the neonate is frequently characterized by oliguria (urine output <0.5 to 1.0 mL/kg/hour) after the first 24 to 48 hours of life and a serum creatinine level of >1.5 mg per dL. Causative factors associated with ARF are divided into the prerenal, intrinsic, or postrenal categories (Table 15-5). Prerenal failure results from renal hypoperfusion and is the most common cause of ARF in the neonatal population. If left untreated, continued renal hypoperfusion may result in intrinsic renal damage. Intrinsic renal failure may also result from the presence of certain congenital disorders or following the administration of nephrotoxic medications. Postrenal failure remains the least common cause of renal failure in the neonate and is the result of obstruction of urine flow.

A. **Diagnosis.** Diagnosis of ARF should begin with a review of the neonate's clinical history with emphasis placed on the identification of risk factors. Attention should then focus on performing a thorough clinical assessment (Table 15-6) and obtaining the necessary diagnostic evaluation (Table 15-7).

B. **Management.** Management of ARF in the neonatal population requires a comprehensive approach and must address the underlying cause. A diagnosis aimed at differentiating between the three types of renal failure should be made, and timely intervention should be implemented so that further compromise to the renal system may be avoided. Table 15-8 outlines the management of ARF.

V. **Clinical pearls.**
- With complete nephrogenesis not occurring until 34 to 36 weeks gestation, the glomerular filtration rate is diminished in infants born prior to this gestation and will remain so until the age when complete nephrogenesis has been reached. This must be taken into consideration when addressing alterations in electrolyte balance and in the administration of potentially nephrotoxic medications.
- Fluid requirements fluctuate widely over the first few days following delivery and close monitoring of laboratory values and clinical findings are important in the maintenance of fluid homeostasis.
- IWL must be taken into consideration upon calculating the total fluid requirements in the neonate.
- A positive sodium balance is necessary to support the growth of new tissue.
- Falsely elevated serum potassium levels may result from red blood cell hemolysis. This is a common occurrence in specimens obtained by heel stick.

Table 15-5. Common causes of acute renal failure in the neonate

Prerenal
Hypovolemia
Hypotension
Dehydration
Sepsis
Asphyxia
Congenital heart disease
Necrotizing enterocolitis
Indomethacin administration

Intrinsic
Bilateral renal dysplasia or agenesis
Polycystic kidney disease
Renal artery or venous thrombosis
Sustained renal hypoperfusion resulting in acute tubular necrosis
Infection and inflammation
Drug induced: aminoglycosides, indomethacin, amphotericin B, radiographic contrast media

Postrenal
Urethral obstruction or stricture
Bilateral ureteral obstruction
Ureterocele
Neurogenic bladder

Table 15-6. Clinical assessment

Body weight
   Note fluctuations in daily weight greater than anticipated based on fluid and caloric intake

Urine output
   Oliguria – less than 0.5–1.0 mL/kg/h following the first 24 to 48 h of life

Presence of edema
Assessment of blood pressure, heart rate, and vascular perfusion
Presence of bladder distention or abdominal mass

Table 15-7. Diagnostic evaluation

Serum
   Electrolytes: hyponatremia, hyperkalemia, hypocalcemia, hyperphosphatemia
   Creatinine: >1.5 mg/dL (or increasing ≥0.3 mg/dL/d)
   Osmolality: increased
   BUN: increased (an increase may be resultant of additional influences, however)
   pH: metabolic acidosis
   Glucose: increased

Urine
   Sodium: may be increased with intrinsic renal failure
   Creatinine: decreased
   Osmolality: decreased
   Urinalysis: microscopic evaluation to assess for casts and tubular cells
   Presence of hematuria
   Proteinuria
   Culture

Radiologic Evaluation
   Ultrasound
   Voiding cystourethrogram
   Radionuclide scintigraphy

Table 15-8. Management of acute renal failure

- Obtain body weight once to twice daily.
- Maintain an accurate record of intake and output. The placement of a urinary catheter will ensure accurate accounting of urine output and may help rule out a lower urinary tract obstruction.
- Observe for signs of dehydration or fluid overload.
- Monitor vital signs especially blood pressure as hypertension may require pharmacologic intervention.
- Monitor serum glucose, electrolytes, acid–base status, and treat imbalances accordingly.
- Follow urine studies closely.
- Fluid restriction.
- Maintain optimal nutrition status; however, restriction of protein to 1 to 2 g/kg/d may become necessary.
- Avoid the use of nephrotoxic medications.
- In the absence of congestive heart failure or fluid overload, a fluid challenge of normal saline (10–20 mL/kg) given over 1 h may be considered, followed by the administration of furosemide. A rapid response is often indicative of a prerenal cause, whereas no response may suggest an intrinsic or postrenal etiology.
- Dialysis or hemofiltration may be considered when conservative management has been proven to be unsuccessful.

BIBLIOGRAPHY

Polin RA, Yoder MC, Burg FD. *Workbook in practical neonatology*, 3rd ed. Philadelphia, PA: WB Saunders, 2001:29–46.

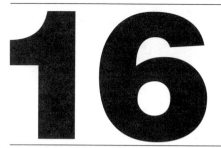

Neonatal Neurology

Deborah K. Sokol and
Gregory M. Sokol

Part 1–Neurologic Examination of the Newborn

I. **Description of the issue.** The neurologic examination is an important part of the evaluation of the newborn infant. The examination is performed in a systematic order, including observation of the newborn and evaluation of the cranium, developmental reflexes, cranial nerves, and motor function.

II. **Observation.** Ideally, the newborn should be examined during the maximal state of alertness, several hours after feeding. General inspection of the body may uncover congenital anomalies such as midline defects in the form of cleft lip and palate, or neural tube defects. Examination of the skin is important owing to the shared embryologic beginnings of the skin and nervous system. A port wine stain over the eyelid and forehead (cranial nerve VI distribution) may suggest Sturge Weber syndrome (Fig. 16-1); café au lait spots may suggest Neurofibromatosis Type 1 (Fig. 16-2).

The normal posture for a term newborn is the flexed position with bilateral flexion at the elbows and knees. The more mature the infant, the greater the flexion, whereas the premature infant will be more lax and extended. The baby should spontaneously extend all limbs at random. Failure to do so may represent hypotonia or hemiparesis. Breathing with the help of intercostal muscles is expected, while the appearance of see-saw chest wall excursion or a "sucking in" of the sternum may indicate spinal muscular atrophy.

Newborns exhibiting seizures frequently have a decreased state of arousal. The clinician may evaluate an infant's state by assessing the levels of alertness, arousal, and responsiveness. Hypoxic-ischemic encephalopathy may present with altered states of consciousness ranging from increased irritability to unresponsiveness. For example, can the infant be brought to the awake state or does he/she remain lethargic or asleep? Likewise, the quality of response to arousal may be assessed. These findings can help classify the presence or severity of encephalopathy from mild to moderate or severe.

III. **Evaluation of the cranium.** The occipito-frontal head circumference (OFC) is a measure of brain growth. The OFC should be measured in all babies and the value should then be plotted on a gender-specific graph. Microcephaly may represent intrauterine growth restriction or infection, maternal drug abuse and poor nutrition, or genetic abnormality. Macrocephaly may represent cephalohematoma, hydrocephalus, or megaloencephaly. The anterior fontanel should be palpated while the child is held in the sitting position. Crying or increased intracranial pressure can cause this fontanel to bulge. The cranial sutures can be overriding for up to 1 week in infants delivered vaginally. Asymmetric, premature suture closure may result in plagiocephaly (misshapen head), but this usually does not present until a few months of age.

IV. **Developmental reflexes.** Developmental reflexes are stereotypic responses that are achieved by certain ages. Three common primitive reflexes present in the newborn are the Moro, the palmer grasp, and the asymmetric tonic neck reflex. They represent integrity of the brainstem and spinal cord. A generalized decrease in these reflexes at birth implies diffuse depression of brain function. Many primitive reflexes are present at birth and then go away as the infant matures. Persistence of these reflexes beyond their expected extinction suggests impaired central nervous system (CNS) function. The Moro reflex usually disappears by 6 months, the palmar grasp by 2 months, and the tonic neck reflex by 7 months. Asymmetry of motor movement during the response also may point to an abnormality such as Erb or Klumpke brachial plexus palsies or fractures of the humerus or clavicle.

V. **Cranial nerves.**
   A. **Cranial nerve 1 – Olfactory.** Virtually all infants over the age of 32 weeks show arrest of arousal and /or sucking activity when exposed to pleasant aromas such as cinnamon or cloves.

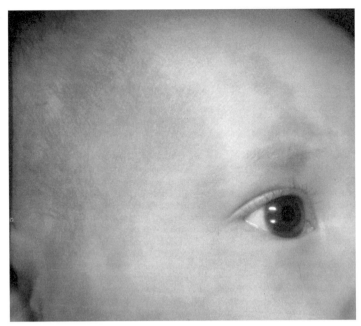

Figure 16-1. Port wine stain in the distribution of cranial nerve VI seen in a neonate with Sturge Weber syndrome.

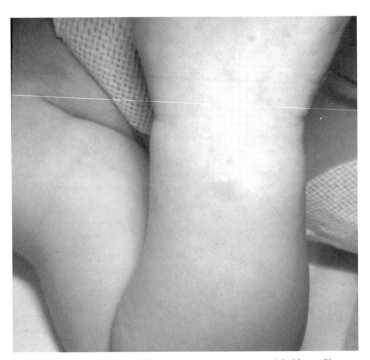

Figure 16-2. Café au lait spot seen on the forearm of a neonate with Neurofibromatosis Type 1.

B. Cranial nerves II, III, IV, VI – Assessment of visual system. The pupils should be symmetric and reactive to light. Babies should be able to visually fix and follow the face of the examiner or a large red target. Infants should blink symmetrically with light flashed into their eyes. The presence of ptosis may indicate congenital myasthenia gravis, myotonic dystrophy, Horner syndrome, Mobius syndrome, or congenital myopathy. Should a metabolic genetic disorder be suspected, a formal ophthalmologic consult should be obtained to look for retinal abnormalities, hypoplastic optic nerves, or cataracts.

The Doll's eye maneuver tests the integrity of cranial nerves III and VI and the brainstem nuclei of these nerves. The examiner gently rotates the infant's head from one side to the other. The eyes should move together in the direction opposite to the rotation of the head.

C. Cranial nerve VII – Facial nerve. Cranial Nerve VII innervates the muscles of the forehead, eyelid, and cheek. Facial movements are readily observed when the baby is crying: the brow is wrinkled, the eye is closed, and the angle of the mouth is depressed. Cranial nerve VII can be damaged by pressure incurred from positioning during labor or forceps application during delivery. An asymmetric cry with lack of depression of the angle of the mouth on one side suggests cranial nerve damage on that side. Agenesis of the motor nucleus of cranial nerve VII is seen in Mobius syndrome and involvement is bilateral. A purely lower lip weakness may be caused by hypoplasia of the depressor muscle of the mouth, unrelated to any cranial nerve VII abnormality.

D. Cranial nerve VIII – Hearing. Due to variability in infant responsiveness to bedside auditory examination, universal hearing screening via brain stem auditory evoked response testing or other automated assessment is recommended.

E. Cranial nerves IX, X, and XII – Assessment of swallow and tongue movement. The infant should be observed while feeding. A gag reflex is present in term newborns and requires normal function of cranial nerves IX and X. The function of these nerves may also be assessed when the newborn is crying. Infants with depressed CNS function may demonstrate an infrequent, weak cry. During crying, the tongue can be inspected for asymmetry or loss of bulk, implying abnormality in cranial nerve XII or its nucleus. The presence of fasciculation may indicate spinal muscular atrophy.

VI. Motor function. Tone is the resistance to passive movement whereas strength is the ability to overcome gravity or resistance to perform a movement. Gentle movement of the infant's limbs while the newborn is supine enables the assessment of muscle tone and strength. Clues from the observation period should direct this assessment by further examination of the strength and tone of the limb or limbs showing decreased movement.

The infant should be held in the horizontal and vertical positions to determine if flexor tone of the limbs is present and symmetric. Horizontal suspension can help determine head control while vertical suspension can detect hypotonia if the infant tends to slide through the examiner's hands. The most common cause of generalized decreased tone is depression of CNS function, which may be due to hypoxic-ischemic encephalopathy, intraventricular hemorrhage (IVH), neonatal sepsis, or metabolic abnormalities. Both tone and strength can be decreased in neuromuscular conditions such as spinal muscular atrophy, congenital myopathy, and neonatal myotonic dystrophy. Muscle tone can be increased in hypoxic-ischemic encephalopathy, IVH, and congenital malformations. Asymmetry of strength and tone, that is, hemiparesis, may indicate a neonatal stroke.

Deep tendon reflexes, elicited with a reflex hammer, can be symmetrically brisk or absent in the normal newborn. Cerebral damage may cause exaggerated, brisk reflexes or, alternately, depressed reflexes, and the findings must be corroborated with the rest of the exam. Asymmetric brisk reflexes on one side may indicate upper motor neuron disease such as a neonatal stroke, whereas asymmetric absent reflexes may represent lower motor neuron disease such as brachial plexus injury. Absent reflexes together with flaccidity of the lower extremities implicates spinal cord damage, a neurologic emergency. Up to eight beats of clonus at the ankles can be seen in normal newborns. Jaw or full body clonus, often a sign of an immature CNS, occasionally can be elicited and should not be mistaken for a seizure.

VII. Clinical pearls.
- The most common cause of decreased generalized tone is central nervous system depression.
- Failure to move and extend an extremity may be a sign of hypotonia or hemiparesis in a newborn.

Part 2–Neonatal Seizures

I. **Description of the issue.** Seizures are the most common overt manifestation of brain injury in the newborn period. Neonatal seizures represent a medical emergency, as they are associated with mortality and neurologic morbidity. Recognition and treatment of neonatal seizures is important, as prolonged seizures, per se, may cause further brain injury.

   A. **Risk factors.** An increased incidence of seizures is found in infants of very low birth weight (VLBW) (<1,500 g) as opposed to heavier infants, and in infants of mothers with fever during labor. In infants experiencing perinatal depression, the following risk factors have been associated with neonatal seizures: 5-minute Apgar score of 5 or less, fetal acidemia, and intubation in the delivery room.

   B. **Clinical manifestations.** The newborn brain is more prone to seizures than is the mature brain, although electrographic seizure activity usually remains localized to one hemisphere. The reason for the lack of electrical conduction of seizures across cerebral hemispheres is the immature connections between brain cells in the newborn brain. Therefore, newborns rarely show well organized, generalized tonic clonic seizures. Four seizure types can be recognized: subtle, clonic, tonic, and myoclonic. The clinical manifestations of seizures are listed in Table 16-1.

   1. **Subtle seizures.** Subtle seizures are most commonly indicated by abnormal eye movements. In premature infants, sustained eye opening is seen; in term infants, horizontal deviation of the eyes is more prominent. Other signs of subtle seizures include unusual repetitive movements such as sucking, chewing, blinking, swimming movements of the arms, or pedaling movements of the legs. Apnea is more likely to be a sign of subtle seizures in the term infant, whereas apnea in the premature infant is more likely to be of nonepileptic cause. Apnea accompanying a seizure is less likely to be associated with bradycardia than is nonconvulsive apnea. The electroencephalogram (EEG) may not detect subtle seizures.

   2. **Clonic seizures.** Clonic seizures are rhythmic jerks (one to three jerks per second) with a focal (one side of the body) or multifocal (several body parts) distribution. These are readily detected via EEG.

   3. **Tonic seizures.** Tonic seizures are characterized by sustained posturing of one or several extremities. These may resemble decerebrate posturing and may or may not be detectable by EEG.

   4. **Myoclonic seizures.** Myoclonic seizures are focal, multifocal, or generalized twitches. They are distinguished from clonic seizures by the more rapid speed of the myoclonic jerk and by their appearance in the distribution of flexor muscles. Myoclonic seizures can be associated with severe neonatal epileptic syndromes and can be detected by EEG.

   Not all repetitive movements are seizures. Jitter, a kind of tremulousness, can be confused with seizures. Differentiation of jitter from seizure can be made at the bedside. In contrast to seizures, abnormal eye movements or autonomic changes such as an increase in heart rate or blood pressure do not accompany jitter. While seizures occur randomly, jitter can be elicited via a noise or handling the infant. Unlike seizures, jitter can be stopped by gentle passive flexion of the affected limb.

   C. **Etiology.** There are a wide variety of causes of neonatal seizures and many require specific treatment. Therefore, determining the cause of the seizure is essential. Hypoxic-ischemic encephalopathy associated with perinatal depression, intracranial

Table 16-1. Clinical manifestations of seizures

Abnormal cry
Apnea
Autonomic disturbances in heart rate and/or blood pressure
Chewing or sucking motions
Complex movements (e.g., "swimming," "bicycling")
Facial twitching
Limpness
Myoclonic jerk
Nystagmus or horizontal eye deviation
Tonic-clonic movements
Tonic extension of limb or body
Vasomotor changes

hemorrhage, intracranial infection, and developmental defects account for the majority of neonatal seizures. Metabolic disturbances, drug withdrawal/toxicity, and idiopathic seizure disorders are less frequent causes, but should also be considered (Table 16-2).

1. **Hypoxic-ischemic encephalopathy.** Hypoxic-ischemic encephalopathy is the most common cause of neonatal seizures in both premature and term infants. Evidence of perinatal depression may be obvious at birth, but the episode may have occurred prior to the intrapartum period. For intrapartum events, umbilical cord blood gases provide insight into the fetal status immediately prior to birth. The severely asphyxiated infant will show stupor with hypotonia followed by hypertonia. Cerebral edema is frequently present. These infants often develop seizures within the first 24 hours of life that can be difficult to control. Multisystem organ dysfunction is frequently present (renal insufficiency/failure, elevated liver enzymes, disseminated intravascular coagulation). Stupor persisting for more than 1 week is associated with poor neurologic recovery.

2. **Infection.** Bacterial or viral infections are the cause of 5% to 10% of neonatal seizures. Approximately 50% of neonates with meningitis develop seizures. The onset of seizures is usually in the latter part of the first week of life. Intrauterine infection with toxoplasmosis or cytomegalovirus may result in seizures within the first 3 days of life. Cerebral calcifications (best visualized on head CT) are seen in both types of infection. A characteristic "blueberry muffin" skin rash is seen with cytomegalovirus infection.

   Herpes simplex encephalitis is usually acquired perinatally and, therefore, the onset of seizures is delayed. Congenital lesions have occurred. A vesicular skin rash should raise the suspicion of herpes, but only one-third of infants present with these findings. Fever within the first week of life or the presence of hepatitis should raise the index of suspicion for herpes. Infants with herpes, cytomegalovirus (CMV), or toxoplasmosis should be evaluated for ocular involvement of disease.

3. **Intracranial hemorrhage.** Intraventricular hemorrhage (IVH) occurs primarily in premature infants less than 32 weeks gestational age and weighing less than 1500 g. Approximately 30% of VLBW infants experience IVH, with most cases occurring in the first 3 days of life. With severe IVH, seizures are generalized tonic, often heralding deterioration, coma, and death. These infants are at increased risk of developing posthemorrhagic hydrocephalus. Subtle seizures also may occur in infants experiencing IVH.

Table 16-2. Causes of neonatal seizures

Acute metabolic disorders
    Hypoglycemia[a]
    Hypocalcemia[a]
    Hypomagnesemia
    Hypo/hypernatremia
    Hyperbilirubinemia/kernicterus
Congenital brain malformations[a]
Drug withdrawal/toxicity
Hypoxic-ischemic encephalopathy[a]
Infection
    Sepsis[a]
    Meningitis[a]
    Encephalitis
    Congenital (e.g. toxoplasmosis, cytomegalovirus)
Intracranial hemorrhage[a]
    Intraventricular
    Subarachnoid
    Subdural
Inborn errors of metabolism
Ischemic stroke
Neonatal epilepsy

[a]Common causes

Birth trauma with or without instrumentation can result in subdural hemorrhage. Infants who experience subdural hemorrhage may present with focal clonic or tonic seizures. Subarachnoid hemorrhage is another intracranial hemorrhage presenting in the newborn period. It is very common and often presents without any clinical manifestations. When seizures do occur, it is usually on the second postnatal day in infants who are otherwise asymptomatic, that is, the "well baby" with seizures.

4. **Intrauterine stroke.** Intrauterine arterial ischemic stroke accounts for a large proportion of stroke in children, as 25% to 30% of pediatric ischemic stroke patients present within the first month of life. The majority of strokes are in the distribution of the left middle cerebral artery. In term infants, seizures associated with strokes present as clonic jerks in the extremities contralateral to the side of the stroke (usually the right arm), without loss of consciousness.

5. **Metabolic causes.** Metabolic causes of seizures usually present in the first 3 days of life. Hypoglycemia, especially of long duration in small-for-gestational-age infants of diabetic mothers, can cause seizures. Seizures are less frequent in hypoglycemic infants of normal or above average birth weight who are born to diabetic mothers than they are in small infants.

Early onset hypocalcemia with serum levels less than 7 mg/dL can occur in premature, sick, or asphyxiated infants and may result in seizures. Late onset hypocalcemic seizures are more commonly caused by endocrine problems or congenital heart disease (DiGeorge syndrome). The ionized fraction of calcium represents the physiologically active component and should be measured if possible. Hypomagnesemia should be considered in an infant with hypocalcemia who is unresponsive to calcium therapy.

Hyponatremia may result after excessive water intake or with inappropriate secretion of antidiuretic hormone that may be associated with pulmonary disorders, IVH, or meningitis. Hypernatremia is more common in the premature infant secondary to excessive fluid losses but also may occur in the term infant with improper mixing or inadequate intake of formulas.

6. **Congenital brain malformations.** Brain developmental abnormalities are responsible for 5% to 10% of cases of neonatal seizures. Congenital infections, chromosomal or metabolic disorders, and drugs can interfere with normal neuronal proliferation and migration in the fetal brain. Some of these malformations may be suspected because of abnormal mid-facial development, microcephaly, or colobomata, while others occur in normal appearing infants. Seizures may begin at any time and are usually difficult to control.

7. **Drug withdrawal/toxicity.** Infants with intrauterine exposure to drugs such as opiates (morphine, heroin, methadone), barbiturates, benzodiazepines, tricyclic antidepressants, or alcohol may display withdrawal from these drugs after birth. Symptoms of withdrawal primarily include irritability, jitter, and hyperreflexia; however, seizures may occur. When present, seizures usually occur within the first 3 days of life, except for methadone, which may occur after 1 to 2 weeks. Narcan should be avoided in infants at risk for intrauterine opiate exposure as it may precipitate a withdrawal reaction.

Seizures can occur after inadvertent administration of local anesthetics ("-caine" type drugs). This occurs from administration of the drug into the fetal scalp or through transplacental delivery after a maternal paracervical or pudendal block during labor. Seizures usually occur immediately but may occur up to 18 hours after birth.

8. **Inborn errors of metabolism.** Inborn errors of metabolism may present with seizures. Defects in organic or amino acid metabolism such as phenylketonuria, multiple carboxylase deficiency, nonketotic hyperglycinemia, propionic acidemia, and urea cycle defects are associated with seizures and a depressed neurologic exam. These conditions are also associated with hyperammonemia and acidosis.

Pyridoxine (vitamin B_6) dependency causes seizures that are refractory to standard therapy. The EEG in pyridoxine dependency shows a distinctly abnormal pattern of high-voltage spike waves that normalize after pyridoxine infusion.

9. **Neonatal epilepsy.** Neonatal seizures that run in families may represent benign familial neonatal seizures. These seizures can occur 10 to 20 times per day, but usually cease by 1 to 6 months of age. While the majority of infants may show normal development, 10% will have epilepsy.

Benign idiopathic neonatal seizures describes an unusual type of seizure disorder that is also known as "fifth day fits." These seizures begin around the fifth day of life and cease within 15 days. The cause is undetermined.

Early Myoclonic Encephalopathy (EMI) and *Early Infantile Epileptic Encephalopathy (EIEE)* are rare epileptic conditions that present in the first weeks of life. EMI is characterized by myoclonic and clonic type seizures, resulting from primary metabolic etiology such as nonketotic hyperglycinemia. EIEE seizures are characterized by "tonic spasms," a burst suppression pattern on EEG, and structural abnormality on magnetic resonance imaging (MRI), such as cortical malformation or hypoxic ischemic changes. Outcome in both conditions is unfavorable.

II. **Evaluation.** An approach to the evaluation of an infant with seizures is shown in Table 16-3. A thorough history and physical examination can focus the direction of further investigation. A history of the pregnancy, maternal health and drug use, and any family history of seizures should be obtained. The circumstances of the delivery and intrapartum period, including heart rate monitoring, medications, anesthesia, instrumentation, and mode of delivery should be recorded. The extent of neonatal resuscitation, Apgar scores, and umbilical cord blood gases should be obtained. The infant should be examined for dysmorphic features suggestive of a genetic syndrome or the presence of hepatosplenomegaly, petechiae, or rashes suggestive of congenital infection. Neurologic examination should include the OFC, state of alertness, strength and tone, and any asymmetry suggestive of a focal brain lesion. Blood should be sent immediately for testing of glucose, calcium, magnesium, sodium, hematocrit, and culture. A lumbar puncture should be performed and the cerebrospinal fluid (CSF) sent for glucose, protein, cell count, culture, and gram stain. In select patients additional CSF studies may be indicated. In patients with a burst suppression pattern on EEG, an elevated CSF glycine may indicate non-ketotic hyperglycinemia while serum glycine may be normal. If herpes is suspected, a viral culture and/or herpes polymerase chain reaction (PCR) should be obtained. If intrauterine substance exposure is suspected, a meconium drug screen should be obtained.

A serum ammonia and urine for amino and organic acids should be performed if disorders of metabolism are suspected. Evaluation for toxoplasmosis, rubella, CMV, syphilis, and herpes may be indicated. An EEG should be obtained; a video EEG, if available, would help ascertain the likelihood of clinical events being seizures. Prolonged or repeated EEGs can be used to follow seizures without clinical manifestation (subclinical seizures) and assess the effectiveness of anticonvulsant treatment.

A head computerized tomographic (CT) scan should be obtained once the patient is stabilized. A head CT can detect intracranial hemorrhage, gross structural abnormalities, and intrauterine stroke. A cranial ultrasound can be used in critically ill infants at the bedside and is reliable in detecting IVH. Once the infant is stable, MRI does a superior job of detecting all forms of brain anomalies. Brain ischemia is best visualized by diffusion weighted MRI 4 days after the event. However, it may miss ischemia before or after this period. Ischemic changes are more apparent on conventional MRI imaging after 3 weeks. MRI spectroscopy, a noninvasive measure of brain chemicals, can be used to detect evidence of ischemia or metabolic conditions as demonstrated by elevation of spectra representing lactate.

III. **Treatment.** Maintaining optimal oxygenation, ventilation, cardiovascular support, hydration, and correction of acid-base disturbance are essential in treating neonates experiencing seizures. Because glucose is the major source of energy for the brain and

---

Table 16-3. Evaluation of an infant with seizures

History and physical examination

Blood glucose, calcium (or ionized calcium), sodium, magnesium, complete blood count with differential and platelets, bacterial culture

Cultures and/or titers for toxoplasmosis, rubella, cytomegalovirus, syphilis, and herpes

Cerebrospinal fluid for glucose, protein, culture, cell count, and gram stain (include glycine, herpes pce, and/or viral culture if indicated)

Serum ammonia

Urine for metabolic screen (organic acids, amino acids)

Meconium drug screen

EEG

CT/Ultrasound of head

MRI of brain

EEG, Electroencephalogram; CT, Computerized tomography; MRI, Magnetic resonance imaging.

hypoglycemia may accompany seizures, the initiation of a continuous glucose infusion ($D_{10}W$ at 100 mL/kg/day) is one of the first steps in the treatment of neonatal seizures. To treat hypoglycemia (blood glucose less than 40 mg/dL), 2 mL/kg of D10W should be administered intravenously promptly and may be repeated. If repeated doses are necessary, consider increasing the continuous glucose infusion rate. If laboratory results reveal hypocalcemia or hypomagnesemia, neonates should be treated appropriately with intravenous calcium and/or magnesium.

Broad-spectrum antibiotic therapy (i.e., ampicillin and gentamicin) should be instituted after blood and spinal fluid cultures have been obtained. These should be continued until culture results are available. If herpes is suspected, acyclovir should be added.

Anticonvulsant therapy consists of phenobarbital and, if necessary, phenytoin/fosphenytoin. Phenobarbital is the anticonvulsant of choice in the treatment of neonatal seizures. Phenobarbital has an extremely variable serum half-life in the newborn (60 to 200 hours). Despite the longer half-life, the neonate requires a relatively larger loading dose of 20 mg/kg to achieve a therapeutic serum concentration of 20 to 30 μg/mL. An additional 20 mg/kg can be given 20 minutes after the first dose to treat status epilepticus for a total of 40 mg/kg. Phenobarbital causes significant respiratory depression; therefore, patient monitoring and the ability to assist ventilation should be available. Maintenance phenobarbital is provided by 3 to 5 mg/kg/day, given in 1 to 2 daily doses. Adjustment in the daily dosage based on serum drug concentration may be required because of the wide variability in clearance in the neonate.

Phenytoin/fosphenytoin is a good second drug of choice in the treatment of refractory neonatal seizures. In term infants during the first week of life, phenytoin has a half-life ranging from 6 to 140 hours. The intravenous loading dose is the same as phenobarbital. Cardiac monitoring is recommended during phenytoin administration by the intravenous route because the drug may cause arrhythmias. The loading dose should be given at a rate of no more than 0.5 mg/kg/minute to avoid disturbance of cardiac function. When given intravenously, care should be taken to avoid extravasation of phenytoin into the tissues as this can cause a substantial chemical burn. Some neonates require a high daily maintenance dose (15 to 20 mg/kg/day) to provide sustained therapeutic levels (10 to 20 μg/mL). Therapeutic concentration may be impossible to achieve by oral administration alone, and clinical response should be followed instead. Serum levels substantially higher than the established therapeutic range may enhance seizures rather than suppress them. Usually phenytoin is needed as a second anticonvulsant only for a limited period of time (days or weeks), after which it may be withdrawn and seizure control maintained by phenobarbital.

Fosphenytoin, a drug designed with properties similar to phenytoin, is a major advance in therapy of status epilepticus in children and adults. It is beginning to be used with good results in the management of seizures refractory to phenobarbital in neonates. Fosphenytoin is less caustic to tissues should intravenous infiltration occur and produces less cardiac disturbance allowing for faster intravenous administration (5 to 10 minutes). Fosphenytoin is dosed in "phenytoin equivalents" of 20 mg/kg and therapeutic level of phenytoin (10 to 20 μg/mL) is attained.

Lorazepam, a benzodiazepine anticonvulsant, can be used as a third agent in infants refractory to phenobarbital in combination with phenytoin. The effective dose is 0.05 to 0.1 mg/kg and the half-life in newborns is 6 to 24 hours. Lorazepam is primarily used to acutely treat seizures, and then the infant is maintained on phenobarbital and/or phenytoin.

If seizures are resistant to the above treatment and the EEG shows continuous discharges or a burst suppression pattern, a trial of pyridoxine may be given intravenously with continuous monitoring via EEG. The usual intravenous dose is 50 to 100 mg.

The optimal duration of anticonvulsant therapy for neonatal seizures has not been defined. The subsequent persistence of neurologic deficits and the results of the EEG help guide decisions about the timing of discontinuation of anticonvulsants. If the infant is neurologically abnormal or has an abnormal EEG at 3 to 6 months of age, it is inadvisable to discontinue anticonvulsants even if the child has been free of seizures since the neonatal period.

IV.   **Prognosis.** Recent evidence shows that the type of neonatal seizure may predict neurologic outcome. Infants with subtle and generalized tonic seizures may be more likely to have epilepsy, mental retardation, and cerebral palsy. Myoclonic seizures are more likely to be seen in epilepsy syndromes that predispose to mental retardation. Infants with more than two seizure types also are at higher risk for epilepsy, mental retardation, cerebral palsy, and abnormal neurologic exam.

The prognosis for neonatal seizures, however, generally relates to the underlying etiology. The prognosis related to brain injury caused by ischemia-hypoxia, intracranial hemorrhage, and meningitis depends on the severity and extent of the injury. The prognosis of those infants with cortical malformations is poor whereas the prognosis for those infants whose seizures were related to isolated, rapidly corrected metabolic derangement is excellent. The infant with an abnormal neurologic examination or delay in attaining developmental milestones has a poorer prognosis.

V.   **Clinical pearls.**
- Hypoxic-ischemic encephalopathy associated with perinatal depression, intracranial hemorrhage, intracranial infection, and developmental defects account for the majority of neonatal seizures.
- Apnea is more likely to be a sign of subtle seizures in the term infant whereas apnea in the premature infant is more likely to be of nonepileptic cause.
- Approximately 50% of neonates with meningitis develop seizures.
- Fever within the first week of life or the presence of hepatitis should raise the index of suspicion for herpes.

BIBLIOGRAPHY

Swaiman KF, Ashwal S. *Pediatric neurology: principles and practice*, 3rd ed. St. Louis, MO: Mosby, 1999.

Volpe JJ. *Neurology of the newborn*, 4th ed. Philadelphia, PA: WB Saunders, 2001.

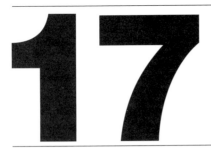

Necrotizing Enterocolitis

Michael Stone Trautman,
Diane Estella Lorant, and
William A. Engle

I. **Description of the issue.** Necrotizing enterocolitis (NEC) is a disease that predominantly affects neonates. The pathology of NEC is necrotizing injury to the intestine. NEC remains the most common gastrointestinal emergency in newborn intensive care nurseries. Although multiple predisposing factors such as prematurity, enteral feeding, hypoxia/ischemia, and infections are associated with NEC, the pathogenesis remains incompletely understood. The presence of numerous predisposing factors suggests that NEC is precipitated by a complex common pathway with multiple causes. This chapter will review predisposing factors, presentation, and treatments for NEC. Newer concepts in NEC's pathogenesis will be presented; however, detailed presentation of emerging scientific research is beyond the scope of this chapter.

A. **Epidemiology.** The incidence of NEC has remained unchanged during the last 20 years, despite significant advances in neonatal care. The incidence is between 3% and 10% in very-low-birth-weight (VLBW) infants (<1500 g), and remains primarily a disease of prematurity. Infants born with extremely low birth weight (<1000 g) at less than 29 weeks gestational age are at the greatest risk for NEC. Term infants who develop NEC often have complex congenital problems such as congenital heart disease, disorders of metabolism, or significant perinatal risk factors (Table 17-1).

B. **Pathogenesis and contributing factors.** Other than prematurity, the most consistent risk factor for NEC is enteral feedings. More than 90% of neonates affected by NEC have been fed. The mechanism by which feeding predisposes to NEC is not well understood. Feedings may contribute to NEC by direct damage to the immature intestinal mucosa, by altering intestinal blood flow, or by providing substrate for pathogenic bacterial growth. Delay in enteral feedings for several days after the birth may be indicated in extremely preterm, critically unstable, or asphyxiated infants. However, prolonged delays in enteral feedings have not been shown to be of benefit and recent evidence for early small (trophic) feedings suggests a significant benefit to the developing intestinal tract without imposing additional risks.

Various feedings strategies have been proposed to reduce the incidence of NEC. However, strategies that consist of initiation of enteral feedings with minimal trophic (10 to 20 cc/kg) amounts and a gradual increase in feeding volumes (20 cc/kg/day) versus more rapid advancement (30 to 40 cc/kg/day) have not been shown to correlate with the incidence of NEC. Early introduction of small trophic feedings (20 cc/kg/day) and the maintenance of this volume for 7 to 10 days may be beneficial in reducing the incidence of NEC.

The first infant formulas available for preterm infants had relatively high osmolalities. Older studies in animal models using theses formulations showed intestinal mucosa injury. Recently, premature formulas have addressed most of these issues and currently there is no consistent data to correlate their use with NEC. The two most effective enteral therapies to reduce the incidence of NEC are the use of a standardized feeding protocol within an individual nursery and, most importantly, the use of human milk.

Human milk feedings have been shown to reduce the incidence of NEC nearly 50% in some studies and have contributed in part to the reestablishment of breast-milk banks. Despite the extensive processing that breast milk undergoes as part of the banking process, meta-analysis of several studies suggests a positive benefit for its use. This reduction in NEC in infants fed human milk has been attributed to a variety of bioactive factors that are not present in premature infant formulas. These factors act to promote the growth of nonpathogenic flora and the maturation of the gastrointestinal system.

Bacterial colonization of the intestinal tract is another factor associated with NEC. The peak incidence of NEC occurs around 3 weeks of age, with reports of its occurrence

Table 17-1. Risk factors for necrotizing enterocolitis

Prematurity
Enteral feeding
Intestinal bacterial colonization
Hypoxia
Ischemia
Cyanotic heart disease

anywhere from several days of age in near-term infants to several months of age in growing premature infants. The intestinal tract is rapidly colonized with bacteria following birth, regardless of age. Nursery epidemics of NEC support the concept of an infectious etiology. However, case-control studies in premature patients have shown no differences in intestinal colonization with pathogenic organisms between those premature infants who develop NEC and control populations (Table 17-2).

Positive blood cultures occur in only about 30% of patients with NEC. Whether these cultures represent the causative agent or nonspecific bacterial translocation across damaged intestinal mucosa is unclear. Because no specific organisms have been consistently associated with NEC, investigators hypothesize that bacterial toxins like lipopolysaccharides (LPS) along with inflammatory mediators, such as platelet activating factor (PAF) and tumor necrosis factor (TNF), act to generate an inflammatory cascade resulting in NEC.

One of many other factors associated with NEC is intestinal hypoperfusion that can cause ischemic mucosal damage to the immature intestine. Most commonly this is seen in the terminal ileum and proximal colon, which are watershed areas of arterial supply. Ischemic bowel necrosis is likely associated with other extrauterine events because *in utero* intestinal ischemia causes intestinal stenosis and atresia rather than NEC. Ischemia may occur in association with birth asphyxia, hypotension, vascular thrombosis, or the "diving reflex." Investigators hypothesize these mechanisms explain the development of NEC in infants who have never been fed or in larger, near-term infants.

II. **Making the diagnosis.** The symptoms of NEC have been staged by Bell and others (Table 17-3). The most frequently encountered early sign is abdominal distention and nonspecific abdominal findings on anteroposterior (AP) views of the abdomen. In Stage 1 NEC, these clinical and radiographic findings are nonspecific and serve more to act as "warning signs" for caregivers rather than true measures of disease. Treatment is conservative, with the patient having enteral feedings discontinued for a period of time and, depending on other clinical findings, an evaluation for sepsis being performed. In Stage II disease, the diagnosis is established by the presence of pneumotosis intestinalis (intramural gas collections), the hallmark of the disease, or portal air on abdominal radiographs. Most infants experience increased gastric residuals, which may become bilious in nature along with abdominal tenderness and absent bowel sounds. Hematest-positive stools occur in 20% to 50% of infants with proven NEC. Although grossly bloody stool occur in less than 50% of patients with NEC, it is an indicator of bowel wall necrosis. Stage III disease is manifested with more advanced disease, including disseminated intravascular coagulation, thrombocytopenia, acidosis, ascites, and anterior abdominal wall erythema and edema. Evidence of intestinal perforation is demonstrated by the presence of pneumoperitoneum (Fig. 17-1).

Table 17-2. Organisms reported associated with epidemics of necrotizing enterocolitis

Klebsiella pneumoniae
Escherichia coli
Clostridia
Coagulase negative staphylococcus
Rotavirus
Coronavirus
Enterovirus

Table 17-3. Modified Bell staging for necrotizing enterocolitis (NEC)

Stage	Systemic signs	Intestinal signs	Radiographic signs
I. Suspected NEC	Temperature instability, apnea, bradycardia	Elevated gastric residuals, mild abdominal distention, occult blood in stool	Normal or mild ileus
IIA. Mild NEC	Similar to stage I	Prominent abdominal distention, +/− tenderness, absent bowel sounds, grossly bloody stools	Ileus, dilated bowel loops with focal pneumatosis
IIB. Moderate NEC	Mild acidosis and thrombocytopenia	Abdominal wall edema and tenderness, +/− palpable abdominal mass	Extensive pneumatosis, early ascites, +/− portal venous gas
IIIA. Advanced NEC	Respiratory and metabolic acidosis, mechanical ventilatory support, hypotension, oliguria, disseminated intravascular coagulation	Worsening abdominal wall edema with induration	Persistent ascites, persistent bowel loops, no free air
IIIB. Advanced NEC	Vital signs and laboratory evidence of deterioration, shock	Evidence of perforation	Pneumoperitoneum

III. **Management.** Prompt recognition and treatment are critically important for an infant with NEC. Extent of assessment and treatment depend on clinical suspicion and severity of illness at presentation (Table 17-4).

   A. **Medical.** When NEC is suspected because of mild abdominal distention or increased gastric residual with no other abnormality suggestive of NEC, the clinician orders that the infant have nothing by mouth (NPO) until symptoms resolve. Abdominal radiographs with AP film and/or left lateral decubitus (left side down) are the mainstay of diagnostic imaging. A complete blood cell count with differential, platelet count, and blood cultures are obtained because the initial presentation of NEC is often indistinguishable from sepsis with ileus. Cerebrospinal fluid cultures may be obtained if meningitis is suspected. Serial physical examinations are performed and serial laboratory assessments monitor for anemia, thrombocytopenia, and acidosis. The management of the infant with highly suspected or proven NEC is more aggressive. These infants are given nothing enterally and the abdomen is decompressed with an

Table 17-4. Signs and symptoms of necrotizing enterocolitis

Apnea
Abdominal distention
Increased gastric aspirates
Bilious emesis
Bloody stools
Lethargy
Increased respiratory distress
Metabolic acidosis

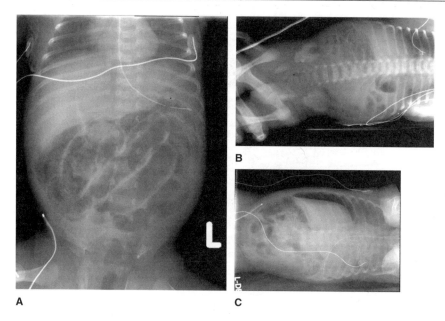

Figure 17-1. Abdominal radiographs of NEC can best be visualized with abdominal radiographs. Panel A is AP film of an abdomen of a patient with NEC. The film reveals multiple distended loops of bowel with areas of *pneumatosis intestinalis* in the lower right quadrant. Panel B is a left lateral decubitus radiograph (left side down) showing areas of *pneumatosis intestinalis* but no obvious indication of an intestinal perforation. Panel C is a left lateral decubitus radiograph showing a large amount of free air within the peritoneal cavity consistent with an intestinal perforation.

oral or nasal gastric tube with multiple side holes. In addition, parenteral antibiotics that provide coverage for both gram-negative and gram-positive organisms (including anaerobes) are administered. Length of treatment varies based on clinical symptoms and index of suspicion and ranges from 7 to 14 days. The circulatory status is frequently evaluated by monitoring blood pressure, urine output, and peripheral perfusion. Infants with NEC may quickly become hypovolemic because of third space fluid accumulation in the damaged intestinal mucosa and other tissues. This third space accumulation of fluid may result in electrolyte and acid-base imbalances (e.g., hyponatremia and metabolic acidosis). Blood transfusions are utilized to maintain an acceptable hematocrit (30% to 40%). Thrombocytopenia and consumption of clotting factors may result from localized or disseminated intravascular coagulation. Coagulation factors and platelets may be replaced with fresh frozen plasma and platelets. Platelets are administered if the platelet count drops below 50,000 to 100,000/mm³, especially with disseminated intravascular coagulation or clinical bleeding. If hypotension persists despite adequate volume expansion, vasopressors such as dopamine are initiated. Oxygen is administered to maintain normal oxygenation (arterial PaO_2 at 60 to 80 mm Hg, saturations >90%). Respiratory support is provided if persistent apnea or hypercapnia ensues. Metabolic acidosis is treated with plasma expanders if hypovolemia is present and with sodium bicarbonate.

B. **Surgical.** The indications and timing for surgical treatment of infants with NEC depend on clinical suspicion of bowel necrosis, occult perforation, or overt intestinal perforation. The following guidelines are generally accepted: (a) bowel perforation, (b) a deteriorating clinical course, and (c) evidence for progression of peritonitis, for example, a tender abdomen with edema or inflammation of the abdominal wall or an abdominal mass. A persistently dilated intestinal loop associated with pneumatosis may be an additional radiographic indicator for exploratory laparotomy. Surgical intervention consists of resecting the affected bowel, which may be extensive, and the placement of an ostomy with or without a distal mucus fistula (Fig. 17-2). Bowel reanastomosis takes place weeks to months later.

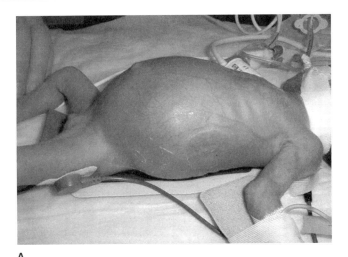

A

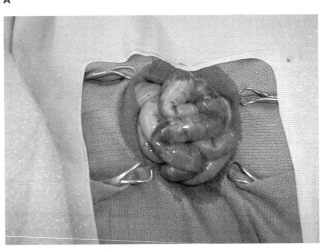

B

Figure 17-2. The marked abdominal distention is shown (Panel A) with a preterm infant with NEC. In Panel B, at the time of exploratory laporotomy, diffuse areas of poor perfusion (darkened areas) is seen with areas of relatively well perfused intestine.

Recently, in VLBW infants (<1000 g) major surgical interventions are often delayed and instead of a laporotomy, a peritoneal drain is placed and the patient is managed medically until stable. An infant with a definite diagnosis of NEC (i.e., pneumatosis intestinalis) but who does not meet surgical criteria is treated medically for 7 to 14 days. Because of the inability to feed during this time, parenteral alimentation is an important adjunct to therapy.

Even without surgery, intestinal strictures—especially in the colon—may occur in 15% to 30% of infants with NEC. Presentation of strictures frequently occurs 2 to 8 weeks following the acute NEC illness. If strictures are associated with bowel obstruction, surgical intervention is indicated. Those infants with intestinal resections often face extended hospital courses with prolonged periods of parenteral nutrition. The most significant postoperative complication is short gut syndrome resulting from large segments of the intestinal tract being resected and loss of the ileocecal valve. Such patients often require a multidisciplinary team approach to their care as it may take several years for the neonatal intestinal tract to grow and adapt.

Table 17-5. Protective factors within breast milk

Immunoglobulin A (IgA)
Macrophages, lactoferrin, lysoyme
Erythropoietin
Platelet activating factor acetylhydrolase
Cortisol
Growth hormone, insulinlike growth factors, epidermal growth factor, hepatic
  growth factor, transforming growth factor
Antioxidants
IL-1 receptor antagonist

IV. **Prevention.** The onset of NEC is often abrupt and overwhelming. It is unlikely that interventions will succeed after the presentation of clinical signs and symptoms have developed. Prevention, rather than treatment, is of the utmost priority. One preventive measure that has been shown to reduce NEC is maternal corticosteroid administration. Antenatal steroids stimulate lung development and maturation of the perivascular bed of the nervous system, and may have a significant maturational effect on the developing intestinal tract. In animal studies, steroids have been shown to increase mucosal thickness, goblet cell number, pancreatic amylase, gastric acid secretion, and the total number of mucosal cells.

The use of human breast milk, as noted earlier, has been shown in recent studies to significantly reduce the incidence of NEC in preterm infants when compared with standard premature formulas. The numerous immunoprotective and maturational factors contained in breast milk are thought responsible for this decrease (Table 17-5). Other preventive modalities have been studied, including the use of probiotics (*lactobacilli* and *bifidobacteria*), prophylactic oral antibiotics, oral immunoglobulin G and immunoglobulin A, and polyunsaturated fatty acid (PUFA). These trials have had small sample sizes and confirmatory studies have not yet been reported, and so these therapies cannot be recommended at this time. Other preventive interventions such as administration of oral antibiotics (e.g., aminoglycosides) have shown efficacy, but the development of antibiotic resistant microorganisms has prevented continuation of this strategy. As research continues and allows a better understanding of the maturing gastrointestinal tract and the mechanisms of inflammation, better strategies may be developed to reduce the incidence of NEC and to better treat its complications.

V. **Clinical pearls.**
- NEC is a multifactorial disorder and enteral feedings, bacterial overgrowth, and hypoxic injury can contribute to the incidence of this disease.
- The onset of NEC can occur insidiously over several days or precipitously with symptoms that mimic overwhelming sepsis.
- Although a patient may recover from NEC without surgery, long-term complications such as stricture may occur in as many as 10% to 30% of patients.
- One of the interesting side benefits of antenatal steroid use to prevent neonatal lung disease is a significant reduction in the incidence of NEC.

BIBLIOGRAPHY

Berseth CL, Bisquera JA, Paje Vu. Prolonging small feeding volumes early in life decreases the incidence of necrotizing enterocolitis in very low-birth-weight infants. *Pediatrics* 2003;111:529–534.

Cland EC, Walker WA. Hypothesis: inappropriate colonization of premature intestine can cause neonatal necrotizing enterocolitis. *FASEB J* 2001;15:1398–1403.

Kamitsuka MD, Horton MK, Williams MA. The incidence of necrotizing enterocolitis after introducing standardized feeding schedules for infants between 1250–2500 grams and less than 35 weeks. *Pediatrics* 2000;105:379–384.

McGuire W, Anthony MY. Donor human milk versus formula for preventing necrotizing enterocolitis in preterm infants. *Arch Dis Child* 2003;88:F11–F14.

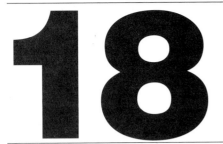

Abdominal Surgical Emergencies

Scott A. Engum and
Jay L. Grosfeld

I. **Description of the issue.** The prompt recognition and stabilization of two categories of common surgical emergencies in the newborn—namely, alimentary tract obstruction and abdominal wall defects—are discussed in this chapter (tracheoesophageal fistula and diaphragmatic hernia are discussed in Chapter 10). Prompt recognition, stabilization, and transfer to a facility capable of handling neonatal surgical problems may be lifesaving in some instances.

II. **Alimentary tract obstruction.** The four cardinal signs of alimentary tract obstruction in the newborn include the following:
   - maternal polyhydramnios
   - bilious emesis
   - abdominal distention
   - failure to pass normal amounts of meconium during the first 24 hours of life

   Any one of these signs suggests the possibility of intestinal obstruction.

   Amniotic fluid in excess of 1500 to 2000 mL is considered polyhydramnios. Twenty-five to forty percent of amniotic fluid is swallowed by the fetus and is usually reabsorbed in the first 20 to 25 cm of jejunum. A high alimentary tract obstruction (e.g., esophageal atresia, pyloric atresia, duodenal atresia, high jejunal atresia) may be associated with maternal polyhydramnios. Any pregnant woman with hydramnios should be studied with a prenatal ultrasound, which may detect an obstructive defect prior to the infant's birth.

   Bilious vomiting is nearly always pathologic and must be investigated. The newborn infant's stomach usually contains less than 15 mL of clear gastric juice at birth. Greater than 18 to 20 mL of clear gastric juice or gastric juice containing bile in the newborn may signify an intestinal obstruction. Bilious emesis may also be seen in a septic infant with an adynamic ileus.

   The normal contour of the newborn abdomen is round, unlike the usual scaphoid appearance of the adult; however, a distended abdomen in the neonate is abnormal. Physical findings associated with distention include visible veins on the abdominal wall, visible intestinal loops with or without peristalsis, and, occasionally, respiratory distress caused by elevation of the diaphragm. In each instance, one should obtain supine and left lateral decubitus radiographs of the abdomen to evaluate the nature of the distention. Distention may be a result of free intraabdominal air (perforated viscus), fluid (hemoperitoneum, chyloperitoneum), or distended bowel resulting from intestinal obstruction or adynamic ileus.

   Normal meconium is composed of amniotic fluid, squames, lanugo hairs, succus entericus, and intestinal mucus. It is dark green or black, and sticky in consistency. Failure to pass normal amounts of meconium during the first 24 hours of life may be pathologic. Infants with low intestinal obstruction (Hirschsprung disease and the meconium plug syndrome) may present with this finding.

   A. **High small bowel obstruction.** High small bowel obstruction may occur at the level of the pylorus, duodenum, or jejunum in the form of atresia (complete obstruction), stenosis (partial obstruction), or volvulus (complete or partial). In the case of atresia or stenosis, the diagnosis is based on several findings. Polyhydramnios is frequently observed. Vomiting (with or without bile), increased gastric contents, and intolerance to feedings are uniformly observed. Resultant fluid and electrolyte disturbances are common if the diagnosis is not made promptly. Persistent or exaggerated jaundice may also occur.

      1. **Pyloric atresia.** Pyloric atresia is an uncommon form of alimentary tract obstruction in the newborn. Familial occurrences have been observed with a probable autosomal recessive inheritance that in some cases may be associated with epidermolysis bullosum. Pyloric atresia can be detected on prenatal ultrasound studies and the α-fetoprotein level in the amniotic fluid may be elevated. These

infants vomit clear (nonbilious) gastric fluid on attempted feedings. A plain abdominal radiograph will show a single upper abdominal gas bubble with no air beyond the stomach.

2. **Duodenal atresia.** Duodenal atresia is associated with Down syndrome (trisomy 21) in one third of the cases. Since 85% of the cases of duodenal obstruction are distal to the entry of the bile duct into the duodenum, vomiting is most often bilious. Because of the high level of obstruction, abdominal distention is not observed. Recumbent and left lateral decubitus radiographs of the abdomen usually document the presence of an air-filled stomach and first portion of the duodenum—the classic "double-bubble" sign (Fig. 18-1). Approximately one third of all cases of duodenal atresia have associated annular pancreas as well as malrotation.

3. **Jejunoileal atresia/stenosis.** Jejunoileal atresia may be isolated or multiple. Infants with isolated atresia or stenosis normally present as vigorous, active babies. The physical findings are minimal, as the abdomen is usually soft, nondistended, and nontender. Diagnosis is confirmed radiologically. An anterior-posterior (AP) x-ray film of the abdomen may demonstrate proximal large bubbles of gas in the bowel but a scanty bowel gas pattern elsewhere (Fig. 18-2A). Atresias occur slightly more commonly in the jejunum than in the ileum. In approximately 90% of cases, the atresias are single (Fig. 18-2B); however, in 10% to 15% of these patients, multiple atresias are observed.

4. **Volvulus.** Volvulus is a surgical emergency in the newborn. It is often associated with malrotation of the intestine and is characterized by twisting of the intestine about the mesentery, which includes the superior mesenteric artery that is the

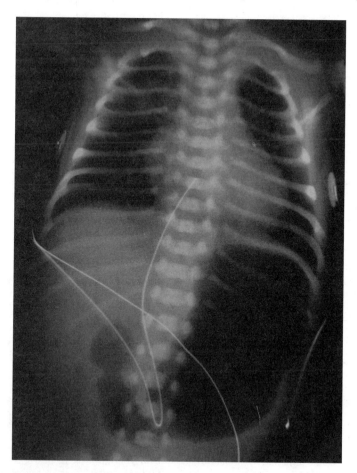

Figure 18-1. "Double-bubble" sign of duodenal atresia.

primary blood supply to the bowel. The result may be vascular compromise to the intestine with partial or complete infarction of the involved bowel. Clinical symptoms and signs may develop at any point during the newborn period or even *in utero*. Such infants become extremely ill over a short period of time, as they develop abdominal distention, tenderness, and rigidity. A metabolic acidosis is often noted, as well as other attendant complications such as fluid and electrolyte imbalance, respiratory distress, infection, and disseminated intravascular coagulation. Radiographic findings are variable, often requiring upper (preferred) or occasionally lower bowel contrast studies to confirm the presence of malrotation of the intestine and the likely presence of congenital Ladd bands with volvulus.

B. Low small bowel obstruction. Infants with low small bowel obstruction present with bilious vomiting and abdominal distention. Recumbent and left lateral decubitus abdominal radiographs demonstrate many dilated loops of bowel (Fig. 18-3). Because the infant colon does not show haustral markings, a barium enema is performed in low intestinal obstruction. The barium enema distinguishes between small and large bowel distention, determines if the colon is used or unused (microcolon) and therefore the level of obstruction (small intestinal or colonic), and evaluates the position of the cecum in regard to intestinal rotation and fixation. It is impossible to differentiate large from small bowel on the basis of flat plate x-rays of the abdomen in the newborn. Therefore, contrast studies are indicated when there is any question regarding the diagnosis.

Occasionally, calcification is seen on abdominal radiographs and signifies the presence of "meconium peritonitis." This is a sign of intrauterine bowel perforation. The two most common causes of low small bowel obstruction are ileal atresia and meconium ileus.

1. Ileal atresia. Infants with ileal atresia present with abdominal distention, bilious vomiting, and failure to pass meconium. Significant small bowel distention and many air-fluid levels are usually seen. The barium enema shows the unused "microcolon" (Fig. 18-4), limiting the obstruction to the distal small bowel.

2. Meconium ileus. Meconium ileus is a unique form of congenital intestinal obstruction that occurs in 10% to 15% of infants with cystic fibrosis (CF). A deficiency of pancreatic enzymes and an abnormality in the composition of the meconium are the factors responsible for the solid concretions that result in intestinal obstruction in this disorder. A careful family history is conducted when this hereditary disorder is suspected.

Other less common causes of small intestinal obstruction in the newborn include intrinsic stenosis and extrinsic compression from congenital bands, bowel duplication, mesenteric cysts, internal hernia through a mesenteric defect, and an incarcerated inguinal hernia.

C. Colonic obstruction. Causes of colonic obstruction in the neonate include meconium plug syndrome, aganglionic megacolon (Hirschsprung disease), colon atresia, small left colon syndrome, and imperforate anus.

1. Meconium plug syndrome. The exact etiology of meconium plug syndrome is unknown, but it is thought to be some factor that dehydrates meconium. The patient presents with distention and failure to pass meconium. A plain x-ray of the abdomen usually shows many loops of distended bowel with some air-fluid levels. A barium enema shows a microcolon up to the descending or transverse colon, at which point the colon becomes dilated, and copious intraluminal material (thick meconium) is observed. The barium enema is often diagnostic and therapeutic. Following instillation of the contrast material, large plugs of inspissated meconium may be passed, and the obstruction completely relieved. Occasionally, a second or third enema (usually Gastrografin) is required to prompt complete evacuation. If any signs of recurrent obstruction do occur, aganglionic megacolon must be considered and a suction rectal biopsy can be performed. In addition, rarely, meconium plug syndrome may be a presenting feature of CF, and therefore a sweat chloride test or DNA analysis looking for the CF genotype should be considered.

2. Aganglionic megacolon (Hirschsprung disease). Aganglionic megacolon (Hirschsprung disease) is a neurogenic form of obstruction in which there is an absence of ganglion cells in the myenteric (Auerbach) and submucosal (Meissner) plexuses. The absence of parasympathetic innervation results in a failure of relaxation of the internal sphincter. The disease begins at the anorectal line and extends proximal to the rectosigmoid in 80% of the cases. In 10% of the patients, the aganglionic segment extends proximal to the splenic flexure and may involve the entire colon and distal ileum or more proximal small bowel. Rare cases of total

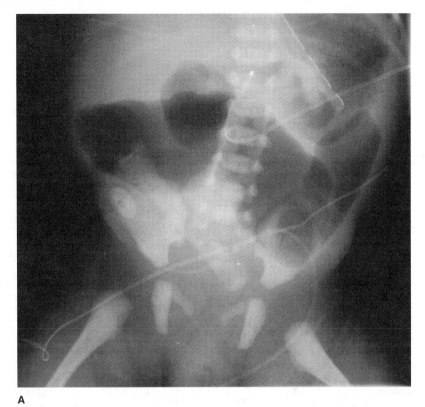

A

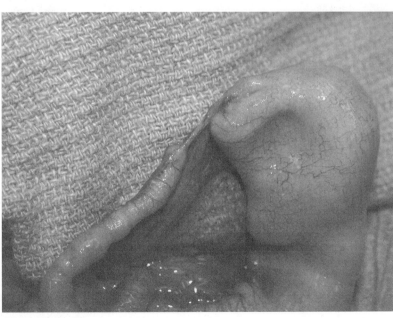

B

Figure 18-2. (A) Dilated proximal bowel loops suggestive of a high small bowel obstruction (jejunal atresia). **(B)** At operation a jejunal atresia. Note the dilated proximal segment and very small distal bowel caliber.

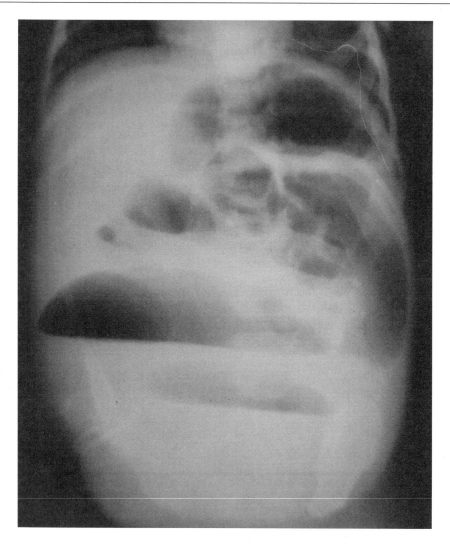

Figure 18-3. Markedly dilated loops of bowel suggestive of lower bowel obstruction.

aganglionosis of the entire gastrointestinal tract have also been reported. The disease has a definite familial tendency.

Most infants with this disorder demonstrate symptoms during the newborn period. Ninety-five percent fail to pass normal amounts of meconium during the first 24 hours of life. These infants usually have abdominal distention and often vomit bile. Distention may be severe, with dilated loops of bowel seen on the abdominal wall. The sigmoid colon is often palpated as a "mass." X-rays obtained in the recumbent and left lateral decubitus positions show dilated loops of distal bowel; the barium enema during the newborn period may not demonstrate a transition zone. The normal infant evacuates barium promptly after a contrast enema. However, neonates with Hirschsprung disease usually retain the barium for greater than 24 hours following a contrast enema. Occasionally, this disorder presents with the triad of abdominal distention, vomiting, and severe diarrhea alternating with constipation. This diarrhea is known as the "enterocolitis" of Hirschsprung disease.

In most cases, a suction rectal biopsy will demonstrate the absence of ganglion cells in Auerbach plexus; however, if insufficient tissue is obtained or the patient's clinical status dictates the need for emergent or urgent evaluation, a

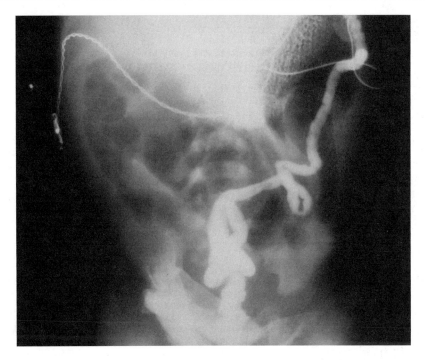

Figure 18-4. Unused "microcolon" in a patient with low small bowel obstruction.

full-thickness rectal biopsy in the operating room with frozen tissue evaluation is the most accurate and timely method of diagnosis.

3. **Colon atresia.** Colon atresia as an isolated entity (not associated with imperforate anus or cloacal extrophy) is a relatively rare anomaly. Failure to pass meconium during the first 24 hours of life, abdominal distention, and bilious vomiting are the usual clinical manifestations. These infants are usually full term and rarely have associated anomalies. Diagnosis is confirmed by a barium enema, which demonstrates a blind-ending distal end of a microcolon and dilated air-filled loops of proximal intestine.

4. **Anorectal anomalies.** There is a wide spectrum of anal anomalies that fit the general category of anal atresia, imperforate anus, and rectal atresia. Anal atresia usually refers to a thin, veil-like membrane covering the normal anal canal and residing within the external sphincter. Eighty-five to ninety percent of infants with imperforate anus and rectal atresia have an associated fistulous tract. These children frequently have associated anomalies in other systems. A careful systems review involving other areas of the gastrointestinal tract, cardiovascular system, musculoskeletal system, genitourinary tract, and central nervous system is carried out during early infancy to delineate these problems and initiate treatment. The detailed management of infants and children with variants of imperforate anus is beyond the scope of this chapter; however, for practical purposes therapy can be divided into high (fistula present above levator ani muscle) and low (fistula present below the levator ani muscle) variants. High imperforate anus typically involves a colostomy until definitive repair is performed, whereas low imperforate anus may be treated with a variety of options that center on an anoplasty. Pediatric surgeons with expertise in the management of these anorectal defects should perform these types of surgeries. The first operation is usually the most important.

Infants who have perineal anoplasty during the newborn period will develop good external sphincter tone and have a bright outlook for developing continence. The higher the rectal atresia, the poorer is the potential outcome of the operation with regard to obtaining fecal continence. Long-term care and follow-up are required in such patients, and the families must be counseled not to expect the normal

progression of bowel training in these children. If the puborectalis sling and external sphincter are preserved at the time of the pull-through operation, most of these
children have a reasonable chance of obtaining socially acceptable forms of continence. This may not be achieved, however, until 6 to 9 years of age, when the child
voluntarily participates in attempts to stay clean and avoid fecal odor.

III.   **Abdominal wall defects.**

A.   **Omphalocele.** An omphalocele (Fig. 18-5) is a covered defect of the umbilical ring
into which the intra-abdominal contents herniate. The sac is composed of an outer
layer of amnion and an inner layer of peritoneum. This defect occurs in approximately 1/5000 births. There is a high incidence of associated anomalies, with more
than 50% of cases having other serious defects involving the alimentary tract, cardiorespiratory, genitourinary, musculoskeletal, and/or central nervous systems.
Many of these infants are premature. Others may be affected by a number of syndromes, including Beckwith–Wiedemann syndrome and chromosomal anomalies.

The size of the defect varies considerably, from as small as 2 cm to as large as
10 cm. The smaller the defect, the better is the prognosis. A small omphalocele may
present as a small knot or discoloration at the base of the umbilical cord; in such
cases, care must be taken when clamping the cord in the delivery room. The contents
of the sac may include only small bowel and colon, although frequently the liver as
well as the entire gastrointestinal tract is within the sac. Since the intestines reside
in the sac and not within the abdomen, the resultant size of the abdominal cavity
may be exceedingly small, making a primary repair rather difficult.

The emergency care of the patient includes insertion of an orogastric tube to decompress the stomach and prevent swallowed air from resulting in bowel distention,
which may interfere with an attempted repair. The lower half of the infant can be
placed in a sterile intestinal bag (these plastic bags are commercially available and
are found in most operating rooms), which is then cinched with the drawstrings
under the arms. This protects the omphalocele sac, helps to maintain body temperature, and minimizes fluid losses. Antibiotic therapy is usually initiated. The patient's overall status is also carefully assessed with respect to cardiorespiratory
status. Because the viscera are covered by the sac, the bowel is usually normal in appearance; fluid needs are reasonably similar to those in normal newborns. The patient
is transported in a thermally neutral incubator in the supine position. Intravenous
therapy is given in the form of 10% dextrose in 0.25% saline unless excessive orogastric losses are encountered.

Prognosis in infants with omphalocele depends on the size of the defect, whether
the infant is premature, whether the sac ruptures (adding the dimension of potential

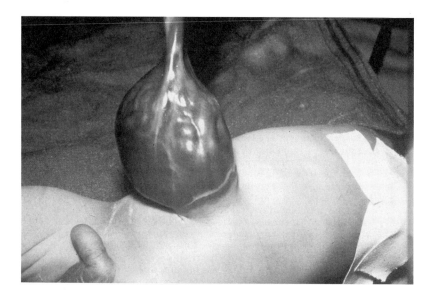

Figure 18-5. Omphalocele with intestines protruding through the umbilical ring.

sepsis and abdominal closure complexity), and the severity of associated anomalies. Mortality may be as high as 35% in the presence of the above-mentioned adverse factors.

B. Gastroschisis. Gastroschisis (Fig. 18-6A), Greek for "belly cleft," is a defect of the anterior abdominal wall just lateral to the umbilicus. The defect is almost always located to the right side of an intact umbilical cord. This anomaly is associated with

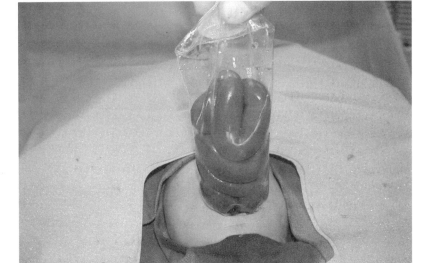

A

B

Figure 18-6. **(A)** Gastroschisis with the majority of the intestine protruding through the defect. **(B)** Gastroschisis with silo in place for a staged bedside reduction.

antenatal evisceration of the gastrointestinal tract. Unlike an omphalocele, there is no peritoneal sac. The irritating effects of amniotic fluid on the exposed bowel wall result in a chemical form of peritonitis characterized by a thick edematous membrane over the bowel, which is occasionally exudative in appearance. The exposed viscera are often congested and foreshortened. Malrotation always accompanies this condition. In contrast to patients with an omphalocele, associated anomalies in patients with gastroschisis are relatively infrequent. The exception to this general rule is that intestinal atresia is noted in 10% to 15% of cases. The liver is almost never eviscerated. Sexes are equally affected, and 40% of patients are either premature or small for gestational age.

Once delivered (via vaginal birth or cesarean section), the infant is subject to a variety of problems caused by the increase in insensible losses related to exposure of the eviscerated bowel. Hypothermia, hypovolemia, and sepsis are the major potential problems. Hypothermia occurs because of increased radiant heat losses from the exposed bowel surface. There are significant "third-space" fluid deficits related to extra- and intra-abdominal sequestration of interstitial fluid. As with the omphalocele, it is recommended to wrap the entire lower half of the infant, including the eviscerated bowel, quickly in a sterile intestinal bag. This is extremely important because, in contrast to the omphalocele, there is no peritoneal sac, and fluid and heat loss from the exposed viscera is exaggerated. In addition, sequestered fluid from the defect collects in the bag and can be measured for fluid replacement. Five percent dextrose in lactated Ringer solution is given intravenously at a rate of 20 mL/kg over 30 to 60 minutes to replace initial fluid losses. Acid-base balance must be closely monitored. Metabolic acidosis is commonly observed as a result of poor perfusion related to hypovolemia. An orogastric tube is placed to prevent air swallowing and to aspirate intestinal contents, as these babies have an associated adynamic ileus. Antibiotics are administered to prevent secondary infection. If cyanosis or respiratory distress is noted, arterial pH and blood gases are determined, and appropriate oxygen and respiratory support are initiated. Because of the often-complicated nature of their care, these patients should be transferred to a tertiary neonatal intensive care facility, where they can be given appropriate pediatric surgical management. In uncomplicated infants, prefabricated silos may be applied at the bedside (Fig. 18-6B) that allow for reduction of the herniated bowel over the course of a few days. This minimizes the necessity for immediate surgery and avoids the potential for acute abdominal compartment syndrome, which has been noted with immediate reduction of the entire bowel into the small abdominal cavity. With appropriate neonatal support, surgical treatment, and nutritional management, the current survival rate in these cases is 90%.

V. **Clinical pearls.**
- Bilious emesis is always pathologic and further investigation is always warranted prior to discharge.
- After making the diagnosis of meconium ileus, one should evaluate for CF.
- Most infants with Hirschsprung disease will fail to pass normal amounts of meconium during the first 24 hours of life.
- An omphalocele is characterized by having a central umbilical defect and a sac and is commonly associated with other health problems.
- A gastroschisis is characterized by an abdominal wall defect to the side of the umbilicus (primarily right) without a sac, and generally few other health problems.

BIBLIOGRAPHY

McCollough M, Sharieff GQ. Abdominal surgical emergencies in infants and young children. *Emerg Med Clin North Am* 2003;21(4):909–935.

O'Neill J, Rowe M, Grosfeld J, et al. *Pediatric surgery*, 5th ed. St. Louis, MO: Mosby–Year Book, 1998.

Pollack ES. Pediatric abdominal surgical emergencies. *Pediatr Ann* 1996;25(8):448–457.

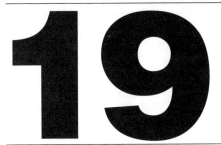

Hematologic Disorders

Mark Lawrence Edwards and
Mervin C. Yoder

I. **Description of the issue.** Blood is a heterogeneous mixture of cells, proteins, and fluids that serves many functions. Red blood cells serve as transporters of vital gases. White blood cells are the primary defense against invading microbes and are the frontline effectors of wound repair. Platelets serve to protect the integrity of the vascular system against large volume losses of blood when a vessel wall is compromised. The most common hematologic abnormalities of consequence in the human newborn infant involve anemia and coagulation disorders.

II. **Anemia.** Anemia is a condition in which the neonate demonstrates a lower than normal number of red cells (erythrocytes) in the blood, usually measured by a decrease in hemoglobin concentration or hematocrit. Cord blood hemoglobin concentrations vary from 14 to 20 g/dL in term infants and may be 1 to 2 g/dL lower in preterm infants. Anemia at birth or in the immediate neonatal period may result from a number of causes with or without associated complications such as circulatory collapse, congestive heart failure, anasarca, respiratory distress, and hyperbilirubinemia. It is imperative to ascertain the underlying cause of the anemia whenever possible. The use of a straightforward algorithm (such as that illustrated in Fig. 19-1) permits classification of anemia into three general causes in term neonates: diminished red cell production, altered red cell survival (hemolysis), or excessive red cell loss (hemorrhage).

A. **Etiologies.**
   1. **Diminished red cell production.** Diminished red cell production is an extremely rare cause of anemia in the neonate. Early diagnosis is important, because prompt treatment may increase the chance of remission. One-fourth of patients with Diamond-Blackfan anemia (Fig. 19-1) present at birth with profound anemia and reticulocytopenia, but other hematopoietic lineages are normal. These patients may display other abnormalities including short stature, triphalangeal or duplicated thumbs, ocular anomalies, or congenital heart disease. Many patients respond favorably to corticosteroid treatment. Fanconi anemia is an autosomal recessive disorder composed of 11 genetic phenotypes. These patients may also display short stature as well as upper limb, renal, and skin anomalies. These patients' cells are hypersensitive to DNA cross-linking agents such as diepoxybutane and mitomycin C, and increased chromosomal breaks in the presence of these agents are considered diagnostic. Aase syndrome also presents as anemia in the neonate with skeletal anomalies. This corticosteroid-responsive anemia may improve with age. Three types of congenital dyserythropoietic anemia have been identified. Though rare, dyserythropoietic anemia should be considered in infants with anemia, jaundice, and hepatosplenomegaly.
   2. **Altered red cell survival (hemolysis).** Hemolytic anemia is characterized by a shortened red cell survival time and is manifested by a decreased hematocrit, increased reticulocyte count, and increased bilirubin levels (Fig. 19-1). The normal life span for a red cell in a neonate is 60 to 90 days, approximately two-thirds what it is in adults. Even shorter red cell survival times (35 to 50 days) are observed in the most preterm neonates. A variety of factors predispose the red cells of the neonate to early destruction, including increased membrane fragility, decreased intracellular enzyme, ATP, and carnitine levels, and enhanced susceptibility to membrane peroxidation. Causes for red cell hemolysis can be divided into isoimmune disorders, congenital red cell defects, and acquired red cell defects.

   More than 60 distinct red cell antigens are capable of eliciting a maternal antibody response when incompatible paternal alleles for the antigen are expressed on the fetal red cells. These fetal cells can be presented to the maternal circulation via transplacental passage and evoke a maternal antibody response. The maternal-derived antibody subsequently enters the fetal circulation transplacentally and a hemolytic anemia ensues as the targeted red cells, which bear the maternal antibody,

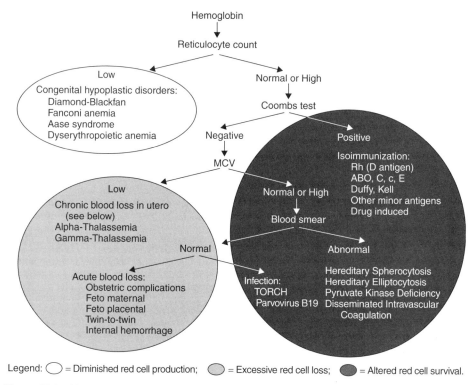

Legend: ◯ = Diminished red cell production; ⬤ = Excessive red cell loss; ⬤ = Altered red cell survival.

Figure 19-1. Algorithm to classify the causes of anemia in the newborn into diminished red blood cell production, excessive red cell loss, or altered red cell survival.

are removed from the circulation and destroyed. The D antigen of the Rh group continues to be a primary target as anti-D antibodies continue to be detected in a significant number of newborn infants despite the use of anti-D γ globulin (RhoGAM) in susceptible women. ABO, C, E, Duffy, and Kell antigens also contribute to hemolytic disease in the newborn. In affected patients, the reticulocyte test is positive, the Coombs test is positive (Fig. 19-1), polychromasia is apparent on the blood smear, and many nucleated red cells are also present. Indirect bilirubin levels may rise rapidly soon after birth, precipitating the need for intensive phototherapy and, on occasion, exchange transfusion. The ability to identify the severely affected fetus *in utero* is now associated with the ability to intervene when necessary with direct intravascular transfusion of packed type O, Rh negative red cells via the umbilical vein. This intervention may result in the isoimmune antibody exposed infant to be delivered with a normal hemoglobin concentration, negative Coombs test, and a relatively normal appearing blood smear. The only apparent abnormality may be the elevated concentrations of direct and indirect bilirubin. Obviously, such an infant must be observed closely to ensure that a late appearing anemia does not emerge as the transfused cells are lost from the circulation with an ongoing low level of hemolysis of the infant's own red cells.

A variety of hereditary defects of the red cell membrane may cause hemolysis in the newborn infant. Membrane defects such as hereditary spherocytosis and elliptocytosis may lead to accelerated destruction as a result of increased membrane fragility and fragmentation. A similar mechanism may be functioning in red cells harboring inherited enzymatic disorders, such as deficiency of pyruvate kinase, hexokinase, or glucose-6-phosphate dehydrogenase. All of these disorders lead to characteristic morphologic abnormalities that may be apparent on the peripheral blood smear (Fig. 19-1). Evidence for increased mechanical destruction of red cells may be present in neonates with disseminated intravascular coagulation as well.

In some instances, hemolysis caused by acquired red cell defects may become apparent during or following bacterial and/or viral infections. Certain TORCH infections (toxoplasmosis, rubella, cytomegalic inclusion disease, and herpes virus) may manifest as hemolytic anemia, hepatosplenomegaly, extramedullary hematopoiesis, thrombocytopenia, jaundice, and intrauterine growth retardation in neonates. In these neonates, the reticulocyte count will generally be elevated, the Coombs test negative, the mean corpuscular volume (MCV) normal or high, and the blood smear will often be normal (Fig. 19-1).

3. **Excessive red cell loss (hemorrhage).** Hemorrhage that produces anemia at birth or in the early neonatal period may be the result of obstetric accidents, malformations of the cord and placenta, hemorrhage from the fetus into the maternal circulation or to another fetus, or internal hemorrhage (Fig. 19-1). A rapid loss of 20% of the blood volume will produce shock. Table 19-1 lists some causes of hemorrhage in the newborn. A review of the obstetric history will often lead the physician to suspect a complication of pregnancy or delivery resulting in acute hemorrhage. A history of vaginal bleeding during the last trimester, placenta previa, abruption, nonelective cesarean section, or difficult delivery can result in an increased risk of blood loss prior to delivery. A newborn who has suffered an acute hemorrhage will be pale and hypotensive without edema or hepatosplenomegaly; cyanosis may be absent, and the child's pallor will not improve with supplemental oxygen.

The fetus may adjust hemodynamically to the blood loss if the fetal hemorrhage has been chronic (days to weeks). Infants born after chronic blood loss may present with pallor and unexplained anemia but be quite vigorous; the blood count may reveal a microcytic hypochromic index reflecting iron deficiency caused by the chronic blood loss. To document fetal-to-maternal bleeding, a Kleihauer-Betke test is performed by incubating unstained slides of the mother's blood in an acidic buffer. Fetal hemoglobin will resist elution and remain within the intact red blood cells, whereas the adult hemoglobin will be eluted from the erythrocytes. After staining, the fetal erythrocytes containing hemoglobin appear as darkly stained cells, whereas the adult erythrocytes are clear and are often described as "ghost" cells. The percentage of fetal cells present can then be used in calculating an estimate of the fetal blood transfused.

Anemia that appears in the first 24 to 72 hours of life and is not initially associated with jaundice may be caused by internal hemorrhages. There may be a history of a traumatic delivery with a large cephalohematoma. Internal hemorrhage may occur in association with vitamin K deficiency. Breech presentation may be associated with hemorrhage into the adrenal gland, liver, kidney, spleen, or retroperitoneal area. An infant with a ruptured liver may appear well for the initial 24 hours and then, as the increasing hematoma ruptures the hepatic capsule, suddenly develop shock. Other less common sites of hemorrhage include the spleen, gastrointestinal tract, and hemangiomas.

4. **Anemia of prematurity.** Physiologic anemia generally occurs between 6 and 10 weeks of life in term and premature infants. During the first week of life, the hemoglobin concentration is generally unchanged or may increase slightly in response to a shift in plasma to extravascular space to compensate for the placental transfusion that may occur with delivery.

Table 19-1. Types of hemorrhage

Obstetric complications
   Rupture of an umbilical cord
   Hematoma of cord or placenta
   Placenta previa
   Abruptio placentae
   Incision of placenta during cesarean section
Occult hemorrhage before birth
   Fetal–maternal
   Twin-to-twin
Internal hemorrhage
   Intracranial
   Giant cephalohematoma
Ruptured viscus (e.g., liver)

After the first week of life, the hemoglobin concentration falls, gradually reaching a nadir between 6 and 10 weeks of life. Factors that contribute to the fall in hemoglobin include a shortened red cell survival, blood sampling, and increasing blood volume with growth. The hemoglobin concentration may fall as low as 7 g/dL in the very-low-birth-weight infant and averages 11 g/dL in the term infant. When the hemoglobin concentration falls low enough to limit tissue oxygenation, erythropoietin production is stimulated, and active marrow erythropoiesis ensues. Most term infants will adapt to the temporary lower hemoglobin concentration to ensure adequate tissue oxygenation. Adaptation may include lowering of the oxygen affinity to facilitate oxygen release to tissue, increasing blood flow to vital organs to maintain delivery of oxygen, and lowering the mixed venous PaO_2 to maintain tissue oxygen extraction.

In contrast, the preterm infant has a limited compensatory mechanism. The higher proportion of fetal hemoglobin with its higher oxygen affinity makes oxygen delivery more difficult. The diminished response of fetal hemoglobin to 2,3-diphosphoglycerate (2,3-DPG) results in an oxygen affinity that cannot easily be lowered. A rebound in fetal hemoglobin production has been noted in the premature infant who has been transfused with adult hemoglobin. Phosphorus depletion may also limit the production of 2,3-DPG, as phosphorus is in great demand for bone mineralization in the growing premature neonate. With a low phosphorus level the production of 2,3-DPG is decreased and the oxygen affinity can increase appreciably.

Accumulation of nutrient stores is greatest during the third trimester, and infants born before term often have nutrition deficiencies that accentuate anemia. Iron, vitamin E, folic acid, and vitamin B_{12} needs must all be met to decrease the severity of anemia experienced by the very-low-birth-weight infant.

When to transfuse an infant experiencing anemia of prematurity is often a difficult question. As many as 40% of anemic, premature infants will display some symptomatology including poor weight gain, apnea, congestive heart failure, tachypnea, tachycardia, pallor, or poor perfusion. Although it is not recommended that every premature be transfused prophylactically at some predetermined hemoglobin level, the clinician must have a low threshold for transfusion when initial signs of poor oxygen delivery develop. In addition, transfusion should be performed earlier when an infant is at higher risk for serious problems related to low tissue oxygenation. Such infants include those with a continued oxygen requirement, apnea, necrotizing enterocolitis, or a patent ductus arteriosus.

Anemia of prematurity is associated with abnormally low erythropoietin concentrations in the face of diminished tissue oxygen levels and signs of anemia in affected preterm infants. Because the erythroid progenitors in these patients are highly sensitive to erythropoietin and because the other growth factors that support erythropoiesis (interleukin-3 and granulocyte macrophage-colony stimulating factor) appear to be present in normal concentrations, numerous clinical trials of the use of recombinant erythropoietin to prevent the need for transfusions in preterm infants have been conducted with variable results. A summary of these results would suggest that recombinant erythropoietin may be safely given by subcutaneous or intravenous routes to preterm infants who are supplemented with oral iron. While this therapy may reduce the number of transfusions required to prevent symptoms of anemia in preterm infants, administration of recombinant erythropoietin is not sufficient to prevent the need for any transfusions in extremely and very-low-birth-weight preterm infants, and is therefore not recommended for routine use in these patients.

B. Diagnosis. Infants with anemia often require prompt treatment, yet it is important to determine the etiology, if possible, before a transfusion is given as the transfused red cells may obscure the diagnosis. A history will provide information regarding the presence of anemia or jaundice in family members as well as information concerning the labor and delivery. Attention should be paid to third-trimester bleeding, placenta previa, abruptio placenta, multiple gestation, and nonelective cesarean section as being associated with acute hemorrhage.

The age of the infant at the time of diagnosis of anemia may also be useful. Anemia present at birth is usually associated with obstetric complications or severe isoimmunization. Anemia occurring after the first day or two of life is frequently caused by hemorrhage (internal or external) or hemolysis.

Initial laboratory evaluation should include a complete blood cell count, reticulocyte count, direct and indirect Coombs test, and a peripheral blood smear. If the anemia has resulted from chronic (weeks) hemorrhage or hemolysis, the reticulocyte count will be elevated, whereas the reticulocyte count may be normal with an acute hemorrhage. A positive direct and indirect Coombs test will identify infants with isoimmunization in the rhesus, ABO, or minor blood group systems.

The peripheral blood smear should be carefully reviewed. If it reveals hypochromic microcytic red cells, iron deficiency should be considered. This might result from chronic blood loss secondary to chronic fetal-maternal hemorrhage or twin-to-twin transfusion. Red blood cell fragmentation might be seen with infections. Spherocytes can be seen in ABO hemolytic disease and infections as well as with congenital spherocytosis. Red cell membrane defects frequently cannot be diagnosed from the peripheral smear in the neonate and require specific laboratory tests (e.g., osmotic fragility testing) as well as evaluation of the peripheral smear after the infant is a few months old.

C. Treatment. Signs of anemia in the newborn usually will not appear until the hemoglobin is <12 g/dL. An acute (minutes to a few hours) blood loss, however, may produce shock and may not be reflected in the hemoglobin concentration for 3 hours or more after the episode. As soon as anemia with hypovolemia is diagnosed, 10 to 20 mL/kg of normal saline or type O, Rh negative, blood should be administered.

Occasionally, a partial exchange with packed red blood cells (PRBC) may be indicated to prevent volume overload in the infant with severe anemia. Once it has been decided to perform a partial volume exchange transfusion, an umbilical venous catheter is inserted. Ideally, the catheter should be placed so that its tip is above the diaphragm. Blood is removed in 10 to 15 mL aliquots from the umbilical vein and an equal amount of PRBC is infused. The volume of PRBC to be given in a partial exchange transfusion may be calculated from the equation:

$$\text{Packed Red Blood Cells required (mL)} = \frac{(\text{desired Hct*} - \text{existing observed Hct}) \times \text{blood volume (mL)}}{75 \text{ or known Hct of donor blood}}$$

$$\text{Hct*} = \text{hematocrit}$$

The hematocrit of PRBC is generally assumed to be 75%. In emergent situations, whole blood obtained from the cord may also be used as an "autotransfusion" in the infant. A 20 mL syringe that has been heparinized by coating the syringe with 0.1 mL of heparin (1000 units/mL) may be used to collect blood from the cord vessels. This should be administered through a blood filter within 1 hour after collection.

In nonemergent situations, type-specific cross-matched blood may be used. Absolute indications for transfusion are impossible to give. The decision to transfuse must be made on the basis of each infant's clinical condition. However, the following guidelines may be helpful:

- Infants requiring cardiorespiratory support should have hematocrit maintained at 35% to 40%.
- Premature infants who are acutely ill should have cumulative records of blood loss. When 10% of the infant's blood volume has been removed, a transfusion with isotonic colloid or crystalloid should be considered.
- Premature infants at the nadir of their anemia should each be evaluated and not transfused unless symptoms of tissue hypoxia are present (e.g., failure to thrive, tachycardia, apnea). These infants should also be started on supplemental oral iron to achieve an optimal intake of 2 to 4 mg elemental iron/kg/day when they are tolerating full volume enteral feedings and are approximately 4 weeks of postnatal age.

The decision to transfuse an infant should always be made with consideration of the risks involved. Transfusion reactions and the risk of transmitting cytomegalovirus (CMV), hepatitis, or human T-cell lymphotropic virus type III (HTLV-III) are potential complications. Air emboli are probably the greatest potential complication of an exchange transfusion. Other risks include portal vein thrombosis, bacterial infection, bleeding, and necrotizing enterocolitis. It may be preferable to avoid feeding an infant who has had an exchange transfusion for 8–12 hours after the procedure. During that time, an intravenous infusion of glucose may be required.

III. Polycythemia. Polycythemia, defined as a hematocrit >65%, occurs in 1% to 5% of all newborns. The clinical signs associated with polycythemia are thought to be related to hyperviscosity. Viscosity is defined as the resistance of one layer of a fluid over another layer of fluid over another layer and is determined by red blood cell deformability, plasma proteins, and the hematocrit. The hematocrit is the most important of these factors. Above a hematocrit of 65%, blood flow becomes increasingly sluggish, and viscosity increases

Table 19-2. Causes of neonatal polycythemia

Increased erythropoiesis (active)
   Small for gestational age
   Chronic intrauterine hypoxia
   Fetal hyperinsulinism
   Trisomies 13, 18, 21
   Congenital thyrotoxicosis
Transfusion (passive)
   Delayed cord clamping
   Maternal–fetal transfusion
   Twin-to-twin transfusion

---

exponentially with the increasing hematocrit. Although most infants with polycythemia with hyperviscosity do not require invasive treatment, this disorder may cause significant morbidity and affected infants may require a partial exchange transfusion.

A. Etiologies. Hyperviscosity may result from (1) polycythemia, the most important cause, (2) decreased red blood cell deformability, and (3) abnormalities of plasma proteins. Polycythemia occurs because of increased hematopoiesis (active) or because of transfusions (passive). The common causes that predispose an infant to polycythemia are presented in Table 19-2. Chronic intrauterine hypoxia is thought to be a major stimulus for increased erythropoietin production. The highest incidence of polycythemia is seen in small-for-gestational-age (SGA) neonates, occurring in approximately 15% of these infants. Post-term infants who are large for gestational age (LGA), especially infants of diabetic mothers, also demonstrate an increased incidence of polycythemia. Hyperinsulinism is associated with increased fetal plasma concentrations of erythropoietin. The offspring of women who smoke have been shown to have elevated hematocrits. Maternal cigarette smoking has been shown to cause an elevation in the carbon monoxide level in maternal and umbilical cord blood as well as decreased uterine blood flow. Both of these factors may contribute to a reduction in the fetal oxygen supply and thereby increase erythropoiesis. Infants with chromosomal abnormalities such as trisomy 13, 18, and 21 also have a high incidence of polycythemia.

Placental transfusions are an additional potential cause of polycythemia. These passive causes of polycythemia may occur as a result of (1) obstetric manipulations such as holding the baby lower than the perineum following delivery or delayed cord clamping, (2) twin-to-twin transfusion, or (3) maternal–fetal transfusion.

Decreased red blood cell deformability contributing to hyperviscosity may occur because of hypoxia, acidosis, hypoglycemia, or a congenital red cell membrane defect. Elevated levels of plasma proteins, fibrinogens, and platelets, and abnormalities in plasma proteins may also cause hyperviscosity. However, abnormalities of RBC deformability and plasma protein as an etiology for hyperviscosity have not been well-defined or studied.

B. Diagnosis. Polycythemia with resultant hyperviscosity causes a variety of symptoms in association with impaired organ perfusion. The cardiac, respiratory, and neurologic systems may be affected. The most common findings include lethargy, poor feeding with inadequate sucking, plethora, jitteriness, tachypnea, jaundice, and hypoglycemia. There have also been reports of thromboembolic conditions resulting in cerebral infarcts, peripheral gangrene, necrotizing enterocolitis, and renal failure.

A frequent abnormality noted in association with polycythemia is hypoglycemia. However, it must be noted that a screening glucose method that relies on a reagent strip tends to underestimate serum glucose concentrations because it measures whole blood glucose; as the hematocrit increases, the discrepancy between the estimate of the whole blood glucose concentration and the plasma glucose concentration becomes greater.

Investigators have found that an umbilical venous hematocrit >63% is frequently associated with hyperviscosity and correlates better with the presence of symptoms than did a peripheral venous hematocrit. However, an umbilical vein catheterization is an invasive procedure, and most clinicians continue to use blood samples from a peripheral vein for a diagnosis of polycythemia. In many nurseries a hematocrit is performed as part of the admitting procedures to the nursery. If the hematocrit is >65% to 70% when obtained from a warmed heel after 1 hour of age, the measurement should be repeated on a free flowing venous blood sample. If the venous hematocrit is equal to or >70%, treatment with a partial exchange transfusion may be indicated. If the venous hematocrit is between 65% and 70% and the infant is asymptomatic, close monitoring of the clinical status is indicated. If the hematocrit is between 60% and 65% and the infant is symptomatic, an exchange transfusion may be indicated.

C. **Treatment.** The partial volume exchange transfusion is performed as described for a partial volume exchange with PRBC, with the exception that blood is removed in 10 to 15 mL aliquots from the umbilical vein and an equal amount of normal saline is infused. The volume to be exchanged is calculated from the equation:

$$\text{Volume of exchange (mL)} = \text{weight (kg)} \times 85 \text{ mL} \times \frac{(\text{observed Hct*} - \text{desired Hct})}{\text{observed Hct}}$$

$$\text{Hct*} = \text{hematocrit}$$

The risks are similar to those described for a partial exchange with PRBC (above). It may be preferable to avoid feeding an infant who has had an exchange transfusion for 8–12 hours after the procedure. During that time an intravenous infusion of glucose may be required.

IV. **Coagulation disorders.** Coagulation disorders in the newborn may be the result of many different factors. Evaluation of bleeding in the newborn begins with the determination of the type of bleeding as well as an assessment of the overall clinical status of the infant. A healthy infant with isolated petechiae is more likely to have an isolated platelet or vascular disorder. A severely ill infant with any bleeding manifestation needs to be thoroughly evaluated for complex coagulation defects.

A. **Etiologies.**

1. **Hemorrhagic disease of the newborn.** Hemorrhagic disease of the newborn occurs in 0.5% to 1% of newborns. In vitamin K deficiency the infant usually appears healthy but will manifest bleeding from the gastrointestinal tract, umbilical cord, circumcision site, or venipuncture sites. Intracranial bleeding has also been reported in association with this defect. It is thought that the hemorrhagic disease is caused by negligible stores of vitamin K, limited oral intake, and absent intestinal flora to produce vitamin K during the infant's first days of life. Bleeding may occur on the first day of life but usually occurs on the second or third day; rarely, it may not present until the second to fourth week of life, particularly in the breastfed infant. Hemorrhagic disease of the newborn is preventable by the administration of 1 mg vitamin K (phytonadione) to the newborn in the first hour of life. For infants born at <32 weeks a lower dose is recommended: 0.5 mg vitamin K for those weighing more than 1000 g, and 0.3 mg vitamin K for those weighing <1000 g. When hemorrhage occurs as a result of vitamin K deficiency, the history should be reviewed to make sure the infant received a prophylactic dose of vitamin K and to evaluate whether the mother was receiving Coumadin or phenytoin during pregnancy. Both of these drugs cross the placenta and impair vitamin K production in the newborn. These infants may require additional doses of vitamin K. Infants who are born at home often do not receive vitamin K and may present with bleeding problems or even seizures secondary to an intracranial hemorrhage.

2. **Anticoagulant deficiencies.** The presence of intracranial hemorrhage in a term newborn may reflect the presence of a cerebral thromboembolic event. Mutations in Factor V Leiden and prothrombin, deficiencies in protein C, S, and antithrombin III, as well as the presence of maternal antiphospholipid antibodies may predispose the neonate to thromboembolism. There are no screening tests for hereditary deficiency of these anticoagulants. A careful family history is helpful but a negative history does not rule out predisposition to thrombosis. Specific tests for the quantitation and functional analysis of the proteins are available. Genetic testing for Factor V Leiden and the prothrombin mutation are sensitive and specific. Complete protein C deficiency may present as purpura fulminans soon after birth. Fresh frozen plasma is an immediate source of protein C and doses of 10 to 15 mL/kg every 8 to 12 hours generally ameliorates the symptoms. Use of anticoagulants to prevent thrombosis in predisposed patients is generally avoided in the neonatal period.

3. **Thrombocytopenia.** There are several causes of thrombocytopenia and platelet dysfunction in the neonate. Table 19-3 lists some of the more common causes of neonatal thrombocytopenia.

   Idiopathic thrombocytopenic purpura (ITP) in the mother results in transplacentally acquired IgG antibodies in the infant that may react with the neonatal platelets and result in their destruction. Infants affected with ITP appear healthy

Table 19-3. Causes of neonatal thrombocytopenia

Infection
Bacterial
Viral
Immune disorders
Isoimmunization
Maternal antibody induced (SLE, ITP)
Bone marrow abnormalities
Aplastic anemia
Congenital leukemia
TAR syndrome (thrombocytopenia, absent radii)
Intravascular coagulation
Peripheral utilization, e.g., giant hemangioma
Hereditary thrombocytopenias
Miscellaneous
Postexchange transfusion
Maternal hyperthyroidism
Thrombotic thrombocytopenic purpura
Maternal drugs (e.g., tolbutamide, thiazides, quinidine)

SLE, systemic lupus erythematosis; ITP, Idiopathic thrombocytopenic purpura.

except for generalized petechiae. The platelet count may be $<10,000/mm^3$. Thrombocytopenia in the newborn may last for several months, although serious bleeding such as intracranial hemorrhage usually does not occur after the first week of life. The use of corticosteroids, platelet transfusions, immunoglobulins, and exchange transfusions to remove immunoglobulin and to increase transfused platelet survival may be indicated.

Occasionally, mothers with thrombocytopenia secondary to systemic lupus erythematosis (SLE) may pass antiplatelet antibodies to the fetus, resulting in neonatal thrombocytopenia.

Infants with neonatal alloimmune thrombocytopenic purpura (NATP) will appear healthy except for bruising and petechiae. Mothers of these infants have no bleeding disorder and will have a normal platelet count. The antibodies in the newborn are maternally derived IgG directed against specific antigens (Pl^{A1} antigen most common) on the infant's platelets that were inherited from the father but are absent from maternal platelets. Both firstborn and subsequent newborns are affected with NATP. If a positive family history is lacking, the diagnosis is often one of exclusion. With this disorder the risk of central nervous system bleeding may be as high as 10% to 15%, although this usually occurs only during the first week of life. Thrombocytopenia may last for 2 to 3 months. Exchange transfusion may be effective in removing some antibody, but it is not likely to result in long-term benefit. Transfusion of washed maternal platelets, which lack the antigen, will have a normal survival in the neonate. Often, only a single platelet transfusion with maternal platelets is required, yielding adequate platelet counts for the first 10 days of life. Prenatal detection of this disorder permits monitoring of fetal platelet counts by percutaneous umbilical blood sampling. Administration of intravenous immunoglobulin prenatally to the mother is effective.

In thrombocytopenic newborns who appear ill, sepsis must be ruled out. Congenital or acquired infection is probably the most common cause of thrombocytopenia in the newborn. Other causes of thrombocytopenia may include congenital leukemia, malignancy including neuroblastoma, inborn errors of metabolism, giant hemangiomas with platelet trapping, and exchange transfusions with platelet-poor blood.

4. **Disseminated intravascular coagulopathy.** Disseminated intravascular coagulopathy (DIC) is a generalized coagulopathy manifested by the intravascular consumption of platelets and various plasma clotting factors. This is a condition that results from predisposing factors such as hypoxemia and acidosis, disseminated viral or bacterial septicemia, or obstetric complications such as abruptio placentae and shock. Infants with DIC appear ill and usually have generalized bleeding

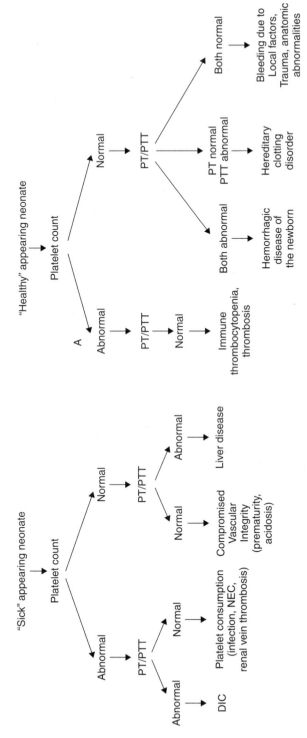

Figure 19-2. Algorithm to classify an approach to make the diagnosis for the cause of bleeding in the newborn based upon an overall clinical assessment of whether the patient is a "sick" appearing infant or a "healthy" appearing infant.

from puncture sites as well as the gastrointestinal tract, central nervous system, and skin. Treatment for DIC requires correction of the underlying etiology. Platelet transfusions and fresh frozen plasma are indicated.

B. **Diagnosis.** If a newborn is bleeding, certain historical data may be helpful. Review of the maternal history may reveal such factors as collagen vascular diseases, idiopathic thrombocytopenia purpura, viral infections, or ingestion of drugs such as salicylates, phenytoin, or Coumadin. A family history may reveal siblings with bleeding problems or neonatal petechiae, and an obstetrical history may reveal a traumatic delivery, delivery outside the hospital, or the need for resuscitation. The birth history should be reviewed to confirm the administration of vitamin K.

The physician must determine whether the bleeding is localized, such as with a traumatic delivery, or more generalized, which might indicate a bleeding diathesis. Scattered petechiae on the head and shoulders of a normal infant must be differentiated from the diffuse petechiae seen in infants with thrombocytopenia. The infant who appears well is more likely to have a platelet function defect, hemophilia, or vitamin K deficiency. An infant who appears ill suggests sepsis, congenital infection, acute infection, or DIC as a cause of bleeding. Hepatomegaly, splenomegaly, and jaundice suggest sepsis or DIC. Absent radii in the thrombocytopenic neonate, chorioretinitis, congenital heart disease, microcephaly, or giant hemangiomata may provide diagnostic clues in the evaluation of infant with a bleeding problem.

The basic laboratory evaluation of the bleeding infant should include a platelet count, prothrombin time (PT), and partial thromboplastin time (PTT). Other laboratory evaluations are indicated depending on the results of these and the clinical appearance of the infant. Fig. 19-2 provides a guide for the evaluation of the results of the PT, PTT, and platelet count.

C. **Treatment.** Treatment of an infant with vitamin K will stop the bleeding within a few hours if vitamin K deficiency was the cause of the bleeding; the PT and PTT will also improve. An empiric trial of 1 mg vitamin K should be considered in any infant with unexplained bleeding. If bleeding is severe or the infant does not respond to vitamin K, intravenous administration of 10 to 20 mL/kg fresh frozen plasma may be indicated. Platelet transfusions are used in those infants with thrombocytopenia. Factor replacement is indicated in the infant with a documented factor deficiency.

V.   **Clinical pearls.**
- Be wary that the pale infant born with a nuchal cord may display significant anemia as a result of an unbalanced redistribution of blood from the newborn into the placenta (umbilical arteries pump blood into the placenta, but the venous blood returning to the fetus is restricted by the tightening of the nuchal cord).
- Remember that infants with hemolytic disease who are treated *in utero* with intravenous transfusions may appear entirely normal at birth but display a "late" hyporegenerative anemia during the first few months of life.
- Insufficient iron supplementation will limit red blood cell production and thereby dampen the ability of the neonate to recover from anemia.
- An infant who appears cyanotic may be suffering from polycythemia with hyperviscosity and can be readily treated with a partial volume exchange transfusion.
- Of all the peripheral blood cell counts, platelet counts may be the most difficult to obtain and an abnormal count deserves to be repeated while therapeutic intervention is considered.

BIBLIOGRAPHY

Christensen RD, ed. *Hematologic problems of the neonate.* Philadelphia, PA: WB Saunders, 1999.

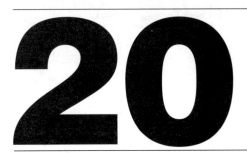

Stabilization and Preparation of the Infant for Transport

Vicki Powell-Tippit

I. **Description of the issue.** Neonatal transport systems were introduced in the early 1970s following the development of neonatal intensive care units. Although most hospitals were equipped to provide basic care to compromised neonates, the need for tertiary referral centers became evident as neonatal care became more complex with advances in the field of neonatology. As the concept of regionalization of perinatal services began to evolve, the need for neonatal transport systems to referral centers with neonatal intensive care capabilities became apparent.

Transport of the compromised neonate is a complex undertaking requiring an organized system of communication, experienced personnel, equipment, and mode of transportation. Ideally, the transportation of critically ill neonates should be performed by the staff of a tertiary neonatal intensive care center. However, because of the time that elapses between recognition of illness in the neonate and the arrival of the transport team, every referring hospital must be able to provide stabilization and continuing care to the ill neonate. It is imperative that the personnel who practice in any hospital that provides obstetrical services become skilled in the recognition of illness in the neonate and in the initiation of stabilizing measures. The ultimate goal of the events that surround neonatal transport is the safe arrival of a well-stabilized neonate to the tertiary center. The success of this goal lies in the capabilities of the referring hospital in the initiation of stabilization, as well as the organization of the transport system.

II. **Making the decision and initiating transport.**

A. **Criteria for transport.** It would be ideal if every infant born at risk for compromise could be delivered at a facility equipped to provide neonatal intensive care. Careful screening for maternal and fetal risk factors can aid in determining instances where maternal transfer prior to delivery would be advised. Unfortunately, even with rigorous screening, it is impossible to predict every infant that will require intensive care. It is therefore essential to have trained personnel who are capable of performing neonatal resuscitation and stabilization and who are readily available in every hospital that provides obstetrical services.

While individual hospitals must determine their own capabilities for caring for compromised neonates, the decision to transport an infant should be made in consultation with the staff at the referral facility. The criteria for consultation, evaluation, and consideration of transport of infants to a referral facility are outlined in Table 20-1.

B. **Initiation of the transport process.** The transport process is initiated when the physician at the referring hospital contacts the physician coordinating transports at the tertiary center. Information about the infant's provisional diagnosis, gestational age, and current status are relayed. The coordinating physician gathers further information and advises the referring physician in ongoing management while the transport team is mobilized. Consideration must also be given to legal and regulatory standards that have been set in place regarding patient transport. These standards vary from state to state and all transport systems must comply with the standards that have been set forth in their particular areas.

Following the transport team's arrival, informed consent for transport and admission into the tertiary center must be obtained. Additional consent forms, such as those for administration of blood products or those for emergency procedures that may be necessary prior to the parent's arrival at the tertiary facility, may be obtained as well. In localities where great distance exists between the referring and tertiary facilities, informed consent for specialized procedures (such as extracorporeal membrane oxygenation) may be obtained via direct consultation over the telephone between the parents and the physician at the tertiary center. Lastly, patient identification needs to be verified and in place prior to the transport team's departure. Additional items that should be included in the transport packet are a copy of the maternal and

Table 20-1. Neonatal indications for possible transfer to a referral facility

Prematurity
    Gestational age ≤34 wk or birth weight <2000 g
Respiratory distress
    Surfactant deficiency
    Respiratory acidosis
    Meconium aspiration
    Pneumonia
    Pulmonary and/or airway malformation(s)
Sepsis/infection
Metabolic acidosis
Congenital heart disease
Shock/hypovolemia
Asphyxia
Seizure activity
Metabolic disorders
    Hypoglycemia
    Hypocalcemia
    Inborn errors of metabolism
Electrolyte disorders
Maternal health issues
    Diabetes
    Substance abuse
    Autoimmune disorders
    Hypertension
Hyperbilirubinemia
    Exchange transfusion necessary
    Hemolytic disease
Congenital malformations

        infant medical records, a detailed perinatal history, and copies of any radiographic studies performed prior to transport.

III. **Stabilizing and preparing the infant for transport.** The stabilization process for transport should include a comprehensive physical assessment (Table 20-2). In addition to the physical assessment, testing and monitoring steps that are usually performed as part of the infant evaluation are outlined in Table 20-3. The following paragraphs identify and present a synopsis of the more common therapies involved during the stabilization process.

    A. Thermoregulation. One of the most important aspects of neonatal care involves the maintenance of an optimal thermal environment (see Chapter 5). Following delivery, the infant should be dried thoroughly and placed under a radiant warmer or in an incubator. The servo-control sensor should be applied to the skin and the controls adjusted accordingly to maintain the infant's temperature within a normal range. The use of a chemical heat mattress can also be useful, especially with extremely-low-birth-weight infants. If supplemental oxygen is administered, it should be heated as well as humidified. Placing the infant directly on cold surfaces, such as scales or x-ray plates, should be avoided.

    B. Glucose homeostasis and intravenous fluid administration. Blood glucose analysis should be performed on all ill neonates. A blood glucose level of <40 mg/dL identifies hypoglycemia and corrective measures should be implemented (see Chapter 7). The infant in need of transport to a tertiary center is usually too sick to feed enterally and, therefore, a peripheral intravenous infusion is necessary. Should difficulty be encountered in establishing peripheral access, umbilical venous catheterization is indicated. The recommended treatment of hypoglycemia is a 2 mL/kg intravenous bolus of 10% dextrose solution followed by a constant infusion containing 10% dextrose at a rate to provide 80 mL/kg/day. This infusion will provide approximately 5 mg/kg/min of glucose, which under most circumstances will maintain the infant's serum glucose within the normal range. Blood glucose analysis should be performed

Table 20-2. Pretransport assessment and evaluation

Weight	
Vital signs	Obtain heart rate and respiratory rate; measure body temperature and blood pressure.
Respiratory	Observe respiratory effort and auscultate clarity of breath sounds; note presence of cyanosis.
Cardiovascular	Auscultate heart rhythm and note presence or absence of murmur; assess skin perfusion; palpate strength of peripheral pulses comparing intensity between upper and lower extremities.
Abdomen	Identify abdominal wall defects; note if distended or scaphoid in appearance; note presence or absence of bowel sounds.
Neurologic	Assess muscle tone; note the presence of lethargy or irritability; observe for seizure activity or tremors; identify neural tube defects.
Genitourinary	Note passage of urine and stool; identify ambiguity if suspected.
Dysmorphism	Identify congenital anomalies and/or dysmorphic features.

frequently to evaluate the infant's response. Increases in the rate of administration of the intravenous dextrose solution may be necessary should hypoglycemia persist.

C. **Oxygenation and ventilation.** Supplemental oxygen should be provided as necessary to relieve cyanosis and maintain the infant's oxygen saturation at greater than 90% (see Chapter 11). It is important to remember that supplemental oxygen should be warmed and humidified during administration to prevent hypothermia, the drying of mucous membranes, and insensible water loss.

On occasion, positive pressure ventilation and endotracheal intubation may be indicated prior to arrival of the transport team. The delivery of positive pressure ventilation, followed by endotracheal intubation, should be considered if the concentration of supplemental oxygen required to maintain acceptable oxygen saturation levels increases dramatically, if the arterial PCO_2 is >55 mm/Hg, or whenever the infant exhibits markedly increased respiratory effort, gasping, or apnea. If someone with expertise in neonatal intubation is unavailable, then bag and mask ventilation should be initiated to deliver 100% oxygen at a rate of 40 to 60 breaths per minute. Once endotracheal intubation has been successfully performed, a chest x-ray to confirm tube placement should be obtained. Additionally, an orogastric tube that is appropriate to the size of the infant should be measured and inserted in all acutely ill infants for the elimination of stomach contents and prevention of gastric distention and pulmonary aspiration. In nonsurgical conditions, the tube may be left to open gravity drainage. If a surgical lesion is present, a decompression tube containing multiple holes should be inserted and placed to low, intermittent suction.

D. **Pneumothorax.** The development of a pneumothorax can be spontaneous or can complicate the course of an infant receiving positive pressure ventilation. Signs and symptoms of a pneumothorax are listed in Table 20-4. Whenever a pneumothorax is suspected, detection and diagnosis should be carried out immediately. Rapid detection of a pneumothorax may be accomplished by utilizing a transilluminator containing an intense fiberoptic light source. A chest x-ray should be obtained to provide a definitive diagnosis if time and the infant's clinical status allow.

Not every pneumothorax requires evacuation. In the absence of respiratory distress or when only mild respiratory distress is present, the provision of 100% supplemental oxygen may be administered. The goal of this therapy focuses on resolution of the

Table 20-3. Common pretransport testing and monitoring

- Oxygen saturation
- Blood culture
- Complete blood cell count with differential
- Blood gas analysis
- Blood glucose analysis
- Chest x-ray/KUB

KUB, kidney, ureter, and bladder.

Table 20-4. Signs and symptoms of a pneumothorax

- Increasing respiratory distress
- Cyanosis
- Hypoxemia
- Hypotension
- Apnea
- Bradycardia
- Shift or change in heart sounds
- Chest asymmetry

pneumothorax via the nitrogen washout principle. Should the infant demonstrate signs of increasing respiratory or cardiac compromise, than evacuation is indicated and should be carried out expeditiously. Chest tubes are discussed in depth in Chapter 10.

E. Shock, hypovolemia, and metabolic acidosis. In the neonatal population, hypovolemia is the primary causative factor in the development of shock. Hypovolemia may result from acute blood loss secondary to placental abruption or placenta previa, or it can result from intravascular fluid losses secondary to dehydration or third spacing. Two other types of shock encountered in the neonatal population include cardiogenic shock and septic shock. The physiology of shock revolves around the development of decreased cardiac output, inadequate tissue perfusion, and the accumulation of lactic acid.

Clinical manifestations of shock include hypotension, pallor, delayed capillary refill time, tachycardia, and metabolic acidosis. The treatment of shock should target the underlying causative factor. In the presence of hypovolemia, volume expansion using 10 mL/kg normal saline should be administered intravenously. If anemia is present, 10 mL/kg emergency neonatal packed red blood cells (O negative, cytomegalovirus negative) or whole blood should be administered following the initial normal saline bolus. Should signs and symptoms of shock persist, additional aliquots of normal saline at 10 mLl/kg may be repeated. The administration of sodium bicarbonate 4.2% (0.5 mEq/mL) at 1 to 2 mEq/kg may be considered following intravenous fluid resuscitation in the treatment of metabolic acidosis once adequate ventilation has been assured. Should hypotension persist following repletion of intravascular volume, the administration of an inotrope such as dopamine at 5 to 20 micrograms/kg/minute should be considered. Whenever septic shock is suspected, the administration of antibiotic therapy should be initiated.

F. Surgical emergencies. The interventions necessary in the stabilization of neonatal surgical emergencies are discussed in great detail in other chapters of this text. Table 20-5 identifies several common surgical emergencies and briefly outlines the interventions necessary in stabilization for transport.

IV. Care of the family. The birth of an infant who is premature or critically ill or who has a serious congenital malformation is often an unexpected event and usually results in an acute emotional crisis within the family. Regionalization of neonatal care has resulted in the transfer of these critically ill infants to tertiary newborn intensive care units, and as a result parents are frequently a long distance from their newly born child. Most neonatal units have developed a family-friendly policy for visitation; however, medical, economical, and transportation issues may hamper the parents' ability to visit regularly.

It is important that parents view and touch their newborn infant prior to transport from the referring hospital. The infant should always be referred to by his or her given name (if named by the time of transport). Photographing the infant is encouraged, in addition to offering personal items such as a footprint or lock of hair. A packet of information concerning the tertiary center, including a parent handbook, should be offered to the parents so that they may familiarize themselves with the unit to which their infant will be admitted. A staff member at the referring hospital should remain present with the parents as information regarding the infant's condition, and subsequent plan of care, is being discussed. This approach will serve to enhance communication and foster comprehension, as the parents often require additional support during this stressful time.

Upon arrival of the infant to the tertiary center, the parents should be contacted and informed of their infant's safe arrival. The parents need to be provided with the names of the infant's attending physician, neonatal nurse practitioner, and primary nurse. Frequent telephone calls from the parents regarding status updates should be encouraged. Early involvement of the social worker at the tertiary center is helpful in addressing the family's financial and transportation needs in a timely fashion.

Table 20-5. Common neonatal surgical emergencies

Surgical emergency	Intervention(s)
Diaphragmatic hernia	Perform endotracheal intubation.
	Insert a 10 Fr orogastric decompression tube with multiple side holes and place at low intermittent suction.
	Administer IV fluids.
Gastroschisis	Place infant into a bowel bag and secure under the infant's armpits.
	Administer IV fluids.
	Insert an orogastric decompression tube with multiple side holes and place at low intermittent suction.
	Place in side-lying position to support the herniated viscera.
	Administer antibiotic coverage.
Omphalocele	Place infant into a bowel bag and secure under the infant's armpits.
	Administer IV fluids.
	Insert an orogastric decompression tube with multiple side holes and place at low intermittent suction.
	Administer antibiotic coverage.
Esophageal atresia or tracheoesophageal fistula	Elevate the head of bed 30–45 degrees.
	Insert an orogastric tube with multiple side holes and place at low intermittent suction.
	Administer IV fluids.
	Administer antibiotic coverage.
Bowel obstruction	Insert an orogastric tube with multiple side holes at low intermittent suction.
	Administer IV fluids.
	Administer antibiotic coverage.
Choanal atresia or Pierre Robin sequence	Place prone.
	Insert an oral airway.
	Provide supplemental oxygen.
	(Infants with Pierre Robin may benefit from having a 2.5 endotracheal tube inserted nasally to rest in the posterior pharynx).
	Administer IV fluids.
	Perform endotracheal intubation if necessary.
Neural tube defects	Cover the exposed lesion(s) with sterile saline-soaked nonadhering sponges and cover with a sterile plastic barrier (bowel bag may be considered).
	Place prone or in side-lying position.
	Administer IV fluids.
	Administer antibiotic coverage.
Extrophy of the bladder	Place infant into a bowel bag and secure under infant's armpits
	Avoid using gauze or sponges on the exposed bladder mucosa.
	Insert an orogastric tube with multiple side holes and place at low intermittent suction.
	Administer IV fluids.
	Administer antibiotic coverage.

V. **Clinical pearls.**
- Stabilization of the neonate for transport is the responsibility of the referring hospital. Factors that directly influence this process include the following:
  - Preparedness and training of involved staff members
  - Availability of equipment and supplies
  - Guidance from the tertiary referral center
- Thermoregulation is of utmost importance. In addition to the utilization of a radiant heat source or incubator, modalities such as a chemical heat mattress may prove valuable.
- Hypovolemia is the primary causative factor in the development of neonatal shock. Normal saline is readily available in most institutions and can be quickly obtained in emergent situations. Additionally, all institutions providing obstetrical services should

have O negative, cytomegalovirus negative, neonatal packed red blood cells readily available.
- The infant's parent(s) should be updated during the stabilization process and allowed to view and touch their infant prior to transport. Should the mother remain hospitalized, regular telephone contact with the tertiary center should be facilitated.

BIBLIOGRAPHY

American Academy of Pediatrics and American College of Obstetricians and Gynecologists. *Guidelines for perinatal care*, 5th ed. Elk Grove Village, IL: American Academy of Pediatrics, 2002.
Karlsen KA. *S.T.A.B.L.E. transport education program learner manual*. Park City, Utah: 2000.

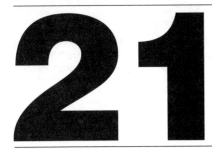

Caring for the Family Mourning a Perinatal Death

Maureen Shea and
James A. Lemons

I. **Description of the issue.** Much of the information provided in this chapter pertains not only to helping parents whose child dies, but also to helping parents of a child whose long-term survival is tenuous or who will have significant physical and/or developmental deficits. Even if a medical problem was diagnosed prenatally, parents experience renewed grief when their child is born and the reality of his or her future becomes more apparent. Parents' grief for the loss of normalcy can be overwhelming and is in many ways comparable to that of parents whose children die.

When parents experience the death of their baby, whether it occurs in a newborn intensive care unit after a prolonged hospitalization, or in the delivery room, their grief is unique. They have lost their child before they have had the opportunity to know him or her. Even if a lethal condition was diagnosed prenatally, parents cannot fully comprehend the finality of their loss until they see their child. They need time to bond with the child and to develop memories. By doing so, parents are able to incorporate their experience on cognitive and emotional levels. Compassionate bereavement care helps parents begin to mourn. As they work through the grieving process, parents redefine their relationship with their baby. Parents begin not to forget, but to relinquish. Mourning is a healing process. A physician's sensitive, considered response at the time of death and appropriate follow-up in the weeks and months afterward will help a family adjust to their loss.

II. **Communication.** For a child who is born prematurely and critically ill, or who develops a life-threatening condition shortly after delivery, there is no presumption of a relationship between parents and their baby's physician. Diagnostic tests must be performed and results shared quickly so parents can participate in decisions about their child's treatment. If a baby is transported from an outside hospital or the baby's mother has had a cesarean delivery, discussions about how aggressively to treat the baby should not occur until both parents can participate, if possible. All appropriate medical care should be provided and treatment discussions delayed until both parents have arrived and have spent time with their baby. Information should be shared in private and with consideration for the parents' level of anxiety. If one or both of the parents is not proficient in English, professional medical translation services should be arranged; it is not appropriate to expect a spouse, an extended family member, or a non-medical hospital staff member to translate and interpret medical information.

A. **Language and information.** Language should be descriptive and clear. Medical terms should be explained. If possible, allow parents to look at x-ray films or ultrasound images and explain to them what they are seeing. If a diagnostic work-up is incomplete, give parents a reasonable estimate of when they can expect more complete information. Even parents who are well-educated and have medical backgrounds can become overwhelmed when their baby is born critically ill. All parents need time to absorb and process information and to place that information in perspective, particularly when critical decisions regarding care are being considered. The necessary time frame parents need to make decisions can vary tremendously between families. Also, it is not unusual, nor necessarily indicative of dysfunction, for one parent to process information more expediently than the other.

B. **Sensitivity.** Whether their child's death is expected or occurs suddenly, when speaking with parents, a physician needs to communicate with sensitivity. Take the baby's family to a comfortable room and speak with them privately. Sit with them; do not stand over them. Make sure that others who can provide additional support are available, even if this means delaying the discussion. Wait for extended family members if the parents request that you do so. Include other members of the medical team who have been closely involved in the baby's care. This may include the baby's primary nurse, respiratory therapist, and social worker. The family should be offered the services of a hospital chaplain, or clergy from a family's own faith community can be invited to participate.

Refer to their child by his or her name. If a baby has not been given a name or if the child's gender has not yet been determined, use the terms "the baby," or "your child." Never refer to a baby as "it." Avoid medical jargon or slang, as in "Your baby was a no-code." In such cases, describe the medical order that precluded resuscitation as distinct from the identity of the child.

Families need to perceive their child's caregivers as competent, sensitive professionals. They need an indication that this particular discussion is different than previous conversations that may have taken place at their child's bedside. Even if you have developed sufficient rapport to address parents by their first names, make a conscious effort to project a more formal tone when discussing the events surrounding their child's death. First names can still be used but parents will appreciate your respectful consideration at this time.

III. **Cultural respect.** Physicians and other care providers for patients in newborn intensive care units encounter families from every ethnic, racial, religious, and socioeconomic background. It is incumbent upon those providers to respond with respect and sensitivity to families from diverse cultures whose values may differ from their own. Even the definition of what constitutes a family unit varies widely. Parents may or may not be married. Siblings may be step- or half brothers and sisters. Single parents may be heavily dependent on extended family. Gay and lesbian parents are now more common.

   A. **Family awareness.** Through experience, physicians develop awareness of families' perceptions and learn to project a non-judgmental attitude. If parents have made choices with which a physician does not agree, either in their lifestyle or regarding their baby, it is inappropriate to address these issues at the time of a child's death.

   B. **Self-awareness.** Self-awareness of one's own cultural bias is essential, because it affects the manner in which one relates to others. For instance, if physicians are insensitive to the discrepancy in the educational level between themselves and their patients' parents, they may be perceived as condescending.

IV. **Preparation for withdrawal of life support.** When all medical therapies have been ineffective and there is no reasonable likelihood of recovery or for a meaningful quality of life, parents and their baby's physician sometimes decide to withdraw life support. This is a well-established practice in many neonatal centers.

   A. **Guiding the family.** Guiding families through this process is one of the most challenging tasks a physician will face. Diagnoses might include, but are not limited to, genetic conditions that are incompatible with life, such as Potters sequence, severe intracranial hemorrhages in extremely premature infants, or advanced multisystem organ failure caused by overwhelming sepsis. In circumstances such as these, death is a predictable outcome and parents, with support from their baby's physician and other care providers, may be motivated by a desire to spare their child further suffering. For a baby who has been in the newborn intensive care unit for several weeks or even months, regular communication with their baby's physicians and other caregivers will have prepared families for these discussions. It is important that a trusting relationship has developed.

   When the option of stopping aggressive therapies and removing life support is introduced, some parents are reluctant to consider such a step. They may feel that by withdrawing aggressive care they are causing their child's death. It is important that they understand the difference between causing a child to die and allowing a child to die. Their baby's condition—not their decision—is the cause of death. Some families will not consider withdrawal of support under any circumstances and the medical staff must respect their decision. Communicating treatment options must be done with objectivity as it is crucial that families not feel pressured or unduly influenced by an individual physician's or other caregiver's bias.

   No matter what their ultimate decision and course of action, most families benefit from supportive counseling, which can be provided by a social worker, family support coordinator, or chaplain. Involving these professionals in care conferences promotes effective family care.

   If there is not a consensus of opinion among the medical staff directly involved in a child's care, or if a child's family requests it, the hospital's ethics committee can be consulted. In most hospitals, ethics committees serve as forums for medical professionals to objectively discuss issues for which there are not always clear answers. Ethics committees discuss whether continuing treatment is in a patient's best interest or is likely to cause additional pain with questionable benefit. Issues such as quality of life and futility of care are considered. The recommendations of an ethics committee are not legally binding but can often validate a family's decision and a physician's recommendation.

B. Preparing the family. If the decision is made to discontinue medical intervention or if death is imminent, parents should be prepared for what they will see and experience at the time of their child's death. Most parents, when given the choice, choose to be present and, if at all possible, to hold their child at the moment of death. Parents should be reassured that their baby will not be afraid or in pain, and that medications can be given to the baby to prevent anxiety or discomfort. If their baby is to be extubated, parents should have an opportunity to spend time at their baby's bedside before extubation occurs. Parents can be encouraged to dress their baby and to take pictures. Whenever possible, siblings and other extended family members should be included in the process. If the parents want their child to be baptized or blessed, this can occur prior to extubation, as well.

After taking the family to a separate room, the medical staff can remove all monitor leads, feeding tubes, and intravenous tubes not needed for pain medication. Following extubation the baby can be brought to his or her family. To assure privacy, most newborn intensive care units and labor and delivery units have a designated bereavement room. The room should be large enough to accommodate several people and should be comfortably furnished and softly lit. Nursing and respiratory staff should be available as needed. Usually, a chaplain and a social worker are also available. Often, family and staff members develop a warm relationship. Parents are comforted by the presence of people who knew and cared for their child.

Before the baby is brought to them, a physician can reassure parents that comfort measures including pain medication and supplemental oxygen are readily available. A physician should also tactfully describe physical changes that may occur during the dying process. Parents should be warned ahead of time that their baby might gasp intermittently for several minutes but this does not mean that their baby is struggling to breathe. Rather, gasping indicates a progressive slowing of respiratory effort and may continue even after there is no detectable heartbeat. Parents should be prepared that their baby's skin might become dusky in color and cool to the touch. After their baby has been pronounced dead, families should be allowed privacy and as much time as they need to stay with and hold their baby.

C. Discussing autopsy. An autopsy is usually offered when the specific cause of death is unknown. The findings could provide a more complete explanation to parents of why their child became ill and may be of value if parents consider another pregnancy. It may also indicate the need for genetic testing or future high-risk obstetrical care. Some families consent to autopsy for the benefit of medical science, feeling that doing so gives value to their baby's life. While this is valid, parents should not feel pressured into giving consent for this reason alone.

Although an autopsy can, and often should be, discussed prior to an expected death, in most states obtaining consent for an autopsy must be done after the baby has been pronounced dead. The physician who requests consent should be sensitive to the family's emotional fragility and the timing of the request should be carefully considered. When parents are holding their baby and saying good-bye, it is not advisable to discuss a postmortem examination. Most parents feel too vulnerable at this point to consider further medical procedures and, even though an autopsy will not harm their baby, parents may feel too protective to consider the issue objectively.

Parents should be advised that an autopsy can usually be completed within 24 hours of death and will not delay funeral plans. If a postmortem examination of the brain is indicated, parents should be advised that the baby would need to wear a bonnet or cap for a viewing at the funeral home. Some families will consider a limited autopsy involving only the particular organs or parts of the body that were malformed or diseased. If a metabolic disorder is suspected and a muscle biopsy is needed immediately after death, special arrangements to transport the baby's body will need to be made prior to death. Parents should be prepared in advance that they will not be able to spend much time alone with their baby in this instance.

D. Funeral planning. Most parents who lose a baby have no experience planning a funeral or memorial service. Some may question the importance of having a service at all. A physician can explain that because their baby was a newborn and was critically ill, many family members and friends did not have an opportunity to see the baby. A funeral or memorial service is a way for parents to publicly acknowledge their baby and to receive support and consolation from people who care about them. Because they are often exhausted by their baby's hospitalization, parents might feel overwhelmed at the prospect of a formal funeral service. Advise them that their clergyman or a funeral director will help them plan a service that is meaningful to them and reflective of their values.

If parents express concern about the expense of a funeral, a social worker should be consulted. Generally, funerals for infants are not as expensive as for adults and some funeral homes offer significantly reduced rates for infant funerals. Public funds for such services may also exist. In any case, families should be informed that, by law, most states require any baby born, alive or dead, after 20 weeks gestation, to be buried or cremated by a licensed mortician. Parents should be assured that it is not necessary for them to complete funeral arrangements on the same day that their baby dies. Even if an autopsy is not done, parents can wait until they have returned home and rested before they begin to make arrangements.

V.   **Counseling families after the death of their baby.** After their baby has died, families typically need some time to regroup before leaving the hospital. At this point it is appropriate for the baby's physician to sit down with parents and initiate a discussion of what they can expect in the days and weeks to come. Parents appreciate a brief description of what feelings they may experience. Having gone through such an emotionally draining event, many parents may initially feel numb, physically exhausted, and even relieved. Parents may have difficulty accepting their new reality; it is not uncommon for parents to think they hear their baby cry after he or she has died. Mothers who have recently delivered sometimes think they can feel their baby move inside them, as if they were still pregnant. Parents should be reassured that such experiences are the mind's way of making sense of what has just occurred. These sensations are normal and will likely pass within a few days.

Parents should be counseled that the death of a child is one of the most significant losses they will ever experience and their pain will not diminish for some time. Bereaved parents should be aware that in the months following their baby's death even a strong, committed relationship could be jeopardized. If communication between parents is affected, professional counseling may be indicated.

Parents should be encouraged to seek support not only from one another but also from their friends, extended family, or faith community. Sometimes parents feel they are imposing on others if they continue to express their grief for more than a few weeks after their baby has died. These parents may benefit from a structured support group but may be reluctant to attend. Physicians can encourage parents to participate, explaining that health care professionals experienced in obstetric or neonatal medicine typically lead these groups. Such groups can provide a safe, nonthreatening environment for parents to talk about their baby and their ongoing feelings of loss.

Increasingly, families are using the Internet as a source of information and support. Numerous websites for grieving parents are available. The anonymity of chat rooms or online support groups may be less threatening for some parents. However, grieving parents are especially vulnerable to those who might take advantage of them. Also, the Internet is not a substitute for, and may even impede, honest communication between grieving mothers and fathers.

Mothers whose babies die within the first few days or weeks after birth may not have had sufficient opportunity to recover from labor and delivery. They are often physically and emotionally exhausted, resulting in increased stress and vulnerability to infection and other postpartum complications. Fathers and extended family members should be advised that the baby's mother might need medical care during this time.

Postpartum depression is a separate clinical issue. If a grieving mother experiences more than the transitory sensations previously described and manifests full-blown audio or visual hallucinations, expresses suicidal thoughts, or attempts to harm herself, immediate psychiatric intervention is needed. Women who have a previous history of depression or other mental illness are at increased risk for postpartum depression.

Fathers are still sometimes referred to as the "forgotten grievers." Increased societal acceptance of expression of emotion by men has helped to lessen the stereotype of the man who must remain strong for others, at the expense of his own emotional health. However, grieving fathers may still need encouragement to express their emotions.

VI.   **Siblings.** Parents may seek guidance from their baby's physician about talking with their baby's siblings. Children react to loss based on their particular developmental stages.

A.   **Infants.** Infants, such as a surviving baby in a set of multiples, can be affected by loss. Though not typical, if an infant's caregiver is incapacitated by grief and unable to care for them, disruptions in the attachment process can occur. A baby reacts to his or her parents' emotional state. When a mother or father is grief-stricken, it is possible that their surviving baby may sense their tension.

B.   **One- and 2-year-old children.** One- and 2-year-old children do not generally have a well-developed capacity for understanding permanent absence. They often mimic behaviors of those around them and may seem to be participating but do not yet understand fully. However, they do have the capacity for memory. As a toddler's vocabulary expands, parents are often surprised when their 2-year-old talks about the baby sister or brother that died 6 months previously and describes events that occurred around the time of the death.

C. **Three- to 5-year-old children.** Three- to 5-year-old children still do not grasp the finality of death. They tend to think that death is reversible and the deceased is going to reappear. They may act their feelings out in regressive behaviors, such as tantrums or bedwetting. Or they may behave as if the event did not happen. They will need reassurance that the baby's death does not mean that they will die or that their parents or other family members will die. What they are really asking is, "Will I be okay? Will someone be here to take care of me?"

Generally, young children should not be excluded from funerals and memorial services. They may resent being left out of the special family gathering and may be traumatized if separated from their parents during this stressful time. In fact, the presence of their children and their natural exuberance can often be comforting to parents.

Choice of language is important when explaining death to young children. Use simple and actual words like death, die, and burial. Phrases such as "your baby sister went to sleep," or "we lost your baby brother" should be avoided, as they may be interpreted literally by a young child. Similarly, euphemisms like "passing away" and "flying up to heaven" are confusing. Vague concepts such as baby brothers and sisters "playing with angels" leave too much to the imagination. When a child this age is left to imagine something they might come to the conclusion that they are somehow responsible for their sibling's death. Magical thinking, typical at this age, leads children to believe that their desire for something causes it to occur. Positive things happen because the child wants or imagines it and, conversely, their thoughts can cause bad things to happen, too.

D. **Six- to 8-year-old children.** By ages 6 through 8, children understand that death is final and they openly express their grief. They might feel anxious about what will happen to them and that they, too, could die. They may have guilt over negative thoughts they had about a sibling who has been ill for a long time and may even feel that their negative thoughts contributed to the death. Children this age are capable of drawing upon happy memories to comfort themselves.

E. **Nine- to 11-year-old children.** Children aged 9 to 11 need a lot of cognitive information. They need to know specifically what happened. They still look to parents and others for emotional support and will still express feelings fairly openly. They will respond to rituals that facilitate mourning.

F. **Older children.** With puberty, ages 12 to 14, comes a natural tendency to withdraw from parents, with children preferring to grieve alone in their rooms. Because the need for peer acceptance is strong at this age, young adolescents may fear displaying too much emotion. Older adolescents aged 15 through 18 are similar to adults in their response. They are able to seek support from others and are more likely to participate in support activities than are younger adolescents. They will seek comfort from their peers. As they move toward greater independence, they may resent it if a parent seems dependent upon them.

Most children return to a normal level of functioning within 1 to 2 years. Just as there are support groups for parents, many areas now offer support groups for bereaved siblings. Children who will not accept support from others and those who become increasingly isolated are at risk for pathologic grief and should receive intensive professional help. Any mention of suicide or self-harm gestures should be taken seriously.

VII. **Loss of one of set of multiples.** Increased success in treating infertility has led to more multiple gestation pregnancies, which can be complicated by prematurity. The loss of one or more babies in a set of multiples is a unique circumstance parents in newborn intensive care units encounter. Parents who have lost one or more of a set of multiples have the difficult task of maintaining attachment to one child while they are grieving for another. They must also return to the setting where their baby died and attempt to remain hopeful for their surviving baby or babies. Well-meaning family members may tell parents they should be grateful because "at least they still have the other baby." Such statements can be interpreted by grieving parents as a diminishment of the significance of the baby they lost. Physicians and other caregivers can express their support for parents by the continued acknowledgment of their deceased child.

VIII. **Mementos and rituals.** Neonatal intensive care units and high-risk obstetrical care centers usually have well-developed protocols for supporting families at the time of their baby's death. These protocols include assembling keepsakes for parents. By taking photographs and making foot and handprints, or molding a plaster cast of their baby's hand, staff members create precious mementos for parents. Because their child was so young, parents may have few specific reminders of their baby. Having pictures of their baby and keeping the clothes they wore facilitates the grieving process. Later, when parents hold and look at these things, they remember their baby and the feelings they had when their baby was alive. Though this can be intensely painful for parents, the act of remembering is an important step in the process of recovering from loss.

Nurses and other members of the hospital unit staff who care for critically ill babies and provide support for their families also grieve when a baby they have cared for does not survive. Creating mementos can be therapeutic. Being able to give families something tangible helps staff members process their own feelings. Part of the culture of hospitals in general, and intensive care units in particular, involves the development of rituals surrounding the death of a patient. The physician's awareness of and participation in these practices is usually welcomed and appropriate.

IX. **Follow-up.** A comprehensive follow-up program includes an opportunity for parents to meet with the neonatal physician who directed their baby's care. This invitation should be extended through phone conversations as well as formal written correspondence. A meeting can be scheduled after a final discharge summary, including autopsy and laboratory findings, is prepared. Even if an autopsy or other postmortem tests were not performed, parents benefit from discussing the events that led to their baby's death. Waiting 1 or 2 months after the event gives parents time to recover and gain some perspective. Although the purpose of this conference is to provide additional information and answer any remaining questions, returning to the hospital where their baby received care often provides some measure of closure for parents.

X. **Clinical pearls.** When counseling families regarding life and death decisions for their newborn infants, it is important to do the following when possible:
   - Include both parents, as well as extended family when appropriate and requested.
   - Include other members of the healthcare team.
   - Speak with the family in a comfortable and private environment.
   - Always refer to the baby by name.
   - Reassure the parents that the team is attending to their baby's comfort.
   - Recognize and respect potential differences in cultural values, lifestyles, educational backgrounds, and socioeconomic resources.

BIBLIOGRAPHY

American Academy of Pediatrics, Committee on Fetus and Newborn. Perinatal care at the threshold of viability. *Pediatrics* 2002;110(5):1024–1027.
Harrison H. The principles of family-centered neonatal care. *Pediatrics* 1993;92(5):643–650.

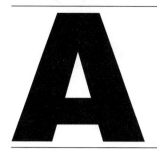

Newborn: Formulary

William F. Buss

Note: As drug elimination in this population is most closely related to the combination of gestational age (GA) and postnatal age (PNA), the term postconceptual age (**PCA**)—which combines GA and PNA—is frequently used to guide drug dosing. (Example: 28-week GA neonate who is 3 weeks PNA is now (28 + 3) = 31 weeks PCA.) For purposes of this table, PCA and PMA (postmenstrual age) will be used interchangeably.

Drug	Dose	Comments
Acyclovir	<33 wk PCA: 10 mg/kg q 12 h** 33–36 wk PCA: 20 mg/kg q 8 h** Term: 20 mg/kg q 8 h IV	Infuse over 1 h, monitor serum Cr; adjust dosage if renal dysfunction. Serial absolute neutrophil count (ANC) twice/wk recommended when giving 15–20 mg/kg q 8 h. **Dosing for preterm infants is controversial; consultation with Infectious Disease Service (ID) and pharmacist is recommended.
Adenosine	50 µg/kg rapid bolus, IV If ineffective, increase dose to 100 µg/kg	Treatment for supraventricular tachycardia (SVT); consult pediatric cardiologist prior to use.
Albuterol	0.25–0.5 mg/kg by **nebulization** q 4–8 h 1–2 puffs by metered-dose inhaler (MDI) q 4–8 h	Tachycardia is common with doses approaching 1 mg/kg. Drug delivery through ventilator circuits is variable. Available in 0.63 mg/3 mL and 1.25 mg/3 mL unit dose as well as 5 mg/mL stock solution MDI is 90 µg/puff. Levalbuterol has no published data supporting use in neonates. Limited neonatal MDI data need to be evaluated before recommendation for routine use can be made.
Aldactone	See Spironolactone	
Amikacin	**INTERVAL** based on PCA: Preterm: **12–15 mg/kg**/dose. ≤**28 wk** PCA: q 36 h **29–32 wk** PCA: q 24 h **33–36 wk** PCA: q 18 h **Term:** **0–7 d:** 10 mg/kg q 18 h >**7 d:** 10 mg/kg q 12 h IV, IM	Levels not needed unless treatment to continue past 3 d; there is renal impairment; or patient received an unusually high dose. Monitor serum concentrations and adjust dosage to achieve post concentrations of 25–35 µg/mL and trough concentrations <10 µg/mL; monitor serum Cr. Give less frequently in infants with **birth depression, congenital heart disease, renal impairment,** or **on inotropic support.**
Amoxicillin	15–20 mg/kg q AM 50 mg/kg × 1, 1 h before procedure	For genitourinary (GU) prophylaxis. For endocarditis prophylaxis.

Drug	Dose	Comments
Amphotericin B	Initial dose 0.5 mg/kg/d IV over 6 h, subsequent daily doses increased by 0.25 mg/kg/d increments until reach 0.75–1 mg/kg/d; Infusion over 2–6 h	Closely assess vital signs during initial dose infusion. Serum potassium, magnesium, and creatinine levels should be monitored. Must be diluted to 0.1 mg/mL for peripheral IV administration. Patients with candida sepsis generally treated to a total dose of 15–30 mg/kg.
Ampicillin	**<1.2 kg:** 50–100 mg/kg q 12 h **1.2–2 kg:** 0–7 d: 50–100 mg/kg q 12 h >7 d: 50–100 mg/kg q 8 h **>2 kg:** 0–7 d: 50–100 mg/kg q 8 h >7 d: 50–75 mg/kg q 6 h IV, IM 0–7 d: 100 mg/kg q 8 h >7 d: 300 mg/kg/d in 4 to 6 div doses	The higher doses are used in meningitis; for other indications, use the lower doses. **Group B strep meningitis**
Ativan	See Lorazepam	
Atropine	0.01–0.03 mg/kg IV, SC, or endotracheal	Severe bradycardia, rarely indicated
Atrovent	See Ipratropium	
AZT (see Zidovudine)		
Beclomethasone metered dose inhaler (40 μg/accuation) QVAR	500 μg/kg/d in div doses for up to 4 wk 500 μg/d MAX Taper used: 500 μg/kg/d × 1 wk; 375 μg/kg/d × 1 wk; 250 μg/kg/d × 1 wk; 125 μg/kg/d × 1 wk; then DC	Neonates requiring mechanical ventilation May reduce subsequent systemic steroid needs or aid in weaning from mechanical ventilation. Preferred over fluticasone because more neonatal efficacy data and no documented hypothalamic pituitary axis (HPA) axis suppression.
Caffeine **Citrate**	**Loading** dose: 20 mg/kg **Maintenance** dose: 5 mg/kg/dose given every 24 h IV, PO	Serum caffeine concentrations of 5 to 20 μg/mL are desired. Check trough level 7 d after starting or dosage changes and then every 1–2 wk.
Calcium Chloride (100 mg/mL)	Emergency use: 0.3 mEq/kg over 2–5 min, IV	Cardiac arrest/severe bradycardia, rarely indicated **Avoid** administration through scalp veins or small peripheral veins. Order in **mEq** 1.4 mEq elemental Ca/mL
Ca Gluconate 10% (100 mg/mL)	Emergency use: 0.45 mEq/kg over 2–5 min, IV (1 mL Calcium/kg) Hypocalcemia: 0.25–0.5 mEq/kg infused over a minimum of 1 h	Cardiac arrest/severe bradycardia, rarely indicated **Avoid** administration through scalp veins or small peripheral veins. 50 mg/mL is max concentration for peripheral IV administration. Addition to maintenance IV fluids and slow administration over 24 h is preferred to faster intermittent infusions. Order in **mEq** 0.45 mEq elemental Ca/mL
Captopril	Neonate: Initial dose: 0.01 to 0.05 mg/kg/dose PO every 6–12 h	Monitor serum potassium in presence of K+-sparing diuretics or K+ supplements. Neutropenia and

Drug	Dose	Comments
Captopril	Slowly titrate as needed up to 0.5 mg/kg/dose.	proteinuria. Begin at lowest dose and titrate. Administer on empty stomach. Contraindicated in renovascular disease. Max neonate dose 2 mg/kg/d. Max infant dose 6 mg/kg/d.
Cefotaxime	All doses are **50 mg/kg/dose** **INTERVAL:** q 12 h: wt <1.2 kg OR 0–7 d old q 8 h: age >7 d old AND wt ≥1.2 kg IV, IM	Not generally used for initial rule-out sepsis course. Some suggest up to 300 mg/kg/d div q 6 h for meningitis in term neonates.
Ceftazidime	All doses are **50 mg/kg/dose** **INTERVAL:** q 12 h: wt <1.2 kg OR 0–7 d old q 8 h: age >7 d old AND wt ≥1.2 kg IV, IM	Reserve for *Pseudomonas aeroginosa* or pathogens resistant to other agents.
Chloral Hydrate	25 mg/kg/dose q 8–12 h PO 50 mg/kg PO	**Sedative** dose **Hypnotic** dose—single use before procedures. Watch for accumulation with repeated doses—especially in preterms. Tolerance to sedation develops.
Chlorothiazide (Diuril)	2–8 mg/kg/d div q 12 h IV	Monitor electrolytes. May cause hypokalemia, hypochloremia, hyponatremia, or alkalosis. Not available PO. Use hydrochlorothiazide if oral administration is desired. For use in renal failure, consult Nephrology.
Cholecystokinin (CCK) Sincalide	0.02 µg/kg bid-tid IV	To promote gallbladder contraction in cholestasis.
Clindamycin	All doses are **5 mg/kg/dose** IV, IM **INTERVAL** **<1.2 kg:** q 12 h **1.2–2 kg:** q 12 h: until 7 d old q 8 h if >7 d old **>2 kg:** 0–7 d old q 8 h >7 d old: q 6 h	May cause severe colitis. Stop drug if significant diarrhea occurs.
Comvax Hib + Hepatitis B	0.5 mL IM	2 mo of age and weight ≥2000 g.
Corticosteroid equivalency approximation	**Glucocorticoid (equivalent mg dose)**	**Mineralocorticoid potency**
	Cortisone 25	+ +
	Dexamethasone 0.4–0.75	0
	Fludrocortisone ----	+ + + + +
	Hydrocortisone 20	+ +
	Methylprednisolone 4	0
	Prednisone 5	+
	Prednisolone 5	+

Drug	Dose	Comments
Cortisone	8–12 mg/m2/d div q 8 h PO/IV	Physiologic replacement.
	20–40 mg/m2/d div q 8 h IV/ PO	Stress dose. BSA(m^2) = (0.05 kg) + 0.05
D10–15W	2–4 mL/kg over 5 min, IV	Hypoglycemia; consult neonatology if must use dextrose concentration >15%.
Dexamethasone (Decadron)	Daily doses are usually div every 12 h:	Numerous dosing regimens are used; consult pharmacist/neonatologist for other dosing regimens.
	10-DAY COURSE: 0.15–0.5 mg/kg/d × 3 d, then reduce dose by 30%–50% every 2 d until DC'd after 10 d IV, PO	Hypertension, hyperglycemia, failure to gain weight, GI ulceration/perforation— especially when concurrent indomethacin, neurologic impact. IV and oral doses are approximately the same.
Diazoxide (Hyperstat)	1–3 mg/kg IV as bolus, may repeat in 5–15 min then q 4–24 h prn IV	Treatment of acute hypertension. Monitor serum glucose; do not use in treatment of compensatory hypertension (coarctation etc.).
Digoxin	**Premature:** 15–20 μg/kg **IV** loading	**Digitalizing** dose; Given over 24 h as 3 div doses.
	4–6 μg/kg/d **IV** div every 12–24 h	**Maintenance** dose; Oral doses 25% more than IV doses. Reduce dose in renal impairment.
Digoxin	**Full Term:** 30–40 μg/kg **IV** loading	**Digitalizing** dose; Given over 24 h as 3 div doses.
	5–10 μg/kg/d **IV** div every 12 h	**Maintenance** dose; Oral doses 25% more than IV doses (IV preparation is 100 μg/mL. PO preparation is 50 μg/mL.) **All orders must be written in mL's and in μg.** Reduce dose in renal impairment.
Dobutamine	5–25 μg/kg/min IV	Less effective at raising BP than Dopamine in premature neonates. Vasodilation at high dose.
Dopamine	2–5 μg/kg/min IV	**"Renal dose"**
	5–20 μg/kg/min IV	**"Inotropic"**and vasoconstrictive dose
Epinephrine	**1:10,000:** 0.1–0.3 mL/kg/dose IV, IT may repeat q 5 min Dilute to 0.5–1 mL with normal saline for ET administration. Continuous infusion 0.05–1.0 μg/kg/min IV	Cardiac arrest, severe bradycardia not responsive to routine resuscitation. Vasoconstriction. Continuously monitor heart rate, blood pressure, and perfusion.
Fentanyl	1–4 μg/kg, may repeat every 2–4 h as indicated	Tolerance may develop rapidly; respiratory depression, withdrawal hypotension, bradycardia, flushing, desaturations, and chest wall rigidity may occur.
	Continuous infusion: Start at 0.5 μg/kg/h and titrate to pain relief. Mean required dose is 0.64–0.75 μg/kg/h (range 0.5–2 μg/kg/h).	Continuous infusion is indicated for severe pain uncontrolled by intermittent administration of opiates in patients intolerant of morphine infusion.

Drug	Dose	Comments
Fentanyl	Higher doses may be required in ECMO patients.	Use of fentanyl in patients where analgesia is not required is NOT indicated. Titrating to sedation (side effect) often results in excessive doses. Benzodiazepines (lorazepam or midazolam) may be a better choice when sedation is the primary desired effect.
Fosphenytoin (Cerebyx)	Loading dose: 15–20 mg PE/kg IV at no greater than 1.5 mg/kg/min; Maintenance dose: 4 to 8 mg PE/kg/d div BID IV, IM	Ordered in PE (phenytoin equivalents). Causes less venous irritation than phenytoin. Consider use in patients with only small peripheral venous access available. Flush line with normal saline before and after infusion. Use with caution in hyperbilirubinemia. Much more expensive than phenytoin. Serum concentrations should be monitored and doses adjusted to maintain concentrations between 8 and 15 μg/mL. Trough levels are most useful. Hypotension and bradycardia possible. Consider checking free phenytoin level if toxicity is suspected or patient is hypoalbuminenic.
Furosemide (Lasix)	1 mg/kg/dose **Preterm:** q 24 h **Term:** q 12 h IM, IV, PO	Monitor electrolytes. May cause hypokalemia, hypochloremia, hyponatremia, alkalosis, dehydration, and ototoxicity. Infuse slowly (>10 min). Oral doses approximately twice IV doses.
Gentamicin	**INTERVAL** based on **PCA:** ≤**28 wk PCA: 3** mg/kg ≤3 wk old: q 36 h >3 wk old: q 24 h **29–32 wk PCA: 3** mg/kg ≤4 wk old: q 24 h >4 wk old: q 18 h **33–36 wk PCA: 3.5** mg/kg ≤2 wk old: q 24 h >2 wk old: q 18 h >**36 wk PCA:** 0–7 d: 3.5 mg/kg q 24 h >7 d: 2.5 mg/kg q 12 h ECMO patients: 3–3.5 mg/kg q 18–24 h	Levels not needed unless treatment to continue past 3 d; there is renal impairment; or patient received an unusually high dose. Monitor serum concentrations and adjust doses to achieve post concentrations of 5–10 μg/mL and troughs <1.5 μg/mL. Give less frequently in neonates with **birth depression, congenital heart disease, renal impairment,** or on **inotropic support.** Consultation with pharmacist for dosing recommendation in renal impairment is suggested. Monitor respiratory status closely in offspring of myasthenics and those exposed to magnesium.
Glucagon	100 μg/kg IM	Maximum 300 μg.
Hepatitis B immune globulin (HBIG)	0.5 mL IM × 1 within 12 h of birth	Indicated for newborns whose mothers have acute Hep B infections or who are HBsAg-**positive** or in preterm newborns <2 kg with unknown HBsAg maternal status.
Hepatitis B vaccine	Maternal HBsAg status positive or unknown: 0.5 mL IM within 12 h of age	See Hepatitis Guidelines above. 0.5 mL Recombivax HB = 5 μg 0.5 mL Engerix B = 10 μg

Drug	Dose	Comments
Hepatits B vaccine	Maternal HBsAg negative: 0.5 mL IM at birth or before discharge.	In preterm infants <2 kg at birth born of HBsAg **negative** moms, delay administration of 1st dose until just before discharge or until 2 kg.
Hyaluronidase (Wydase)	1 mL of 15 unit/mL solution as 5 separate 0.2 mL subcutaneous/intradermal injections.	Use within 1 h of extravasation of hyperal/other solution—NOT for pressors. Inject around periphery of extravasation. Consult Plastics service if affected area is >1 cm.
Hydralazine	**ORAL:** 1 mg/kg/d div q 6–8 h; may slowly increase as needed to MAX of 7 mg/kg/d **IV:** 0.1–0.2 mg/kg/dose q 6–8 h. May slowly increase to MAX of 1 mg/kg/dose.	**Chronic** hypertension. Oral doses approximately twice IV doses. **Hypertensive crisis**
Hydrochlorothiazide	2–4 mg/kg/d div q 12 h PO	May cause hypokalemia, hypochloremia, hyponatremia, or alkalosis. Monitor electrolytes. Only available PO.
Hyperstat	See Diazoxide	
Indomethacin (Indocin)	CLOSURE OF A PATENT DUCTUS	To be used under direction of neonatologist/pediatric cardiologist; monitor platelet count and serum creatinine. q 24 h dosing may be preferred in the most premature infants. Dose must be reduced in renal dysfunction.

CLOSURE OF A PATENT DUCTUS

Age 1st dose	Dose(mg/kg) q 12–24 h IV		
	1st	2nd	3rd
<48 h	0.2	0.1	0.1
2–7 d	0.2	0.2	0.2
>7 d	0.2	0.25	0.25

Drug	Dose	Comments
	PROPHYLAXIS OF IVH 0.1 mg/kg/dose IV q 24 h × 3 doses	For premature infants ≤1250 g birthweight requiring ventilator support for respiratory distress syndrome (RDS). Give first dose ASAP and within 12 h of birth.
Ipratropium	25 μg/kg q 6–8 h nebulized into the ventilator circuit	Tachycardia
Isoproterenol	25–200 ng/kg/min IV	Treatment of bradycardia Continuous ECG and blood pressure monitoring, essential to watch for hypertension and tachycardia
IVIG	400–1000 mg/kg/d for 2–5 d	For alloimmune thrombocytopenia Administer 5% solution at 0.5 mL/kg/h and gradually increase to maximum of 4 mL/kg/h if tolerated. Availability of drug is limited.
Kayexalate	0.5–1 g/kg/dose PO or PR every 6 h as needed. Rectal may be given more frequently if needed. Approximately 1 mEq potassium is removed per 1 g of resin.	Use sorbitol as diluent (oral 3–4 mL/kg of 10% sorbitol soln; rectal 2–3 mL/kg of 25% sorbitol soln) Avoid commercially available suspension.
Lorazepam (Ativan)	0.05–0.1 mg/kg/dose IV or PO every 6–12 h as needed for sedation	Use the longer intervals in prematures. Tolerance may develop; respiratory and cardiac depression, withdrawal, hypotension, bradycardia, myoclonic movements, and desaturations may occur. Potential for drug accumulation with frequent dosing.

Drug	Dose	Comments
Magnesium Sulfate	Hypomagnesemia: 0.1–0.25 mEq/kg IV, IM	Calcium gluconate should be available as an antidote; monitor serum concentrations.
	Dilute to 0.5 mEq/mL and infuse over 2–4 h	Addition to maintenance IV fluids and slow administration over 24 h is preferred to faster intermittent infusions.
Metoclopramide (Reglan)	0.1 mg/kg/dose every 6 h	Irritability; dystonic reactions possible. Give before feedings. Some references suggest up to 0.8 mg/kg/d.
Midazolam (Versed)	0.05–0.1 mg/kg/dose; may repeat every 2–6 h as needed. Continuous infusion: start at 20 µg/kg/h and titrate to sedation. Mean required dose is 30–60 µg/kg/h.	Use the longer intervals in prematures. Tolerance may develop; respiratory and cardiac depression, withdrawal, hypotension, bradycardia, myoclonic movements, and desaturations may occur.
		Potential for drug accumulation with frequent dosing.
		Lorazepam is preferred because it has no active metabolites, doesn't require continuous infusion, and is less expensive.
Morphine	0.05–0.1 mg/kg/dose repeated every 4–8 h IV, IM as needed PO dose is 2 to 5 times the IV dose.	Use the longer intervals in prematures. Tolerance may develop; respiratory depression, withdrawal, hypotension, flushing, bradycardia, and desaturations may occur.
	Continuous infusion: 10–30 µg/kg/h	Continuous infusion indicated for severe pain not controlled by intermittent dosing of opiates. Use in a setting where analgesia is not required is NOT indicated.
		Titrating to sedation (side effect) often results in excessive doses. Benzodiazepines (lorazepam or midazolam) may be a better choice when sedation is the primary desired effect.
Nafcillin	**0–7 d:** 25 mg/kg q 12 h (≤2 kg) 25 mg/kg q 8 h (>2 kg) **>7 d:** 25 mg/kg q 12 h (<1.2 kg) 25 mg/kg q 8 h (1.2 to 2 kg) 25 mg/kg q 6 h (>2 kg) IV	Venous irritation.
Narcan (Naloxone)	0.1 mg/kg/dose IV, IM, SC, IT	May be repeated every 3–5 min; contraindication: maternal narcotic addiction.
Nitroglycerine	Initial: 0.1–0.5 µg/kg/min IV Usual dose: 1–3 µg/kg/min	Titrate to effect. Vasodilator—reduces preload. Continuously monitor blood pressure, heart rate, oxygen saturation.
Oxacillin	**0–7 d:** 25 mg/kg q 12 h (≤2 kg) 25 mg/kg q 8 h (>2 kg) **>7 d:** 25 mg/kg q 12 h (<1.2 kg) 25 mg/kg q 8 h (1.2 to 2 kg) 25 mg/kg q 6 h (>2 kg) IV	Venous irritation.
Pancuronium Bromide(Pavulon)	0.04–0.1 mg/kg/dose q 30–120 min PRN IV	Monitor blood pressure and heart rate. Reduce dose in renal dysfunction.

Drug	Dose	Comments
Pediarix DtaP + Hepatitis B + IPV	0.5 mL IM	2 mo of age and weight ≥2000 g
Penicillin G	**<1.2 kg:** 25,000–50,000 units/kg q 12 h **1.2–2 kg:** 0–7 d: 25,000–50,000 units/kg q 12 h >7 d: 25,000–50,000 units/kg q 8 h **>2 kg:** 0–7 d: 25,000–50,000 units/kg q 8 h >7 d: 25,000–50,000 units/kg q 6 h IV, IM 0–7 d: 250,000–450,000 units/kg/**d div** q 8 h >7 d: 450,000 units/kg/**d div** every 6 h	The higher doses are used in meningitis; for other indications, use the lower doses. For **Group B strep meningitis**
Phenobarbital	Initial loading dose: 15–20 mg/kg IV over no less than 20 min Subsequent loading doses: 5–10 mg/kg Maintenance dose: 3–5 mg/kg/d IV, IM, or PO as a single dose	Trough level should be monitored to maintain concentrations between 15 and 35 µg/mL. Check level at point of seizure resolution and weekly thereafter. Some patients may require more frequent level monitoring. May be div q 12 h if single daily dose not tolerated. Use the lower maintenance dose in patients with history of birth depression or prematurity.
Phentolamine (Regitine)	For vasopressor infiltrate: Infiltrate affected area with multiple small subcutaneous injections of a 0.5 mg/mL solution. Change needles between injections.	Use ASAP after pressor extravasation. Dilute with normal saline. Not for hyperal extravasation. Hypotension with large doses or doses given IV. Do not administer more than 2.5 mg total.
Phenytoin (Dilantin)	Loading dose: 15–20 mg/kg IV at no greater than 0.5 mg/kg/min; may be diluted in 0.9% **NaCl only** to a concentration of <6 mg/mL. Maintenance dose: 5–8 mg/kg/d div BID IV, PO. Higher oral doses may be necessary to maintain therapeutic levels.	Loading dose should be administered with continuous ECG monitoring; infuse through a 0.22 micron filter; serum concentrations should be monitored and doses adjusted to maintain concentrations between 8 and 15 µg/mL. Trough levels are the most useful. Hypotension and bradycardia possible. Check free phenytoin level if toxicity is suspected or patient is hypoalbuminemic. Consider fosphenytoin if only small peripheral venous access is available. Can only be infused with normal saline. Flush with saline before and after administration. Not compatible with heparin.
Piperacillin	**<36 wkGA:** ≤7 d: 75 mg/kg/dose q 12 h >7 d: 75 mg/kg/dose q 8 h **>36 wkGA:** ≤7 d: 75 mg/kg/dose q 8 h >7 d: 75 mg/kg/dose q 6 h	Adjust dosage in renal impairment.

Drug	Dose	Comments
Propranolol	**IV:** 0.01 mg/kg/dose by slow IV push q 6–8 h prn. May increase slowly to MAX of 0.15 mg/kg/dose. **PO:** 0.25 mg/kg/dose every 6–8 h. May increase slowly to MAX of 5 mg/kg/d.	For arrhythmias, hypertension Avoid in patients with respiratory compromise.
	0.15–0.25 mg/kg/dose IV	For tetralogy spells.
Prostaglandin E1 (Alprostadil)	Initial dose of 0.1 μg/kg/min IV, wean to 0.025–0.05 μg/kg/min as tolerated.	To be used under direction of neonatologist/pediatric cardiologist.
Protamine	0.5–1 mg IV for every 100 units of heparin in the previous hour (50 mg/dose maximum).	Bleeding with excessive doses.
Ranitidine	**Preterm:** 1 mg/kg/d IV div q 12 h 2 mg/kg/d PO div q 12 h **Term:** 4 mg/kg/d IV div q 8 h 4–6 mg/kg/d PO div q 8 h	
Regitine	See Phentolamine	
Reglan	See Metoclopramide	
Sodium Bicarbonate	1–2 mEq/kg over 5 min 1–2 mEq/kg over 2 h	Cardiac arrest Metabolic acidosis Use concentration of 0.5 mEq/mL(4.2%).
Spironolactone (Aldactone)	1–3 mg/kg/d PO div q 12 h	Monitor serum potassium especially when used with captopril or potassium supplements. May take several days to see maximal effect.
Survanta (Beractant)	RDS: 4 mL/kg/dose IT div into 4 aliquots. Repeat doses are given at least 6 h later if indicated. Up to 4 doses in the first 48 h of life if indicated.	Use only under direction of neonatologist. Consult neonatologist for other possible uses such as congenital diaphragmatic hernia, persistent pulmonary hypertension, hyaline membrane disease (HMD) in greater gestational age neonates.
Synagis (Palivizumab)	15 mg/kg IM q.mo during RSV season	Consult neonatologist. Premature neonates <32 wk gestation or 32–35 wk EGA with risk factors. Administer prior to discharge only. Not for prevention of nosocomial infection.
Tobramycin	Same as "Gentamicin"	
TPA (tissue plasminogen activator, Alteplase)	Using a 5-mL **syringe,** gently and slowly instill a volume of 1 mg/mL TPA **equal to or less than the internal volume of the catheter.** Do **not** force the TPA into the catheter. If device does not allow infusion or aspiration, a gentle repeated push-pull action can be used to instill the TPA.	For **clearing an occluded line** Allow solution to dwell in line for 30–60 min; then attempt to aspirate TPA from the catheter with a 5-mL syringe. If unsuccessful, wait an additional 30 min before trying again to aspirate solution. Once patency is restored, aspirate, and discard 1–2 mL of blood. Replace this volume with normal saline. For clot dissolution unrelated to occluded lines, consult neonatologist.
Ursodiol	25–30 mg/kg/d div TID	For cholestasis.

Drug	Dose	Comments
Vancomycin	**INTERVAL** based on **PCA** and postnatal age. **DOSE: 15 mg/kg:** **≤28 wk** PCA: ≤2 wk old: q 36 h >2 wk old: q 24 h **29–32 wk** PCA: ≤2 wk old: q 24 h >2 wk old: q 18 h **33–36 wk** PCA: ≤2 wk old: q 18 h >2 wk old: q 12 h >**36 wk** PCA: q 12 h	Intravenous therapy reserved for species of *Staphylococcus* and *Enterococcus* resistant to other agents. Levels not needed unless treatment to continue past 3 d; there is renal impairment; or patient received an unusually high dose. Postlevel should be 25–40 µg/mL and trough level 5–10 µg/mL. Give less frequently in infants with birth depression, congenital heart disease, renal impairment, or on inotropic support. Nafcillin is preferred drug if coagulase-negative staphylococcus (CONS) is susceptible to both vancomycin and nafcillin.
Vaponephrine	0.25–0.5 mL nebulized × 1	2.25% racemic epinephrine.
Vecuronium	0.1 mg/kg/dose every 1–2 h as needed	Monitor blood pressure and heart rate. Less likely to cause hypertension and tachycardia than pancuronium. Consider vecuronium when these side effects become problematic.
Versed	See Midazolam	
Whole Blood or 5% protein solution	5–20 mL/kg IV	History of blood loss, shock, hypotension.
Zantac	See Ranitidine	
Zidovudine (AZT)	**Preterm** (≤34 wk GA): ≤2-wk old: 1.5 mg/kg PO/IV q 12 h until 2 wk old >2-wk old: 2 mg/kg PO/IV q 8 h **Term:** 2 mg/kg PO q 6 h OR 1.5 mg/kg IV q 6 h	Do not give IM. Monitor critical blood cell profile (CBC) with diff and hemoglobin. IV infusion to be over 1 h at ≤4 mg/mL concentration in D5W.

Index